Clinical Methods and Practicum in Speech-Language Pathology

Singular Textbook Series
Series Editor: M. N. Hegde, Ph.D.

Clinical Methods and Practicum in Speech-Language Pathology

Third Edition

M. N. Hegde, Ph.D.
Deborah Davis, M.A.

SINGULAR PUBLISHING GROUP, INC.
SAN DIEGO · LONDON

Singular Publishing Group, Inc.
401 West "A" Street, Suite 325
San Diego, California 92101-7904

Singular Publishing Group, Ltd.
19 Compton Terrace
London, N1 2UN, UK

Singular Publishing Group, Inc., publishes textbooks, clinical manuals, clinical reference books, journals, videos, and multimedia materials on speech-language pathology, audiology, otorhinolaryngology, special education, early childhood, aging, occupational therapy, physical therapy, rehabilitation, counseling, mental health, and voice. For your convenience, our entire catalog can be accessed on our website at **http://www.singpub.com**. Our mission to provide you with materials to meet the daily challenges of the ever-changing health care/educational environment will remain on course if we are in touch with you. In that spirit, we welcome your feedback on our products. Please telephone (**1-800-521-8545**), fax (**1-800-774-8398**), or e-mail (**singpub@singpub.com**) your comments and requests to us.

© 1999 by Singular Publishing Group, Inc.

Typeset in 10/12 Palatino by So Cal Graphics
Printed in the United States of America by Bang Printing

Library of Congress Cataloging-in-Publication Data
Hegde, M. N. (Mahabalagiri N.), 1941–
    Clinical methods and practicum in speech-language pathology / M.N.
Hegde, Deborah Davis. — 3rd ed.
       p.   cm. — (Singular textbook series)
    Includes bibliographical references and index.
    ISBN 0-7693-0016-2 (softcover : alk. paper)
    1. Speech therapy—Study and teaching.   I. Davis, Deborah, 1951–
      II. Title.   III. Series.
    [DNLM: 1. Speech-Language Pathology—education. 2. Communication
Disorders—therapy.   WM 18H462c 1999]
    RC428.H44   1999
    616.85'506—dc21
    DNLM/DLC
for Library of Congress   98–41693
                                   CIP

Contents

Preface to the Third Edition

The extensive changes in the practice of speech-language pathology prompted the third edition of this text. However, the primary motivation for continuing to update and expand this book came from the students and their devotion to excel and help their clients, the clients and their amazing resilience and dedication to hard work, and the paid and volunteer staff with whom we work and their professionalism and expertise. All have enriched our lives and taught us much about the practice of speech-language pathology.

In writing the third edition, we emphasized the students' responsibility in successfully mastering the academic and clinical competencies necessary to provide effective services. Also, we introduced information on distance learning and the Internet and their impact on clinical practicum. We updated ASHA requirements for certification and clinical practicum in speech-language pathology and audiology and revised information about IDEA mandates. In addition, we expanded on such areas as general preclinic requirements, health and safety precautions, assessment of individuals from diverse cultural or linguistic backgrounds, and service delivery in schools, hospitals, and correctional facilities.

We have attempted to provide comprehensive, but concise information on clinical training and hope that students and instructors will find this text beneficial. This text has been adopted by many training programs and we appreciate the continued feedback regarding the strengths and weaknesses of the book. As always, we look forward to receiving comments and suggestions.

PART I
Clinical Practicum

When you have completed certain courses in communicative disorders, your advisor may tell you that you are ready for clinical practicum. This means that you have acquired some basic knowledge about communication and its disorders. Yet, you may not know much about the practicum itself. Therefore, in Part I of the text, we have described the organization of clinical practicum, various rules and regulations you must follow, the relationship with your clinical supervisor, and some basic principles of working with clients. Read this part of the text carefully to understand what practicum is and how to prepare yourself for it.

In Part II of the text, we have described the basic clinical methods of treating clients with communicative disorders. We have given an overview of commonly used treatment techniques with an emphasis on working with families of your clients to achieve maintenance of treatment gains.

1

Clinical Practicum in Speech-Language Pathology

S peech-language pathology is a profession with scientific and academic bases. To be a speech-language pathologist, you need to gain both academic and scientific knowledge through course work and practical experience in working with clients who have communicative disorders. Therefore, speech-language pathology degree programs at colleges and universities include two types of training.

The first type of training is offered through **academic course work**. You learn about speech, language, communication, and communicative disorders by taking various academic courses. Some academic courses are a prerequisite to beginning clinical practicum and others may be taken in conjunction with clinical practicum. The academic portion of the training program provides you with a theoretical basis and foundation for clinical practicum.

The second type of training is offered through **clinical practicum**. Clinical practicum gives you the opportunity to apply and practice what you have learned in academic courses. The combination of academic course work and practicum provides you with well-rounded training in speech-language pathology.

Occasionally, students try to rate the importance of academic classes versus practicum assignments. However, there is no comparison, because each is equally important. Without a strong academic background, students would not know how to assess and treat people with communicative disorders. Without practicum, you would not learn the skills you must have to be successful speech-language pathologists. Therefore, from the beginning, avoid making judgments in favor of one or the other and apply yourself fully and equally to your academic courses and practicum assignments.

Although reference may be made to academic course work, this text emphasizes clinical practicum. If you have any questions regarding specific academic requirements, contact your advisor. Questions regarding clinical practicum requirements should be referred to your advisor, clinical supervisor, or your clinic director.

Clinical Practicum: An Overview

Clinical practicum is an exciting component of your educational experience. You will have opportunities to work with a variety of professionals and clients, apply much of what you have learned in your academic courses, and expand on your knowledge of communication and its disorders. Your clinical practicum is a supervised experience in which you learn professional skills of assessing and treating people with communicative disorders. In some assignments you learn to work independently and in other assignments you learn to work as a member of a team. Your clinical practicum experiences are designed to prepare you for your future role as a professional speech-language pathologist. Enrollment in clinical practicum is a required part of the curriculum in programs accredited by the American Speech-Language-Hearing Association (ASHA). Clinical practicum provides you with the necessary opportunities to apply and expand the information learned in academic courses. Your **enthusiasm, dedication, and hard work** are important variables that influence the degree to which you will benefit from your clinical assignments.

Students generally enroll in clinical practicum during their senior year as undergraduates or during their first semester as graduate students. In some universities, students are allowed to participate in clinical practicum earlier in the training program. This early experience may be limited to observing graduate students providing clinical services and assisting with a client or two toward the end of the semester. For example, you may be assigned to observe a student clinician for a semester prior to being assigned your own clients. You will be involved gradually in the treatment process. You may be required to assist in charting responses, developing stimulus materials, and eventually working with a client for one or two sessions as the primary clinician.

As much as a university clinic's caseload allows, a beginning student clinician is assigned clients with less complex disorders. In most universities, student clinicians are assigned clients based on the academic courses they have completed. For example, during your first semester of graduate work, you may enroll in a course in articulation and be assigned articulation clients only. As you complete course work on other disorders of communication, you may be assigned clients with those types of disorders.

Other universities take a more gestalt view of clinical experience and provide a student clinician with a variety of clients each term, based on the student's individual level of expertise, previous educational experience, and the supervisor's expertise. For example, as a first semester graduate student, you may take a seminar in articulation, a seminar in language, and a seminar in research methods. However, in your clinical practicum, you may be assigned a fluency client based on your undergraduate class in fluency and the expertise of your clinical supervisor.

You will participate in clinical practicum assignments at the university clinic and various off-campus clinical sites. Many universities require student clinicians to complete a certain minimum number of clinical hours before they are assigned to off-campus practicum sites. Your clinical practicum may include hospital, school, or various other clinical sites.

As you progress through your clinical and academic programs, you are given more responsibility in planning, evaluating, and treating clients. As a beginning student clinician, you will not be expected to have all the answers; your clinical supervisor will help you find those answers. Although you will be supervised throughout your clinical practicum, as you gain clinical experience, you will be expected to perform more independently in most of your clinical responsibilities. Eventually, you will be expected to conduct most of your clinical duties with minimal supervisory input.

General Preclinic Requirements

In addition to a solid academic foundation, good writing skills are necessary for success in clinical practicum. Equally important is your ability to talk to people from all walks of life and of all ages. Finally, there are less tangible, personal characteristics without which you cannot successfully complete your clinical practicum. For example, you must be conscientious and reliable. You should be able to organize your schedule and allocate sufficient time to your clinical responsibilities. You are expected to be committed to providing the best quality of client care possible. You are not expected to enter clinical practicum with all the necessary skills, but you should be able to learn from your experiences and interactions with your supervisor.

Academic Requirements

Preclinic academic requirements are completed both at the undergraduate and graduate levels. At the **undergraduate level,** one of your first courses may be an introduction to communication sciences and disorders. You will then probably take courses on phonetics, anatomy and physiology of speech and hearing mechanisms, speech science (perception and production of speech), and those courses related to normal acquisition of speech and language. Some clinical courses, especially those related to disorders of articulation, language, voice, fluency, and hearing, also may be taken at the undergraduate level.

Graduate courses provide you with more advanced information on all aspects of communication sciences and disorders and on assessment and treatment of various disorders. These courses are more research based than the undergraduate courses. Graduate courses build on the information offered at the undergraduate level and emphasize specialized information. For example, besides taking advanced courses in articulation and language, you also take courses in stuttering, aphasia, cleft palate, augmentative communication, and neurologically based speech disorders. Also, at the graduate level, most universities offer courses in assessment and treatment of swallowing disorders (dysphagia). At the graduate and postgraduate levels, some universities offer courses in administration and supervision.

Although **course requirements and sequences vary** from university to university, students are expected to have minimally completed introductory courses in normal and abnormal speech and language development and courses in speech and hearing science before beginning clinical practicum. You should discuss the specific requirements with your advisor well in advance of the time you plan to begin your clinical practicum.

General Writing Requirements

Student clinicians are required to write **numerous clinical reports, treatment programs, lesson plans, and progress notes**. You will discover that different clinical settings have varying writing requirements. Regardless of the specific requirements, at each of your assignments you will be expected to have good basic writing skills. In many instances, your reports may be read by other people including clients' family members, physicians, teachers, and other speech-language pathologists. Therefore, it is important that you develop your writing skills prior to your enrollment in clinical practicum. Unless you have had a course on professional writing in communicative disorders, you are not expected to know the specific formats for reports and some of the technical terms before clinical enrollment, but you should be able to write clearly and concisely. You should be able to organize your thoughts coherently and write grammatically correct sentences. Your writing should be free from spelling errors and easily understood by the intended audience.

If you are concerned about your general writing skills and your program does not offer a course on professional writing, discuss your problem with your advisor as early in your program as possible. Your advisor can assist you in overcoming your writing problems. You may need to take a writing course, or you may need just additional practice in writing. You may practice professional writing skills in a book that is designed for self-teaching. One such book is by Hegde (1998a) and provides many examples of scientific and professional writing and gives you frameworks for practicing writing skills. Take these and other steps that will prepare you for meeting clinical writing requirements.

Oral Communication Skills

Effective oral communication skills are essential to the practice of speech-language pathology. As a student clinician, you will communicate with many clients with varied educational, socioeconomic, and cultural backgrounds. Also, you will interact with many professionals. You may discuss your clients' evaluation, treatment, and progress with physical therapists, physicians, nurses, teachers, audiologists, psychologists, and other speech-language pathologists.

Regardless of the client, professional, or family member you communicate with, you must speak so that individual will understand you. With some clients, you will need to use simple, brief language; with other clients you may use technical terms, advanced vocabulary, and present complex concepts. At times, to establish a shared basis of understanding, you may need to use some professional jargon. For example, you may introduce the term "apraxia" and explain exactly what you are referring to when you us that term. At another time you may refer to a "SST" (student study team) meeting, and explain the meaning of that initialism. You should develop the flexibility to speak at whatever the level the communicative situation requires. In all instances, you should **clearly and concisely articulate** information. You should learn to communicate in whatever the way that maximizes comprehension for the listener. Your department or one of the other departments in your university may offer a counseling course that teaches specific interpersonal communication skills. Consider taking such a course and discuss this with your academic advisor.

Personal Characteristics

In addition to academic preparation and good written and oral communication skills, there are some personal characteristics that are required for successful clinical work. Responsible behavior is probably one of the most important characteristics.

Student clinicians are expected to **act responsibly** in all areas of clinical involvement, including preparation for treatment sessions, meeting with clients, report writing, and interactions with office staff and clinical supervisors. You will have deadlines for various clinical assignments, including scheduling of clients, completion of various reporting forms needed by clinic administrative staff, and submission of diagnostic reports, treatment plans, and lesson plans. Regardless of other academic or personal commitments, you must be well prepared for all your diagnostic and treatment sessions.

As a graduate student, you will have many obligations and it will be important for you to organize your time. Typically, this means you must **establish priorities and prepare in advance**. You may have an examination scheduled and a new client to evaluate on the same day a major paper is due. Obviously, to accomplish all these well, you must have allowed for sufficient preparation time.

Student clinicians work with many people and your ability to **empathize with your clients and their families** is essential. You must combine your technical knowledge with care and regard to your clients' living situations and their personal concerns. For example, it probably would not be useful to expect clients living alone in private care facilities to be able to find people with whom to practice a speech assignment. However, knowing this, you might talk with cooperative nursing assistants and ask them to help your clients practice their speech. Many **external and internal factors** influence your clients' progress. It will be important for you to know and understand the interactions among your clients' disabilities, their living situations, and support systems and how they affect your clients' speech therapy.

Student clinicians should learn to work independently within their level of experience. For example, as a beginning clinician, you are expected to rely on your supervisor for assistance more than experienced clinicians do; however, you still must be prepared to research material independently and, with your supervisor's help, evaluate the efficacy of your clinical sessions, determine areas of needed change, and implement appropriate modifications that your supervisor suggests to you. You will be expected to demonstrate systematic **progress toward working independently**. See Chapter 4 for more on student clinician responsibilities.

Knowledge of the Profession and Related Agencies

In addition to your university's requirements, several agencies and professional organizations affect your training and career as a speech-language pathologist. As you prepare to enroll in clinical practicum, you should have at least a basic knowledge of the various accrediting and licensing agencies and regulations related to the profession of speech-language pathology. Two agencies affect your training and professional career the most: The **American Speech-Language-Hearing Association (ASHA)** and, if your state has a licensure law, the **Board of Examiners for Audiology and Speech Pathology** (or other licensing agency in your state).

The American Speech-Language-Hearing Association. The American Speech-Language-Hearing Association (ASHA) is the national professional organization representing speech-language pathologists and audiologists. Students and student clinicians in departments of communication sciences and disorders or speech-language pathology will repeatedly hear references to ASHA and its various activities, guidelines, and requirements that affect the profession. Student clinicians will constantly be told of ASHA's requirements on how to complete their clinical practicum. Also, students will be expected to become members of ASHA's student organization, the National Student Speech-Language-Hearing Association (NSSLHA).

As you probably know, ASHA is a scientific and professional organization with a long history of contributions to communication sciences and disorders. This national organization is the major force that shapes our scientific and professional discipline. The organization acts as an advocate for individuals with communicative disorders and the professionals who provide services to these individuals. ASHA (*ASHA Membership & Certification Handbook*, 1997) has identified seven goals to:

1. **Encourage basic scientific study** of the processes of individual human communication with special reference to speech, language, and hearing;

2. **Promote appropriate academic and clinical preparation** of individuals entering the discipline of human communication sciences and disorders and to promote maintenance of current knowledge and skills of those within the discipline;
3. **Promote investigation and prevention** of disorders of human communication;
4. **Foster improvement of clinical services and procedures** addressing such disorders;
5. **Stimulate exchange of information** among persons and organizations thus engaged and to disseminate such information;
6. **Advocate for the rights and interests** of persons with communication disorders; and
7. **Promote the individual and collective professional interests** of the members of the Association (p. 1).

ASHA works in various ways to help maintain high standards of clinical competence of speech-language pathologists and audiologists. It has a governing body of elected members from each of the 50 states, the District of Columbia, and other areas. ASHA sponsors conferences and workshops to encourage continuing professional education. It collects and disseminates data related to research, clinical service delivery, education, and career opportunities. It has a policy on the scope of practice for speech-language pathologists and audiologists and has established accreditation and certification procedures that outline minimal standards of education and clinical service delivery. These standards are outlined in the form of academic and clinical preparation guidelines and include required compliance with the ASHA Code of Ethics. These standards are designed to protect consumers and the professionals who serve them.

ASHA Accreditation.   University training programs that meet ASHA standards may receive accreditation from ASHA. ASHA accredits academic programs and clinical services through two of its agencies. The **Council on Academic Accreditation in Audiology and Speech-Language Pathology (CAA)** accredits academic programs and the **Professional Services Board (PSB)** accredits clinical services.

A university must request accreditation of its academic program, its clinical services, or both. When it does this, the university may seek accreditation for its speech-language pathology program, audiology program, or both. ASHA will then send a team of trained professionals to evaluate the educational programs and one to two professionals to evaluate the clinical services offered by the university. ASHA accredits only programs offering advanced degrees.

The team evaluating educational programs looks at the quality and number of faculty teaching the courses, the curriculum offered by the department, physical facilities and instructional equipment and laboratories, the library and other resources of the university, the administrative support, and such other factors that affect the education of future speech-language pathologists and audiologists.

The professionals evaluating clinical services offered by a department looks at the qualifications and certification status of clinical supervisors, financial resources and management, adequacy of clinical facilities and equipment, and all other factors that affect the quality of clinical services offered to the public. The teams may schedule meetings to discuss the training program with current students as well as graduates of the program. After the site visit, each team submits a report to the ASHA board or council to which it is responsible (CAA or PSB). Based on these reports, a final decision on whether to accredit the program is made.

Both CAA and PSB requirements directly influence you and your training program. First, if you are attending a program accredited by ASHA, you are assured that the department has met ASHA's standards. Second, if you completed your course work and practicum after January 1, 1994, you must have initiated and satisfactorily completed at least 21 graduate semester hours of academic course work and 250 graduate hours of clinical practicum (in the area in which certification is sought) at a CAA-accredited program to be eligible for the Certificate of Clinical Competence.

ASHA Certification. ASHA certifies both audiologists and speech-language pathologists. The **Certificate of Clinical Competence** is more commonly referred to as the **CCC** (pronounced "sees"). The **Clinical Certification Board (CCB)** awards the CCC to speech-language pathologists and audiologists who have successfully met ASHA's academic, clinical, and ethical standards. The CCC indicates that individuals have met a certain level of professional competence. Under ASHA's guidelines, individuals with their CCCs may supervise student clinicians, support personnel, and professionals who do not hold certification. When you complete a program of study and clinical experience approved by ASHA you may receive this certification. This certificate may be in audiology or speech-language pathology. To be eligible for certification, you must satisfy the following requirements.

1. **Earn a graduate degree.** You must have earned a master's (MA or MS) or doctoral (Ph.D.) degree in the area in which you are applying for certification. In addition to specific academic course work, professional course work, and clinical practicum requirements, ASHA requires that all CCC applicants satisfactorily complete at least 21 graduate semester course work hours and at least 250 graduate clinical practicum clock hours at CAA-accredited programs in the areas in

which certification is requested. Approval of your academic course work and clinical practicum is automatic, if your master's degree was earned at a CAA-accredited program, the program director verifies your satisfactory completion of all requirements, and your application is received at the ASHA national office within 3 years of the time you received your degree (ASHA Clinical Certification Board, 1994).

2. **Complete a Clinical Fellowship Year (CFY).** The purpose of the CFY is to help you transition from student clinician to independent professional. During your CFY you will learn many skills specific to service delivery in your employment setting and improve and hone the skills you learned as a student clinician. The CFY consists of paid (or volunteer) experience supervised by a professional holding current ASHA certification in the same area in which certification is sought (speech-language pathology or audiology). The CFY is not part of a university clinical training program. Although your supervisor will regularly evaluate your clinical work, no grades are given at the end, because your CFY is outside the scope of a university program. As a general rule, your university and former professors are not involved in your CFY. Typically, after you graduate, you will obtain employment as a speech-language pathologist. Often, your employer can supply CFY supervision. In fact, during your pre-employment interviews, it is a good practice to ask if CFY supervision will be provided and by whom. However, you and your supervisor need not work in the same setting. You may request a qualified speech-language pathologist from outside your work setting to supervise your CFY. Once you begin work and have a CFY supervisor, you will file a Clinical Fellowship Registration Agreement with ASHA. This form must be completed before, or within 4 weeks of beginning your CFY. The CFY can be completed in 9 months of full-time work (at least 30 hours per week) or up to 36 months of part-time work (15–19 hours per week). Less than 15 hours of work per week does not meet ASHA's CFY requirements (*ASHA Membership & Certification Handbook*, 1997).

3. **Pass the National Examination in Speech-Language Pathology and Audiology (NESPA).** The NESPA is a comprehensive assessment of an individual's knowledge in the area of speech-language pathology or audiology. Although the NESPA can be taken any time before you complete your CFY year, many individuals take the NESPA soon after they have completed their academic courses or taken their final comprehensive examinations at the university. Studying for comprehensive exams helps some students review for the NESPA. Also, there are books available and review courses offered on studying for the NESPA (Payne & Anderson, 1991; Roseberry-McKibbin & Hegde,

in press). The NESPA is administered as part of a *Specialty Area Test* of the *Praxis Series* by the Educational Testing Service (ETS). It consists of objective questions and can usually be taken through your university's testing office. Also, the ETS has a site on the World Wide Web. You can obtain information from this web site and from your university testing center.

4. **Know and adhere to the ASHA Code of Ethics.** The ASHA Code of Ethics is vital to the practice of speech-language pathology. It presents guidelines and standards for the protection of clients and clinicians. All individuals (students and graduates) seeking ASHA certification must agree to abide by the ASHA Code of Ethics. Chapter 3 contains a more detailed discussion of the Code of Ethics.

5. **Submit your application for certification and pay your membership fee.** ASHA publishes a Membership and Certification Handbook that contains application forms as well as detailed information regarding academic, practicum, CFY, and membership requirements. Contact ASHA to obtain the latest version of this handbook. If you have been a **NSSLHA** member (**National Student Speech-Language-Hearing Association**), you may be eligible to receive a discounted application fee. This information is also detailed in the Membership and Certification Handbook.

Although the CCC does not confer any legal status, it is nationally recognized as a requisite for practice in most employment settings excluding public schools. As you now know, the CCC indicates that you have met minimum proficiency standards set by ASHA to practice speech-language pathology, and it sometimes assists you in establishing credibility with new patients and associates. Many state licensure requirements are based on the CCC requirements and holding the CCC may make it easier for you to obtain a license in certain states.

State Licensure Board. Depending on where you live and what setting you practice in, you also may need to meet state licensure and credentialing requirements. In states that have a licensure law, ASHA's CCC is not sufficient to practice speech-language pathology or audiology. For example, regardless of their certification, credentials, or degrees, private practice speech-language pathologists in California must be licensed by the state before they can provide clinical services.

Licensure is regulated by a state government agency (e.g., Board of Examiners for Audiology and Speech Pathology). The majority of states in the United States now have licensure requirements for speech-language pathologists. With the exception of only a few states, the state licensure requirements are compatible with those of CCC. Many states also have licensure reciprocity with the CCC (Lynch & Welsh, 1993). Commonly exempt from licensure requirements are speech-language pathologists providing services in the public schools or federal government agencies.

Your university will coordinate your training so that you are meeting the minimum requirements of your state licensure board as well as ASHA certification requirements. However, if you are planning to move to another state after you graduate, you should contact the licensure board of that state to ensure you will have met their licensure requirements. Usually, the March reference issue of the *Asha* magazine contains each state's licensure board's name and address.

Department of Education. The speech-language pathologist who plans to work in the public schools must obtain an educational **credential** or certificate from the state's department of education. A credential is a document that verifies that you have met certain requirements and have obtained certain competencies. To practice speech-language services in the schools, the clinician need not have the state licensure or ASHA's CCC; but many clinicians have them anyway because the credentials indicate a certain level of commitment to the profession and its standards of excellence. A majority of states require a master's degree and a credential to practice speech-language pathology in the public schools. **IDEA (Individuals with Disabilities Education Act)**, one of several amendments to P.L. 94-142, is a federal law that requires speech-language pathologists working in the schools to meet the state's standards for speech-language pathologists practicing in nonpublic school settings. For example, if in your state a master's degree is required for licensure so you can work in a hospital, then you also must have a master's degree to practice in the public schools. In your educational practicum you will hear this referred to as **"highest state standards."** (Chapter 5 contains more information on IDEA regulations.) Educational and practicum requirements of most educational credentials are similar to those of CCC and state licensure. However, each state may have some unique requirement for the educational credential.

In addition to the course work required for the master's degree, a student seeking a school credential often needs to take courses related to public school speech, language, and hearing programs. Additional courses related to public school education also may be required. A student internship in the school setting is a typical credentialing requirement. Certain states require the speech-language pathologist to also have certification as a classroom teacher (Lowe, 1993).

Several states offer more than one educational credential for speech-language pathologists. One credential may allow you to teach a class with students who are communicatively handicapped. In these special classes, you may teach academic courses, physical education, art, and music, while emphasizing intervention for each child's communicative needs. Another credential may allow you to offer clinical services on an individual or small group basis to children with communicative disorders. Many of these services are provided in a private speech therapy room. However, a recent trend is to offer speech and language services in the classroom itself, with emphasis on integration into the class curriculum. Each state has its own educational credential laws for speech-language pathologists.

Because of this diversity and unique educational requirements for state public school credentials, you must consult on this with your advisor early in your clinical training. As you continue in your training program, you will become more familiar with the various requirements in your state.

The National Student Speech-Language-Hearing Association.
The National Student Speech-Language-Hearing Association (NSSLHA) is a national organization affiliated with ASHA. An excellent source of professional information in your department might be the local chapter of the NSSLHA. **Local chapters** of NSSLHA are run by students with the help of a faculty advisor. The NSSLHA is a national organization affiliated with ASHA. Its main purpose is to help students in speech-language pathology and audiology programs get involved with their future profession.

Your local chapter is an association of supportive fellow students who organize fundraising activities, social events, and professional workshops and seminars. Therefore, early in your undergraduate program, become a member of the local chapter of NSSLHA. This membership will help you keep current with all aspects of your profession.

NSSLHA membership dues are a fraction of the ASHA dues, and yet you receive many of the same benefits offered to full dues-paying professional members of ASHA. Members of NSSLHA receive all ASHA journals. These journals are a valuable source of scientific and professional information you cannot do without. As a graduate student, you will appreciate having your own collection of journals, which you frequently will be asked to read. NSSLHA also publishes its own journal that is distributed to its members free of charge. NSSLHA members are eligible to attend certain state and national conferences at reduced rates. Besides, NSSLHA gives students the opportunity to begin developing a social and professional affiliation with individuals having similar interests.

ASHA Special Interest Divisions.
ASHA's Special Interest Divisions (SIDs) are subgroups of ASHA composed of individuals who want to focus on specific areas of interest. For an additional fee, ASHA members

may join certain SIDs. These divisions include such areas as Administration and Supervision, Neurophysiology and Neurogenic Speech and Language Disorders, Speech Science and Orofacial Disorders, and Language Learning and Education. As of 1998, there were 15 divisions. Division members network among other professionals with similar interests. The special interest divisions may publish newsletters, sponsor continuing education, offer specialty certification, and influence the scope of practice for their division areas.

State Speech-Language and Hearing Associations. Many states have speech-language and hearing associations. These associations provide **local support** for speech-language pathologists, audiologists, and individuals with communicative disorders. The state organizations often sponsor workshops and conferences, help disseminate information, and, in conjunction with ASHA, develop professional guidelines. Involvement at the state level allows you to be active in state legislation, organization of state and local conferences, and networking with other professionals in your vicinity. Often members of state organizations also are ASHA members.

Related Professional Organizations. Although ASHA represents the profession of speech-language pathology as a whole, there are many specialty areas in the practice of speech-language pathology. Speech-language pathologists specializing in a certain area of service delivery, such as augmentative communication, may belong to ASHA and other related organizations. Examples of related professional organizations are the *United States Society for Augmentative and Alternative Communication, American Academy of Private Practice in Speech-Language Pathology and Audiology, Society of Hospital Directors of Communicative Disorders Programs,* and *Academy of Neurologic Communication Disorders and Sciences.* Names and addresses of some related professional organizations are published in the March issue of *Asha.*

ASHA Guidelines on Practicum

To ensure that students receive a broad but comprehensive training program, ASHA has established guidelines on clinical practicum. You satisfy the clinical practicum and internship requirements by earning the required number of clinical clock hours under the supervision of an ASHA-certified speech-language pathologist or audiologist. ASHA mandates requirements for both students and supervisors. This section of the text emphasizes the requirements for students.

Clinical Observation

Clinical observation offers students a nonthreatening introduction to the clinical process. It allows you to begin your preparation for clinical practicum by observing the work of more experienced clinicians. **Observation** is your opportunity to find out how what you have learned through your academic course work is applied in a clinic. By observing other clinicians, you begin to understand the assessment and treatment process. To maximize learning and meet ASHA's observation requirements, observe:

1. **A minimum of 25 clock hours.** ASHA requires students to obtain a minimum of 25 clock hours of supervised clinical observation before they begin their clinical practicum. Remember this is a minimum requirement. To enhance learning and ease your transition to active clinical involvement, you will want to observe as many evaluation and treatment sessions as possible.

2. **Live or videotaped clinical sessions.** Most students will observe live clinical sessions. However, observation of videotaped sessions or of live sessions on closed-circuit television monitors is also acceptable.

3. **A variety of clinical sessions.** Observation hours may be obtained for treatment and evaluation of individuals with communicative disorders. Observations may be of children or adults. The 25 hours may be a combination of audiology and speech-language pathology observation; it is not 25 hours of audiology or 25 hours of speech-language pathology. However, many universities specify that students' majority of observation hours be obtained in their area of professional emphasis (speech-language pathology or audiology). Other universities require a fairly equal distribution of observation hours between speech-language pathology and audiology. Typically, you will be directed to observe sessions relevant to your first clinical experience. Also, you may want to observe some clients over a period of time to note the progression of treatment, while you sample a variety of other clients and disorders. Regardless of the required distribution of observation hours, the 25 hours are a minimum requirement, and additional observation hours are strongly advised.

4. **Supervised by an ASHA-certified professional.** You may observe professionals and other student clinicians. All observations must be under the supervision of an ASHA-certified professional. Your supervisors and the clinic director will examine the observation log and reports to verify your observation hours. Observations may be made simultaneously with the supervisor, or the student observer may submit

reports to the supervisor for review and approval (ASHA Clinical Certification Board, 1994).

5. **With a purpose.** It is important to critically evaluate what you observe. It is not sufficient to just "watch" a clinical session and expect to gain much useful knowledge. Your supervisor will help you note the many variables that influence service delivery. To maximize the observation experience, you should take notes and describe specific components of a session. If possible and with the supervisor's approval, you should review the client's file or discuss the session with the clinician prior to observing. Ideally, after you have completed an observation, you should be able to answer the questions:

1. What type and severity of communicative disorder did the client exhibit?
2. What were the objectives of the session?
3. What were the target behaviors?
4. How did the clinician greet the client?
5. How was the session structured?
6. How did the clinician close the session and dismiss the client?
7. How was the room arranged?
8. How were the client and the clinician seated in relation to each other?
9. What types of materials and activities were used?
10. What did the clinician do to teach the target behaviors?
11. What types of cues were used (e.g., visual, tactile, etc.)?
12. What types of reinforcers were used and on what schedule?
13. How were undesirable behaviors decreased?
14. How were responses charted?
15. What activities seemed to be most effective?
16. What activities seemed to be least effective?
17. If you were the clinician, what changes might you make for the next session?

Responsibilities of Student Observers. Remember, as a student observer you are a representative of your university and are expected to demonstrate responsible and ethical behavior. When observing at both on- and off-campus sites, you should comply with the guidelines:

1. **Arrive on time for observations.** Regardless of how unobtrusive you try to be, if you arrive late for a scheduled observation you may disrupt the evaluation or treatment session. You also will not have a chance to discuss the client with the clinician prior to the session. If you do not know how the sessions started, you may have trouble under-

standing what you observe. Arriving late for a scheduled observation is irresponsible behavior. Clinical supervisors may not allow late arrivals to observe a session.

2. **Introduce yourself and request permission to observe.** Clinical supervisors are responsible for their clients' rights to privacy and for ensuring that you derive the greatest benefit from your observations. Although the observation may have been scheduled previously, there may be reasons to disallow a particular observation. For example, the client may have, for whatever reason, decided against being observed; the clinical supervisor may have determined that the observation area was too crowded or that the observation would not be beneficial for you or the client.

3. **Observe the entire clinical session.** This is necessary to obtain the greatest benefit from your observation. Each treatment and evaluation session contains certain sequenced events and procedures. If you arrive late or leave early, you get only a glimpse of the clinical process and, hence, you do not get the total picture. You may observe some isolated techniques while missing out on the rationale, antecedents, or consequences of certain techniques.

4. **Always respect the client's right to confidentiality.** All client information is confidential. As a student you will discuss with or report to others on your observations. These follow-up discussions, reports, or both will help enhance your learning. However, be careful to protect each client's privacy. Never discuss clients in public areas. If you have a report to make regarding your observation, you may refer to the person observed as "the client," "the individual," or, in some cases, you may use an alias for the client's name.

5. **Privately discuss a client with the clinician or the supervisor.** Discuss the client only when confidentiality is assured. Do not discuss the client when there are other people who may overhear your conversation.

6. **Do not interrupt the session or waste the clinician's time.** Clinicians need time to prepare for their sessions and the few minutes they have between clients are important for them. Ask appropriate questions when the clinician has time to respond, but do not converse about unrelated topics. Arriving on time for your observations and observing entire sessions should help provide opportunities for you to talk with the clinician.

7. **Do not remove clinical files from the clinic area.** In most cases, you will be able to review a client's file to obtain background informa-

tion. While reviewing the files, do not write in them or remove anything from the files. Take only notes that are helpful to your observation (e.g., medical history, therapy history, and so on). Once again, remember that all client information is confidential. Do not discuss with others any personal or clinical information you read in client files.

8. **Increase your observation skills.** To accomplish this, phonetically transcribe utterances, chart correct and incorrect productions, and take note of test results. This practice may help sharpen your observational skills as well as increase your recording skills. The more you learn during your observations, the more skills and confidence you will have to bring to your first practicum experience. The time you spend observing is for your benefit, so use it profitably.

9. **Complete an observation report form for each client.** Do this as soon as an observational session ends. Request the clinical supervisor to sign the observation report. Without a signature, observation hours are not valid. Observation reports should be turned into the clinic director or clinical supervisor. These reports will be used to substantiate your observation hours prior to your admittance to clinical practicum. Each university requires different reports and documentation. Follow the specific guidelines of your training program.

10. **Present yourself as a professional.** There will be clients, family members of the client, and other professionals at your observation site. You need to dress and behave like a professional. Therefore, follow the clinic dress code. Professional attire is considered appropriate dress. If you have doubts as to whether something is appropriate to wear, do not wear it. Communicate appropriately with the clinician, clinical supervisor, other student observers, clients, and clients' family members. Careless comments may easily be misinterpreted by others, especially clients and their families. Avoid judgmental remarks and unnecessary questions.

Various clinical sites may have additional rules and procedures. It is your responsibility to know the guidelines for observers at your site. It is also your responsibility to follow ASHA's Code of Ethics (American Speech-Language-Hearing Association 1994a). The Code of Ethics is described in Chapter 3.

Clinical Practicum

After you have taken the preclinic academic courses and completed supervised clinical observation requirements, you are qualified to begin your clinical practicum. Clinical practicum clock hours are earned for screening, evaluation, and treatment of communicative disorders. Some hours may also be earned from clinical staffings. You will gain experience with both children and adults and practice in a variety of settings. You will have some experience with audiologic patients; of course, most of your experience will be in speech-language pathology. To ensure quality training of speech-language pathologists and audiologists, ASHA has developed minimum requirements for students and supervisors.

Supervision Requirements of Clinical Practicum. The ASHA Clinical Certification Board (1994) describes the following supervision standards.

1. **The clinical supervisor must hold a current CCC in speech-language pathology or audiology.** Many states have licensure and credential requirements that clinical supervisors must also meet.

2. **Supervision may be provided only in areas in which the supervisor is qualified.** Speech-language pathologists may supervise all aspects of speech-language pathology service delivery, including evaluation and management. They also may supervise aural habilitation and rehabilitation services and audiologic screenings (nondiagnostic) for the purpose of initial identification of communicative disorders, or as part of a speech or language evaluation. Audiologists may supervise all audiological services, and aural habilitation and rehabilitation services. They also may supervise speech and language screenings for the purpose of initial identification of communicative disorders. Under no circumstances should individuals supervise clients they believe they are not qualified or prepared to supervise.

3. **A *minimum* of 25% of treatment sessions and a *minimum* of 50% of each diagnostic session must be supervised.** This rule must be followed regardless of a student clinician's level of experience. Additional supervision may be provided with beginning student clinicians and with more complex clients.

4. **A clinical supervisor must be available to consult with the student.** The supervisor must hold a current CCC and be available for consultation during all service delivery.

5. **The clinical supervisor should provide direct observation, instruction, and feedback.** Supervision also may include activities such as indirect observation via closed circuit television or videotapes, review of written reports, and conferences with the student clinician.

Number of Clinical Clock Hours Required. Individuals submitting applications for the CCC in Speech-Language Pathology postmarked January 1, 1993 or after must comply with the academic and clinical standards adopted by ASHA October 23, 1988 (ASHA Clinical Certification Board, 1994). These standards require students to complete a minimum of 375 clock hours that include:

1. **A minimum of 25 supervised clinical observation hours.** These hours must be completed prior to beginning clinical practicum and must be supervised by the university training program or its affiliates.

2. **A minimum of 350 total clinical practicum clock hours.** A total of 250 of these hours must be earned at the graduate level in the area in which the certificate is sought (audiology or speech-language pathology). The 250 hours in speech-language pathology may include working with clients with disorders of voice, fluency, articulation, dysphagia, or language. Clock hours may also be earned in clinical staffings.

3. **A minimum of 50 clock hours earned in each of three types of clinical settings.** The clinical settings must offer distinctly different clinical experiences, but may or may not be within the same institution. For example, the university may have special voice and augmentative communication clinics. Although they are located at the same address, they offer unique clinical experiences. Public schools and hospitals also may provide more than a single clinical experience. You also may participate in practicum at three or more different locations. For instance, your practicum may include assignment at an acute care hospital, a public school, and your university clinic.

4. **A minimum of 80 evaluation hours.** Of these, a minimum of 20 evaluation hours must be obtained in each of the categories: speech disorders in children, speech disorders in adults, language disorders in children, and language disorders in adults. The majority of these hours should not be obtained in screening. Speech disorders include voice, articulation, fluency, and dysphagia. Motor speech disorders such as apraxia and dysarthria also are counted. Aphasias are reported under language disorders. Disorders of meaning, syntax, morphologic features, and pragmatic use are counted under language disorders. Phonological disorders are language disorders; however, if you target specific sound productions as part of your treatment, it may be more appropriate to count those hours under speech. Your supervisor will direct you regarding how specific hours should be reported.

5. **A minimum of 80 treatment hours.** Of these, a minimum of 20 treatment hours should be obtained in each of the following areas: speech disorders in children, speech disorders in adults, language dis-

orders in children, language disorders in adults. Typically, you will earn many more than the minimum number of treatment hours. The minimum hour guidelines help ensure that you have experience with a variety of communicative disorders. Although these guidelines do not ensure that you obtain clinical practicum hours with clients who have specific disorders (such as voice disorders, fluency disorders, or apraxia), ASHA accreditation standards recommend that students receive appropriate training to work with a varied caseload. Therefore, if you find you are not obtaining a variety of clinical experiences or you are not obtaining clinical experiences in specific areas, talk with your clinical director or supervisor.

6. **A minimum of 20 hours in audiology.** These 20 hours may include evaluation, screening, or treatment of individuals with auditory disorders. Treatment may include speech-language therapy, auditory training, speech reading and clinical management, or counseling for individuals with hearing impairment.

7. **A maximum of up to 20 clock hours in a related disorder.** These hours are optional and may include a variety of experiences. For example, activities may be related to the development and maintenance of optimal communication or to the prevention of speech or language disorders. ASHA recommends that accent modification be counted under the category of related disorders.

8. **A maximum of up to 25 clock hours in clinical staffings.** These hours are optional and may be obtained from participation in staffings in which you discuss your client's assessment, treatment, or your recommendations with your supervisor and other student clinicians (ASHA Clinical Certification Board, 1994).

Individuals applying for the **CCC in Audiology** between January 1, 1993 and December 31, 2006 may choose to follow standards developed in 1988 by the Council on Professional Standards. Briefly, the clinical requirements include:

1. A minimum of 25 supervised clinical observation hours.
2. A minimum of 350 clock hours with at least 250 of the hours earned in audiology practicum at the graduate level.
3. A minimum of 50 clock hours earned in each of three types of clinical settings.
4. A minimum of 40 clock hours earned in each of the following categories: evaluation of hearing in children and evaluation of hearing in adults.

5. A minimum of 80 hours earned in the selection and use of amplification and assistive devices, with a minimum of 10 hours each with children and adults.

6. A minimum of 20 clock hours earned in the treatment of hearing disorders in children and adults.

7. A minimum of 20 clock hours earned in speech-language pathology. These hours must be unrelated to hearing impairment and can include evaluation, screening, and/or treatment of children or adults with various speech or language disorders. (*ASHA Membership and Certification Handbook, Audiology,* 1997)

As part of the 350 practicum hours, audiology students may earn up to 20 clock hours in related disorders. For instance students may earn hours for activities related to hearing conservation programs (ASHA Clinical Certification Board, 1994). For details on clinical methods and practicum in audiology, see Kelly, Davis, and Hegde (1994).

The 1997 Standards for the CCC in Audiology imposed significant changes in the requirements. These include:

1. A minimum of 75 graduate level semester hours that culminates in a master's or doctoral degree. These hours may include academic and practicum courses.

2. The 75 semester hours are effective for individuals who apply for certification after December 31, 2006. The doctoral degree is required for individuals who apply for certification after December 31, 2011.

3. Training initiated and completed at a CAA accredited program.

4. A minimum of 12 months of full-time, supervised clinical practicum.

The total clock hours required by ASHA are the minimum number of practicum hours. Because ASHA's requirements may change and your department may have additional practicum hour requirements, check with your advisor to ensure that you meet the requirements of ASHA and your university.

What to Count As Clinical Clock Hours. Sometimes there is confusion on what types of activities can be counted as clinical clock hours and what category the clock hours should be counted under. Use the following guidelines in recording your clock hours.

1. Clock hours may be earned in conjunction with a class assignment and during clinical practicum. For example, if as part of a class assignment in a course on aphasia, you are required to evaluate a client with aphasia, you may earn diagnostic clock hours even when not enrolled in clinical practicum. However, to earn those hours, your practicum assignment must be preapproved and you must be supervised by an individual who holds a CCC in speech-language pathology.

2. **Evaluation hours are earned for screening and assessments of communicative disorders.** Typically, the student clinician may earn screening hours at local preschools, at area public and private schools, at health fairs, and at the university clinic. Speech, language, and hearing screenings also may be performed at facilities serving the elderly. Evaluation hours may be earned while you are enrolled in a section of the clinic designated solely for diagnostics. Formal reevaluations may also be counted. For example, you also may acquire diagnostic hours as part of the assessment of your clients at the beginning of a treatment period. Readministering specific tests or other assessment procedures at the end of treatment to document the status of the client also may be counted as evaluation hours. However, administering probes during the treatment period should not be counted as evaluation hours. Time spent administering probes can be counted with treatment hours.

3. **Clock hours are earned for counseling clients or counseling or training family members.** Such counseling, of course, is closely relative to the communicative disorder of a client. For example, providing treatment for a client with a diagnosis of aphasia might include not only direct language intervention with a client, but sharing information with the client's family. It might be necessary for you to explain to the family members what aphasia means and how they can help the client regain some of the lost communicative behaviors. Or, your articulation treatment for a preschool child might included a home training program. In that case, you need to train the parents to ensure that they are able to carry out the home assignments.

4. **Clock hours are credited for the time spent in obtaining or giving assessment and treatment information.** You can count the time you spend taking a case history, interviewing the client, the client's family, or both. You can also count the time you spend discussing your diagnosis and recommendations with the client or client's family.

5. **Clock hours are earned for treatment and evaluation of a variety of disorders.** For example, clock hours earned in language treatment may include treatment of individuals with aphasia, language

delay, or traumatic brain injury. Management of phonological disorders may be counted under language or speech depending on the intervention emphasis. Hours earned in speech may include treatment provided for individuals with articulation disorders, apraxia, or dysarthria. Hours earned in voice disorders may include treatment of individuals with dysarthria or treatment of pitch, intensity, or resonance disorders. Time spent treating individuals with laryngectomy or hearing impairments also may be counted under voice. Hours earned in fluency may include time spent treating individuals with any type of disordered rhythm. As you know, hours earned in articulation, voice, and fluency disorders are reported under the category of speech disorders. Also, ASHA recognizes evaluation and treatment of dysphagia under the category of speech disorders.

6. **In the cases of multiple communicative disorder, you can count separately the time spent in treating each disorder.** A child with a cleft palate may have disordered articulation, voice, and language. An individual with dysarthria may present both an articulation and a voice disorder. An individual with aphasia may have concomitant apraxia. An individual with a hearing impairment may have an articulation, voice, and language disorder. In all such cases, divide your clock hours according to how much time was spent in diagnosing or treating each of the disorders.

7. **Clinical staffings may be counted as clock hours.** Clinical staffings may include activities such as meetings with other professionals to discuss your client's treatment. For example, in certain settings the team of professionals providing rehabilitation services for a client may meet to discuss the client's treatment, progress, prognosis for further gains, and recommendations for future treatment. A maximum of 25 clock hours may be acquired from participation in client staffings with or without the client present when evaluation, treatment, or recommendations are discussed. Routine meetings with your clinic supervisor cannot be counted as clinical staffings.

8. **Count time spent on certain clinically related activities.** These include activities performed to prevent communicative disorders or to develop, maintain, or maximize communication skills. For example, you may be in a setting where you will train certain staff members to communicate more effectively with your client and to assist your client in communicating more effectively with the staff. ASHA suggests that accent modification be counted in this category. A maximum of 20 hours may be counted in this category.

9. **Do not count preparation time as clinical clock hours.** Although you will spend much time in gathering materials or ideas, writ-

ing reports and lesson plans, scoring tests, or transcribing language samples, you cannot count clock hours for these activities.

Remember that most clinical practicum clock hours are earned for direct client contact time only. The exceptions are the 25 staffing hours that can be counted, counseling and training a client's family directly related to a client's communicative disorder, and up to 20 hours in a related disorder. Your clinical supervisor will answer any questions you have regarding how to count, record, or report your clinical hours.

Payment for Clinical Services. According to ASHA guidelines, student clinicians may have a paid clinical practicum. Financial incentives may be in the form of wages, stipends, grants, or scholarships. Although some sites pay students, many do not. Regardless of whether the sites provide students' monetary reimbursement, each site must adhere to ASHA's guidelines on student practicum and supervision. Your advisor and the financial aid office at your university can give you information on financial assistance available to you.

Clinical Practicum as a Learning Experience

Clinical practicum is designed to give you an exceptional learning experience. The practicum gives you an opportunity to gain experience with a wide variety of individuals with communicative disorders. Under the supervision of qualified speech-language pathologists, you learn to evaluate and treat clients with fluency, voice, language, and articulation disorders of various severity and etiological factors. You will gain experience in many different clinical settings including acute care hospitals, rehabilitation facilities, psychiatric hospitals, skilled nursing facilities, private practices, and public schools.

Initially, you may be somewhat apprehensive about beginning your practicum. This is a normal response, but as you gain more experience and confidence, you will discover that clinical practicum is exciting and rewarding. You are encouraged to experience as many types of clients and clinical settings as you can.

Remember, you are a student and are not expected to perform like an experienced professional. What is expected of you is that you demonstrate consistent progress in each of your practicum assignments. Speech-language pathology is exciting partly because there is always something new to learn.

Now you have a general idea of the personal and academic requirements for a successful clinical practicum. You also know ASHA's require-

ments for types of practicum hours and clinical settings in which to acquire them. This is your chance to apply information learned in academic
classes and explore some of the possibilities the profession of speech-language pathology has to offer.

2

Organization of Clinical Practicum

linical practicum is organized on a hierarchy of clinical experiences and expectations. Typically, clinical practicum begins at a university clinic, where beginning student clinicians are assigned one or two clients. As student clinicians gain experience, become more confident, and are able to make more independent decisions, their client caseload is increased and varied. The student clinicians then may be assigned to off-campus clinical settings for clinical internships.

Distance learning programs may have clinical practicum requirements designed specifically for students in that program. Those requirements must meet ASHA's minimum requirements. Students enrolled in distance learning programs take academic classes through such different methods as Internet, videotaped, and televised courses. However, their clinical practicum is done in a more traditional manner. An ASHA certified supervisor must be available.

Regardless of the type of program you are enrolled in, after you have completed the required hours of supervised clinical observation, prerequisite course work, and other departmental requirements, you may begin your clinical practicum. Many clinical practicum settings are available for the speech-language pathology student clinician. Following is an overview of a few of the different clinical settings.

On-Campus Clinical Practicum

University Clinic

The university clinic strives to provide high quality clinical services in conjunction with appropriate educational experiences for student clinicians. Typically, the clinic is designed and equipped to facilitate clinical training and promote clinical research. As a student clinician you may be involved in research activities, providing direct client services, or both.

Prerequisites.   As pointed out earlier, prerequisites for clinical practicum include **completion of 25 supervised observation hours** and certain **preclinic academic courses**. Your university may have additional requisites such as a health clearance, acceptance into the graduate or clinical practicum program, faculty recommendations, and so on. Beginning student clinicians are not expected to work without guidance from a supervisor. However, they are expected to apply information learned in academic course work, implement supervisor recommendations, ask questions, and, as the semester progresses, expand on supervisor suggestions. Together with your clinical performance, these are some of the behaviors your supervisor will use to judge your ability to succeed in future clinic assignments.

Supervision.   Regular observation and supervision are integral components of your university clinic assignment. Supervision at the university clinic may be provided by the university teaching faculty, full-time supervisory faculty, part-time supervisory staff, or a combination of the three. You may have one supervisor per term or more than one supervisor, based on the departmental policy and clinical schedule. Most departments tend to assign a single supervisor to beginning clinicians. All supervision in ASHA-accredited programs should be in compliance with the ASHA guidelines on supervision. The amount of supervision provided also may be adjusted upward depending on your level of clinical experience, your clinical skill level, the complexity of your client's disorder, or a combination of these factors.

University clinical facilities are arranged to maximize observation of sessions with minimal distractions. Many clinics are equipped with observation windows for viewing and with an audio system for listening. Student clinicians providing clinical services at a university clinic should be prepared for frequent observations by supervisors, family members of clients, and other students. Although some beginning student clinicians find it unsettling, it is not unusual for supervisors to enter the treatment room to observe a session or to demonstrate a specific treatment technique. Too, your sessions may be videotaped for later observation or class demonstration. Once you get over the embarrassment of seeing yourself on TV, self-evaluating your clinical session by reviewing a videotape of a session is an excellent learning tool. Your sessions also may be recorded by a television camera for a closed-circuit television monitor. This allows supervisors to view clinical interactions from a central location without interfering with the evaluation or therapy sessions.

Your supervisor frequently evaluates your clinical skills. You may get both written and verbal feedback. You may have weekly meetings with your clinical supervisor, weekly staffing, or discussions after each clinical session. At the minimum, you will receive a written final evaluation; most departments provide written midterm evaluations as well. If your progress in the clinical practicum is unsatisfactory, you will be notified and counseled regarding your continued participation in the program. If you feel you are not getting sufficient feedback from your supervisor, prepare appropriate questions, make an appointment with your supervisor, and meet with your supervisor to discuss your questions and concerns.

Clinic Schedules. Typically, a university clinic is operated on an 8 a.m. to 5 p.m. weekday schedule. Some universities also have evening hours to accommodate individuals who cannot attend the clinic during regular business hours. Some university clinics provide services only during the academic year. This schedule is not optimal, as it disrupts services offered to clients who often need sustained and continuous treatment. To provide more continuous services, some clinics operate 12 months of the year, with professional staff providing services during the intersessions.

Clients receiving speech-language pathology services usually are scheduled for two to three sessions per week, with each session lasting 30 to 60 minutes. Evaluation sessions are sometimes scheduled for larger blocks of time. Most clients are scheduled for individual treatment sessions; however, some clients may be scheduled for group sessions. Generally, you will be allotted 5 to 10 minutes between clients to organize your materials. It is important to be prepared for your sessions in advance; the few minutes between clients is obviously not the time for planning assessment or treatment activities. This is the time for you to finish with one client and greet the next client in the clinic waiting room.

As a student of speech-language pathology, you will also complete a **practicum assignment in audiology**. As with speech-language pathology clients, the appointments for audiology clients vary with the needs of the client. Generally, appointments for a standard hearing evaluation will be 1 hour. Additional time may be allotted for less experienced student clinicians or clients with more complex disorders.

At the beginning of the semester, you will receive your clinical assignment. You will be given your clinic schedule, and your supervisor or clinic director will assign you appropriate clients. At many universities, the student clinician is responsible for telephoning the client and confirming the client's clinic schedule.

Routinely check with the clinic secretary to verify clinic appointments and note any changes in your clinic schedule. Each university has different methods for scheduling clients and communicating the scheduling to student clinicians. To avoid confusion, missed appointments, or last-minute preparations, adhere to the procedures of your university.

Prior to meeting your client, you must review the client's clinical file, develop a plan for the first meeting with your client, and discuss the plan with your clinical supervisor. You should also discuss any evaluation plans with your supervisor and notify your supervisor of the time the evaluation is scheduled. For additional information on working with clients, refer to Chapter 5.

Types of Clients. A wide range of ages and communicative disorders are represented in the university clinic's caseload. The university caseload is influenced by demographic factors and the availability of other speech-language pathology services in the community. For example, if there is a large rehabilitation agency in the area, the clinic may enroll fewer clients with diagnoses of aphasia; if there is a pediatric hospital offering speech and hearing services, the clinic may serve a limited number of children. Economic factors also affect the types of clients typically seen at the university clinic. Compared to private practices or hospitals, a university clinic often has a reduced fee scale and, because of this, may attract clients with limited incomes or no insurance coverage.

Other factors influencing the university client caseload are the expertise of faculty members and the department's relationship with allied health professionals. For instance, if your department has faculty members well known for their expertise in fluency disorders, the clinic may attract a large number of clients with fluency disorders. In addition, if your university is affiliated with a medical center, your clinic may provide outpatient or follow-up services for its clients.

Report Writing and Record Keeping. University clinics have varying policies and terminology regarding writing assignments. Most universities require some type of written description of how you plan to help remediate your clients' disorders. This may be in the form of **daily lesson plans**, **weekly lesson plans**, or **semester treatment plans**. You may be required to submit typed plans, handwritten plans, or computer-generated plans. Whatever the format, your supervisor will review all your plans. Throughout the term, you will be required to **regularly document your clients' progress** and any changes in your treatment plans. At the end of the term, you will be required to write a **final summary** or progress report. The final report should describe the client's status at the beginning of treatment, the treatment goals, the treatment procedures, and the progress made by the client.

Your clinical supervisor will give you instructions regarding the format and timelines for all written work. Report writing and record keeping are discussed in greater detail in Chapter 5.

Off-Campus Practicum Sites

Off-campus practicum sites vary from region to region and from university to university. Common off-campus practicum sites include public schools, hospitals, skilled nursing facilities, rehabilitation agencies, psychiatric hospitals, preschool programs, correctional facilities, and private speech and hearing centers.

As you know, the first semester (or quarter) of clinical practicum typically is completed in a university speech and hearing clinic. Student clinicians may begin off-campus practicum anytime after their first term of clinical practicum. Off-campus practicum usually is supervised by an ASHA-certified speech-language pathologist who works at that site, with consultation provided by the university supervisor. All off-campus sites must comply with ASHA's regulations on the frequency and type of supervision.

Student clinicians usually are required to follow the holiday schedule of the off-campus site instead of the schedule of the university. Student clinicians also must comply with the site's requirements regarding professional responsibility and conduct. University grading policy and the department's criteria of acceptable performance dictate the grading. However, the site supervisor evaluates the student's performance and suggests a grade. The off-campus supervisor's judgment of the student's performance greatly influences a student's final grade.

Public Schools

Typically to work in the public schools, a credential (or certificate) issued by the state's department of education is required. A **credential** is a document that indicates certain competencies have been met and authorizes the individual holding the credential to provide services according to its parameters. For example, you might earn a credential authorizing you to provide individual speech therapy services in the schools, a credential authorizing you to teach in a classroom, or a credential authorizing you to do both. In many states, to obtain a credential or certificate to work as a speech-language pathologist in the public schools, student clinicians must complete a practicum experience in a school setting.

A university seminar may accompany the school clinical practicum assignment. Although the practicum provides experience in assessing and treating children who are communicatively handicapped in the school, a seminar held at the university provides a forum for discussing issues and exchanging ideas. In such a seminar, historical and current issues affecting the school speech-language pathologist and the organization and administration of speech-language pathology programs in the public schools may be discussed. Also, seminars offer student clinicians an opportunity to share their practicum experiences and exchange ideas.

Prerequisites. The prerequisites to internship in the public school depend on the university and state credential requirements. Although it may be helpful for beginning your public school practicum, you need not have experience working with groups. However, you will need to have completed course work relative to childhood speech and language disorders, and you will need to have worked with children of different ages and disorders. Prior to enrolling in your public school clinical practicum you may be required to enroll in your university **credential program**. To verify that you have met the requisites to begin a public school practicum, the credential program's personnel reviews your records, required test results, grade-point average, and so on. Certain states may require you to pass a competency examination. Also, in California, in conjunction with the credential application, individuals are required to obtain a character and identification clearance that includes submission of fingerprint identification cards to the FBI. In addition, credential applicants must show evidence of having passed a recent tuberculosis (TB) test. Review your school's prerequisites with your advisor.

Supervision. The student clinician completes an **internship** assignment (popularly known as a *student teaching*) under the supervision of a school speech-language pathologist who is credentialed and ASHA-certified. Supervision is provided in accordance with ASHA guidelines. Generally, the supervising speech-language pathologists give student clinicians a midterm and final evaluation that is aligned with university grading policy. A supervisor from the university training program coordinates this arrangement and may periodically meet with the student and supervisor or communicate with them by telephone or e-mail.

School Internship Schedules. These generally are full-day assignments, 3 to 5 days a week, perhaps in conjunction with a weekly seminar. The school day usually is from 8 a.m. to 3 p.m., but you should be prepared to spend additional time for writing reports, planning sessions, attending meetings, and preparing materials.

Although basic diagnostic and treatment principles do not vary from those appropriate in other clinical settings, several scheduling and service delivery models may be unique to the school setting. For example, your previous experience in working with children may have followed only the clinical model; school-based speech services may be provided through different service delivery models. You may provide both direct and indirect services. To compound scheduling issues, many students with mild to severe disabilities are **fully included** in a regular education class (McCormick, Loeb, & Schiefelbusch, 1997; Meyen, Vergason, & Whelan, 1996). That is, they receive instruction in a regular education classroom with peers of their age. This setting is referred to as an **inclusive** setting. Typically, support is provided to fully included students by different educational specialists, who provide services in the classroom, make suggestions to the teacher, or both. Other schools and parents may determine that separate special education classes better meet the needs of their students. Regardless of the format followed at your school setting, you should have the option of providing a **continuum of services**.

Direct services are services in which the speech-language pathologist works with a student individually or with other students. These services may be provided by following the traditional clinical format in which a clinician works with individual children or children in small groups. In the **pull-out model**, children are served in the speech-language pathologist's office or a clinical room set aside for this purpose. Students generally attend treatment sessions one to two times per week. Treatment may include stimulus material unrelated to classroom curriculum; however, more and more school curriculum is being incorporated into treatment when it is appropriate to the student's speech or language needs. Also, functional treatment goals and objectives reflecting educational benchmarks are written. This model commonly is referred to as the pull-out model because students are taken out of their classes to receive speech-language services.

You also may provide direct speech-language services in the student's class on a one-to-one or small group basis. This is sometimes referred to as **pull-in** services (Merritt & Culatta, 1998). In this case, you may provide treatment for one or more students in a separate area of the classroom while the rest of the class continues other activities. When classroom instruction is divided into **learning stations**, you may treat children at one of the stations. The classroom teacher and aide may be responsible for two other learning stations and another station may be for independent study. Students rotate from one station to the next, typically spending 10 to 15 min at each station. This type of scheduling may be common in kindergarten and special day classes. Special day classes are classrooms where education is provided to students with specific educational needs by teachers who have specialized training to meet those students' academic needs. Generally, students are in the special day class for much of the day, but participate in regular education for designated times during portions of the day.

A different model of whole class intervention is more commonly used at the secondary level. In this model, the school speech-language pathologist teaches one period of the day and students attend the class as they would their mathematics or history classes. This may be a language laboratory or a **language and speech class**. In some schools, this class may fulfill the students' requirements for English language.

Direct speech-language services in the schools also may be provided within a **collaborative instruction model**. In this model, the speech-language pathologist and classroom teacher coordinate their lessons and work together to provide students with appropriate learning opportunities.. Collaborative models have been identified in various ways. Merritt and Culatta (1998) described three methods that are fairly universal: supportive learning, team teaching, and complementary instruction:

- **Supportive learning** allows the primary instructor to teach a lesson while the coinstructor provides supplementary teaching or activities. In one lesson, the speech-language pathologist may teach a lesson with the classroom teacher offering supportive activities. In another lesson, the teaching roles may be reversed, with the classroom teacher instructing the class and the speech-language pathologist providing supplementary and supportive activities. In this model, you might present language lessons to all the students in the class. During the lesson, you also work on the speech and language objectives of the students enrolled on your caseload. Occasionally, you may teach a subject, such as mathematics, to demonstrate to the teacher how changing the language in a lesson can benefit children with language disorders.
- **Team teaching** is a model in which the teacher and speech-language pathologist share in the responsibilities of planning and teaching a lesson. Typically, the lesson is divided into segments, with each professional teaching certain parts of the lesson.
- **Complementary instruction** is similar to team teaching. Together, the speech-language pathologist and teacher instruct a lesson. The teacher focuses on such content areas as science, social studies, math, and so on. The speech-language pathologist teach-

es such language-related skills as mapping of ideas, selecting main ideas, outlining, and taking notes.

Sufficient planning time is critical to the success of collaborative instruction. When you develop your schedule, you must allow time, not only for teaching a lesson, but for planning with the teacher. In the collaborative instruction model, the speech-language pathologist and classroom teacher discuss the needs of the class and the specific needs of the students enrolled for speech or language services. The speech-language pathologist models an appropriate language and learning environment for students with communicative disorders. The teacher and speech-language pathologist share effective methods of teaching and obtain new ideas by observing each other. In addition, students with communicative disorders receive services in a natural communicative setting that emphasizes classroom curriculum and assists with generalization of skills. Chapter 5 contains additional information on working collaboratively with the classroom teacher, parents, and other professionals.

Indirect speech-language pathology services is another service delivery option used in the public schools. Indirect services are provided under a **consultative model** in which the speech-language pathologist works with the student's parents, teachers, or other professionals to address the needs of the student. In this model, the speech-language pathologist is a consultant who does not directly treat the child. You may assist the teacher by providing suggestions for working with certain students who are not on your caseload. In other cases, you may determine that certain students who were receiving treatment for a language disorder no longer require direct services. You discuss with the teachers and parents ways to modify communication to maximize a student's performance. The students remain on your caseload for a few months as you monitor their progress. During this monitoring stage, you may make suggestions to the parents and teachers. In some instances, you may determine that a student should be re-enrolled for direct services.

All of these models have a place in the delivery of speech-language pathology services. However, each should be viewed on a continuum of need. Some students require intensive, direct services. Others require less direct intervention and benefit from modification of teaching strategies. You must view each student's needs separately. Your public school practicum is an opportunity to learn when and how to effectively implement the various service delivery models.

Scheduling sessions, as you might imagine from the variety of service delivery options, can be difficult. A new experience in the public school setting is that you also may be required to serve a large number of students. At the university speech and hearing clinic, you may be used to working with two to three clients per term. In your school practicum, it is likely that you will be asked to gradually assume a caseload of a full-time clinician. The actual number of children on a public school clinician's caseload varies from state to state. You usually will see each student at least once a week. ASHA has recommended a caseload size ranging from 8 to 40 students for speech-language services offered in the schools (ASHA Committee on Service Delivery in the Schools, 1993). Unfortunately, few school speech-language pathologists have caseloads at or below ASHA's recommended size. A reduced and manageable caseload size is a goal that is yet to be realized in all of the nation's public schools.

Group treatment sessions is another new experience you may have in your public school experience. Because of the large number of students, public school speech-language pathologists typically serve students in small groups. Often, the number in each group depends on the total caseload of the clinician. The larger the caseload, the bigger the group size.

Different options for scheduling and grouping children are available. Some clinicians group students with similar disorders together. This is **called homogeneous grouping**. Other clinicians prefer **heterogeneous grouping** that may allow one student to model for another student. For example, a child with a language disorder may provide an excellent model for production of /r/. The child who mispronounces /r/ may model different language structures. Given the choice of grouping children of widely different ages (e.g., 5–12-year-olds) and those of different disorders, it may be better to group according to age, so that the students share certain comprehension and attention levels.

In addition to scheduling specific students, you must allow time in your day to communicate and collaborate with such other professionals as the classroom teacher, school psychologist, and school nurse. Also, you will want to have specific blocks of time allocated for testing students, writing reports, making telephone calls, and meeting with parents. More specific information regarding scheduling of clients is discussed in Chapter 5.

Types of Clients. As one might expect from the wide range of ages offered services in the public schools, the caseload for student clinicians participating in clinical practicum in that setting can be varied enough to satisfy almost anyone's professional interests. In addition to the different age groups, children with a wide range of disabilities are served in public schools. Depending on the school assignment, your caseload could include children who have a single articulation error to those with multiple errors resulting in unintelligible speech. You will work with many children exhibiting speech and language disorders of unknown etiology. You also might work with students with multiple physical and sensory disabilities. Children who have speech or language disorders associated with traumatic brain injury, cerebral palsy, emotional disorders, cognitive handicaps, hearing impairment, or cleft palate also are served in public schools. You will discover that your school internship gives you the opportunity to work with children exhibiting a variety of disorders. A caseload at a kindergarten through sixth-grade school may consist of students with fluency, language, articulation, and voice disorders. There are also schools that specialize in serving a specific population. For example, a residential school for children who are deaf may focus on oral communication and another may focus on sign language for communicating.

Federal and state laws govern public school services. Speech-language pathology services in the public schools are designed to meet the needs of all individuals who are communicatively handicapped and eligible for school services as mandated by federal legislation, the **Education of All Handicapped Children Act (EHA), Public Law 94–142** (P.L. 94–142) was passed on November 25, 1975 and provided for educational services for all handicapped children (Dublinske & Healey, 1978). Although several amendments to the EHA have been made over the years, it remains the cornerstone for special education services. The discretionary programs of the EHA were reauthorized in 1990. At that time, the name was changed to the **Individuals with Disabilities Education Act (IDEA)** (ASHA Governmental Affairs Review, 1990). In 1997, IDEA again was reauthorized and amendments added.

The EHA Amendments of 1986, P.L. 99–457 (now Part C of IDEA, 1997), established funds for states to provide services for children from birth through 2 years of age who have disabilities. Services to the families of these children also were included in P.L. 99–457. In addition, the 1986 EHA Amendments included legislation (Part B of EHA) on personnel standards. Part B of P.L. 99–457 required state education agencies to develop and maintain personnel standards based on the highest requirements in the state. For speech-language pathologists, including school speech-language pathologists, in many states this standard is the master's degree.

The school speech-language pathology services are governed by several other federal laws and guidelines. State laws and regulations on special education also affect speech-language pathology services provided in the public schools. School speech-language pathologists must know and follow all guidelines affecting their school sites.

In addition to mandating age requirements, P.L. 94–142 outlined the scope of speech-language pathology services in the public schools. The speech-language pathologist is responsible for providing the services of:

1. **Identification of students** with speech or language disorders through such activities as whole class or individual screenings.
2. **Assessment** of speech and language.

3. **Treatment** of students with identified communicative disorders.
4. **Consultation** with parents, teachers, and others regarding communicative disorders.
5. **Referral** to other professionals for service necessary for the remediation of a communicative disorder (Dublinske & Healey, 1978).

The **eligibility criteria** for public school students to receive speech-language pathology services differ from those used in most university clinics. There are both federal and state eligibility guidelines regulating admission to a school speech-language program. These guidelines do not always coincide with the commonly accepted practices in speech-language pathology. For example, in California, a child who has only a single articulation error may not be eligible to receive services through the public school until 7 or 8 years of age (California State Department of Education, 1989). Whereas, the same child might receive treatment at a much younger age at a university clinic.

Report Writing and Record Keeping. In addition to providing assessment and remediation services, school speech-language pathologists have many administrative duties of report writing and record keeping. You will learn to organize and maintain records for all of the students on your caseload according to each of their **individualized educational programs (IEP)**.

The IEP is a contract between the parents and the school that outlines a child's current level of performance, needs, objectives, and intervention that will be provided. Because students receive speech and language treatment in the public schools to maximize their educational opportunities as much as possible, your speech and language objectives should be tied to educational benchmarks. The IEP is one of the cornerstones of service delivery in the public schools and is discussed in greater detail in Chapter 5. In addition to learning more about the IEP and how to write one, you will learn other new terms in your school practicum. Appendix A contains a list of acronyms and abbreviations used frequently in the educational setting.

Working With Parents and Professionals. As a student intern in the public schools, you may schedule and conduct meetings with parents and other professionals. You will learn to communicate effectively and work cooperatively with them to enhance your students' learning. Collaboration with other professionals is an important component of your school-based treatment experience. (Chapter 5 contains additional information on this area.) On occasion you may work closely with or refer your students to school nurses, physicians, audiologists, social workers, psychologists, principals, or special and regular education teachers. You also may be called to provide staff and parent inservices.

Hospitals

Hospital speech-language pathology covers a gamut of services. When completing a clinical practicum in a hospital setting, you may work with patients in the acute care phase, subacute care facility, inpatient rehabilitation units, outpatient departments, or at the home of the patient under the home health care provisions. The activities of your practicum will depend both on the organization of the hospital and the requirements of your individual practicum assignment. The following sections are only an overview of some of the experiences you may gain in a hospital setting. In a comprehensive medical setting, you will encounter a wide range of stimulating and challenging learning opportunities.

Prerequisites. Ideally, before you begin your clinical practicum at a hospital, you will have completed academic courses in **aphasia**, **voice**, **dysphagia**, and **neurological-based speech disorders**. You will have refreshed your knowledge of anatomy and physiology of speech and hearing mechanisms. You also will have had some experience in assessing and treating clients with communicative disorders associated with medical conditions. Because you can expect a large percentage of patients with swallowing disorders to be on a hospital-based speech-language pathologist's caseload, even if it is not required at your university, you will want to complete a course in dysphagia. If your university does not offer this course, you can attend a workshop or complete some independent readings.

Supervision. As a student intern, you gradually will assume the responsibilities of the staff speech-language pathologist under the supervision of a licensed and certified speech-language pathologist on the hospital staff. The staff clinician who supervises in a hospital must follow the ASHA guidelines. Supervision may increase to 100% for patients with complex or unusual disorders. For example, for patients with swallowing disorders, a student clinician may provide limited evaluation and treatment and only after extensive training and with close supervision. The clinic director or a university supervisor will coordinate this internship, routinely communicating with your supervisor at the hospital.

Hospital Schedules. Hospital-based speech-language pathologists typically work an 8-hour day, 5 days per week. In some cases, their day begins at 8 a.m. and ends at 5 p.m. In other cases, to cover swallowing treatment at the patients' breakfast or dinner, the day may begin earlier or later. Unlike programs in the public schools, individual treatment sessions are the most frequent sessions in hospital settings. An exception might be some group language meetings. The clinician typically works with a patient in his or her office or individual treatment rooms. However, bedside evaluation and treatment are sometimes provided for patients with more acute medical conditions. For example, a patient just recovering from a stroke may not be medically stable enough to leave his or her hospital room. However, it still may be necessary for you to perform an assessment to determine the patient's communicative status and need for intervention.

Hospitalized patients may receive speech and language services 5 or 6 days per week. Outpatients are usually seen less frequently and may be seen in the office or as part of home health services. Hospital patients may be seen more frequently than those attending university clinics, but they may receive services for a shorter duration. Because of health care costs, most hospitals discharge patients as soon as possible, with due regard to the patient's well-being. Consequently, you may think that you are just beginning to know a patient or observe some progress when that individual is discharged from the hospital.

Videofluorographic and bedside evaluation of the swallowing mechanism is a large part of the job for many hospital-based speech-language pathologists. Videofluorographic evaluation is an objective procedure in which the client's swallowing mechanism is recorded on a moving picture (that is, video). The speech-language pathologist gives the patient foods or beverages containing radiopaque (barium) material. The radiologist records images of the patient's swallow using a fluoroscopy camera. During and following the examination, the speech-language pathologist can examine the patient's ability to safely swallow foods of various textures. Student clinicians often observe and assist with this procedure, but rarely independently perform the evaluation.

The bedside evaluation is less objective and more controversial regarding the validity of the results. During the bedside swallowing evaluation, the speech-language pathologist notes the patient's medical and swallowing history, oral secretion and awareness levels, general cognitive level, nutritional status, motor control, presence of normal and abnormal reflexes, oral sensory level, and ability to safely eat selected foods. Your internship in the hospital will give you experience working with many patients with swallowing disorders.

Rotating schedules are used in many hospitals. The hospital clinician may be assigned a rotating schedule that includes home health services, alternating weekends, or both. For example, the clinician may work 4 months in the hospital, 4 months with home health, and 4 months with outpatients. Too, the speech-language pathologist may be required to work some weekends to cover required 6 day per week treatments. In addition to hospital-based clinicians, in-home speech services may be provided by private agencies or individual speech-language pathologists contracting for these services.

Types of Patients. The speech-language pathologist providing services in the acute care setting is responsible for the speech and language evaluation and treatment of patients with many medical conditions. Although, you will encounter patients with **neurological diseases** and **traumatic brain injury (TBI), those recovering from a cerebrovascular accident (CVA)**, and **patients facing or recovering from a laryngectomy**, the large majority of your caseload will **involve evaluation and treatment of dysphagia**. Also, and more frequently in the rehabilitation or outpatient setting than in the acute care setting, you may be involved in assessing the need for and training in the use of augmentative communication equipment.

In most hospital and rehabilitation facilities, patients of all ages may be served. An exception is a pediatric setting in which student clinicians work exclusively with children.

The speech-language pathology department is an integral part of a hospital's rehabilitation services. A speech-language pathologist serves as a member of a **multidisciplinary team** and provides assessment and intervention for patients admitted for rehabilitation services. The multidisciplinary team is a group of professionals and family members who work together to determine and provide optimal patient management. In the hospitals, some team members you may work with include a nurse, physician, physical therapist, occupational therapist, family caregiver, and social worker. For additional information on allied health professionals and working on a team, refer to Chapter 5.

Some patients are transferred to the rehabilitation department after discharge from the acute care setting. Other patients are discharged from the hospital for convalescence and may later be readmitted when they become candidates for rehabilitation.

In a hospital rehabilitation setting, you may have the opportunity to work with patients over a longer period of time than you will with most of the patients in acute care settings. You will establish both short-term and long-range communicative objectives for your patients and help them to regain their independent living skills.

Individuals are sometimes discharged from the hospital acute care or rehabilitation setting before they have completed their speech or language treatment. These individuals may be served in the hospital outpatient setting or in their homes via home health services. Patients who are too ill to travel to the clinic outpatient facilities are seen in their homes.

Home health service may be provided to individuals after they are discharged from the hospital. As a home care provider, you may travel extensively because assessment and treatment are provided in patients' homes. Service delivery in the home enables you to evaluate patients' functional communication skills within their natural environments. In the homes, you also can assess the interactional patterns between the patient and his or her family and provide treatment in the natural environment. The speech-language pathologist is one of several home care providers, including nurses, physical therapists, and occupational therapists.

Treatment may be enhanced by working with the patient and his or her family in their home, but there are several factors you must consider. Because you are working in an individual's home, you must be aware of cultural or traditional characteristics of the home. For example, members of a family may remove their shoes before entering the home; other families do not readily accept strangers into their homes. You also must be aware of safety factors such as the type of neighborhood a home is located in (e.g., high crime area), the presence of an aggressive and unfriendly dog in the home, the possibility of substance abuse in the home, and the overall safety of the home. Also, while in a patient's home, there are many distractions from other family members, doorbells, and ringing telephones.

As is the case with speech-language pathologists working in the schools, hospital-based speech-language pathologists and their services are regulated by several agencies, including the federal government. The sort of clients on your caseload and the frequency, duration, and type of service largely may be influenced by private insurance company's policies and the federal government's Medicare programs.

Report Writing and Record Keeping. As you will find in all your practicum assignments, the speech-language pathologist in the hospital is responsible for carefully documenting assessment results, treatment plans, and patient progress. In addition, you will learn to complete different insurance and Medicare forms. In many cases, accurate and appropriate documentation will determine if your hospital receives reimbursement for your services from an insurance company. You will frequently hear and read the acronym: **FIMS (functional independence measures)**. FIMS are similar to the objectives you will have learned to write in your initial clinic experiences; however, FIMS are written with the emphasis on a patient's ability to perform functional tasks (e.g., tell when he or she is ill) with as little assistance as possible. Your supervisor will assist you with the specific requirements at your hospital practicum site.

One of the frequently utilized means of communication among professionals in hospitals is through notations in the patients' charts. Refer to Chapter 5 for additional information regarding progress notes. When reading your patients' charts, you will encounter many abbreviations, symbols, and acronyms with which you may be unfamiliar. Some of the commonly used medical abbreviations and symbols are listed in Appendix B.

Working With Families and Professionals. Counselling the hospital patient and the patient's family concerning the communicative disorder is a major responsibility of speech-language pathologists. Through counselling and consultation, the speech-language pathologist educates the family and the patient about the communicative disorder and assists them in learning to deal with the disorder during the rehabilitation process.

To deliver the best care for your patients, you will work with other professionals such as physical therapists, nurses, occupational therapists, and physicians. (The specific roles of these professionals are discussed in Chapter 5.) As you know, together with the speech-language pathologist, these professionals often serve as part of a multidisciplinary team. The assessment and treatment decisions you make are likely to involve other team members. In addition to multidisciplinary teams, many hospitals are promoting **transdisciplinary teams**. Transdisciplinary teams are composed of different professionals and paraprofessionals who may provide some services for another team member. For example, if one of your patient's goals is to communicate when in discomfort, during nursing activities the nurse may work on this goal.

Multiskilling is similar to the idea of transdisciplinary teams. In multiskilling, you might be trained to take a patient's temperature and blood pressure during management of a swallowing disorder. Generally, multiskilling is not popular with most hospital personnel, but is being offered as a cost-saving alternative by some insurance and research groups. ASHA has published a position on the use of multiskilled personnel that you will want to read before you begin a medical internship (ASHA, 1997a).

In **hospital rounds**, you and other care providers meet with the physician in charge and share information about the patient or ask questions about the results of the various assessments and treatments. Rounds may be performed in the patient's room or in a separate conference room. You will participate in rounds and learn how each team member contributes to the overall care and habilitation of the patient.

Skilled Nursing Facilities

Skilled nursing facilities (SNF) are designed to provide services for individuals requiring convalescent care for many medical reasons. These services are provided following discharge from the hospital and before the patients return home. The SNF also provides services for individuals who need long-term medical care. Generally, patient services in the SNF are similar to those in a hospital.

Nursing care in the SNF involves regularly monitoring the patient's vital signs (such as temperature, pulse, respiration), giving medications, and other types of medical care. These patients also may receive services from such other professionals as a physical therapist, speech-language pathologist, occupational therapist, recreational therapist, and social worker.

Prerequisites. As in other medical practicum settings, it would be ideal for you to have completed **courses in aphasia**, **voice**, **dysphagia**, and **neurologically based speech disorders** before beginning practicum in a SNF. A course in **gerontology** is highly desirable. Also, a knowledge of the SNF's general structure, function, and clinical and administrative procedures is helpful, although much of this is acquired during the practicum.

Supervision. Many SNFs do not employ their own speech-language pathologists. Instead, the SNFs contract with private practices to provide services such as speech-language pathology, physical therapy, and occupational therapy. Therefore, although your supervisor is responsible for service delivery at the SNF, he or she may not be an employee of the site. Supervision is provided by the on-site speech-language pathologist. The university supervisor monitors the practicum experience by routinely consulting with the supervisor and the student. The university supervisor also may make periodic site visits.

Schedules. Individual treatment sessions are common in SNFs, although some group sessions may be held. Group sessions are helpful in promoting social communication skills in an environment where social interactions sometimes are limited. Too, group sessions are used to monitor patients' swallowing abilities as they progress to independent eating. In a SNF, you will soon find that many patients fatigue quickly and the length of both the evaluation and treatment sessions depends on the patients' health.

Typically, work in the SNF is 5 days a week for 8 hours each day. For certain patients, speech-language pathology services are provided 6 days per week. In those cases, you may work some Saturdays. To manage patients' swallowing, speech-language pathologists sometimes begin at 6:30 a.m. or arrive later and work until 7 p.m. If you are treating a patient for a swallowing disorder, you may often work with the patient during meals. For example, to work with patients during their breakfast, you may arrive early, work with patients through lunch, take your own lunch break and leave at 4 or 4:30 p.m. As with most clinical practicum assignments, you will follow the schedule of your clinical supervisor unless other arrangements are agreed on.

Types of Patients. In a SNF, student clinicians work primarily with elderly patients. The communicative disorders of the patients you work with often are associated with **cerebrovascular accidents**, **head injury**, **carcinomas of the head and neck**, **hearing loss**, and a variety of neurological diseases.

Although speech-language pathology services in a SNF include assessment and treatment of communicative disorders, the majority of the caseload is with patients who have dysphagia. However, because of liability issues and different degrees of training, student clinicians may be involved on a limited basis with the evaluation and treatment of patients with swallowing disorders.

Report Writing and Record Keeping. Basically, report writing and documentation of treatment sessions in the form of progress notes will be similar to the hospital setting. In the SNF you may be involved in telephoning physicians for orders to evaluate or treat an individual. You also may be directly involved in billing private and federal insurance and in appealing decisions of third-party payers (e.g., insurance companies) who deny payment for services. As in all cases, your documentation and report writing should be accurate and appropriate to the patient and the clinical setting.

Working With Families and Professionals. In addition to direct patient contact, the speech-language pathologist provides indirect services through consultation with the SNF staff. A significant part of this indirect service is to educate the staff (nurses and aides) regarding communicative and swallowing disorders. You may train the staff to help identify and refer patients who appear to have communicative disorders. You need to train both the staff and the patient's family on ways to optimize communication with the patient. The patient's family can be invaluable in accurately evaluating and treating the patient. In addition to providing patient history, family members also may be actively involved with carryover of some treatment activities.

For your patients who have swallowing disorders, you will work closely with the dietitian and nursing staff. You will assure that your patient has the correct diet and that there are staff trained to appropriately and safely feed your patient.

Rehabilitation Facilities

Rehabilitation facilities provide comprehensive services to the individual disabled by an accident or illness. The goal of rehabilitation is to maximize the individual's recovery and to minimize any residual dysfunction.

Rehabilitation facilities may be a part of community hospital services or a private agency. There are also an increasing number of rehabilitation hospitals that specialize in treating persons with disabilities. Both **inpatient and outpatient services** are provided by the members of a multidisciplinary team. The speech-language pathologist is an important member of the rehabilitation team. You will find participating in practicum at a rehabilitation site an interesting and rewarding learning experience.

Prerequisites. To derive the greatest benefit from your practicum experience in a rehabilitation facility, you should have completed course work in aphasia, dysphagia, neurological speech disorders, and voice.

Supervision. As in other medical settings, direct supervision of student clinicians is provided by a staff speech-language pathologist with coordination of the clinical practicum by the university supervisor. Again, supervision must meet ASHA's minimum standards for supervision of student clinicians.

Schedules. Patients served in rehabilitation facilities receive intensive treatment, sometimes two times per day, 5 to 6 days per week. Usually, treatment is offered between 8 a.m. and 5 p.m.; however, this schedule may vary depending on the needs of the patient. As in other medical settings, if you are treating a patient for a swallowing disorder, your treatment may cover mealtime.

Types of Patients. A large percentage of the population served in a rehabilitation facility includes patients who have suffered head injuries resulting from automobile or motorcycle accidents. **Head injuries** may be called traumatic brain injury (TBI), closed head injury (CHI), or acquired brain injury (ABI). Speech and language disorders of this population include **apraxia**, **dysarthria**, and **aphasia**. It is not unusual for speech-language pathologists also to have patients with dysphagia or cognitive disorders on their caseload.

Patients recovering from cerebrovascular accidents (CVA), or strokes, with associated speech and language disorders often are seen in rehabilitation facilities. Patients recovering from a CVA also may exhibit aphasia, apraxia, dysarthria, dysphagia, and cognitive disorders.

In addition to providing services for individuals recovering from head injury or stroke, some rehabilitation facilities serve individuals with orthopedic handicaps. For example, children with cerebral palsy benefit from several rehabilitative services including physical therapy, speech and language treatment, and vocational therapy.

The clinician may be involved in assisting the patient with relearning daily living activities and functional communication and memory skills. The clinician also may teach the use of assistive communicative devices to patients with poor prognosis for verbal communication.

Report Writing and Record Keeping. Documentation requirements in a rehabilitation facility are similar to those of many hospitals. Follow the requirements of your site.

Working With Families and Professionals. The rehabilitation team often includes a physiatrist, physical therapist, speech-language pathologist, occupational therapist, nurse, neuropsychologist, and social worker. **A physiatrist is a physician trained in rehabilitative medicine** and often serves as the team leader. There is close communication among team members whose services are interrelated. For example, based on information obtained during patient staffing, the speech-language pathologist may find that a specific patient cannot reach across midline. During speech therapy, the clinician will be careful to place pictures the patient is required to point to within the patient's reach. In another instance, the physical therapist consults with the speech-language pathologist and discovers that a patient who has been nonverbal during physical therapy sessions is able to produce single-word utterances; consequently, the physical therapist prompts the patient to respond to questions verbally during treatment sessions.

The rehabilitation team also works closely with the patient's family. The family members take an active part in rehabilitating the patient. A psychologist or social worker may counsel family members to help them deal with the emotional adjustments required. The speech-language pathologist also counsels the family members and works with them to reestablish a patient's communicative skills.

Psychiatric Hospitals

Psychiatric facilities often are state operated and designed to serve individuals who are mentally ill or developmentally disabled (mentally retarded). Most of these facilities offer speech and hearing services. Although residential care is part of psychiatric hospitals, outpatient services also are available. In recent years, there has been an increased emphasis on mainstreaming those who are mentally ill or have developmental disabilities. You may work closely with the client's family, teachers, or employers. You may work in more or less restrictive facilities including state psychiatric hospitals, outpatient clinics, or schools.

Clinical practicum in a psychiatric setting offers you an opportunity to work with unique cases. You will interact with many different professionals. You will learn to work as a member of a **multidisciplinary team**, to resolve many behavioral issues, and to evaluate and treat individuals with communicative disorders associated with mental illness, developmental disability, or both.

Prerequisites. In addition to a strong background in speech and language disorders, student clinicians preparing for an internship in a psychiatric hospital will want to have a good understanding of principles of behavior management. Some sites also may utilize assistive technology. At these sites, computer literacy and a course in augmentative communication are useful.

Supervision. As is the case in many off-campus placements, a staff speech-language pathologist of the psychiatric facility will supervise your practicum in accordance with ASHA guidelines. To coordinate your practicum assignment, the university supervisor communicates regularly with the off-campus supervisor. Because of the emphasis on mainstreaming and serving clients in their natural environment, your clinical practicum at the psychiatric hospital may include accompanying clients to locations away from the hospital. If you leave the hospital with a client for treatment, your supervisor will always accompany you.

Schedules. The frequency and length of treatment sessions will vary, depending on the needs of the patient, the specific setting the patient is seen in, and the financial resources of the patient and the agency. The length of a session also is dependent on the amount of time the patient can effectively be involved in treatment. Some psychiatric patients benefit from a 45-minute treatment session, whereas other patients may need a shorter session because of limited attention span.

Types of Clients. In psychiatric facilities, the speech-language pathologist provides services to both children and adults. In addition to working with individuals with speech or language disorders, the clinician may work with patients who have behavioral disorders as well. Frequently, the speech-language pathologist is requested to evaluate a patient's communicative disorder that might be contributing to his or her problem behavior.

Report Writing and Record Keeping. Documentation of assessment and treatment sessions is very important; however, each facility's requirements are different. Generally, as with other sites, you will be required to write clear, comprehensive assessment reports and regularly chart the results of treatment sessions. If you are at a site that a government agency operates, you may be required to complete specific forms for that agency. Your supervisor will explain the report writing and record keeping requirements at your site.

Working With Families and Professionals. Team work is typical in psychiatric settings. Therefore, the speech-language pathologist often works as a member of a multidisciplinary team, which may consist of a psychiatric nurse, psychologist, social worker, psychiatrist, and other professionals.

Because of the attempts to integrate individuals who are mentally ill or developmentally disabled back into their communities, clinicians may see them in different settings. Depending on the setting, you may work closely with a client's family, teacher, or employer.

Preschool Agencies

Preschool programs typically serve **children ages 3 to 5 years**. However, preschools now are expanding to include infants and toddlers. Although many preschools are privately operated, the primary agencies offering the services of a speech-language pathologist are government programs such as Head Start, state preschools, economic opportunity programs, and local school districts. The latest revision of P.L. 94–142, IDEA 1997, mandates that services be provided in a natural environment. This could be in the home or school, but should represent an environment familiar to the child.

Prerequisites. To work in a preschool setting, you should have a good understanding of normal and disordered speech and language development, infant speech perception and production, and techniques of early intervention. A general knowledge of child development will be helpful.

Supervision. The speech-language pathologist responsible for serving the children on site will provide supervision. Since the passage of P.L. 94–142 and its later amendment P.L. 99–457, public schools are providing many preschool services for children with special needs. In many communities, clinicians providing speech and language services to preschool children in the public school setting are employees of the school district. In other communities, usually because of limited resources, either of finances or of personnel, the school district contracts with a private practice to provide mandated services for preschool children with speech-language disorders. Regardless of who the service provider is, he or she will supervise you according to ASHA guidelines on supervision of clinical practicum.

Preschool Schedules. In public schools and Head Start programs, the speech-language pathologist most frequently works as an itinerant clinician who travels from one location to another. The population served at each preschool setting is relatively small. Consequently, you will find that the itinerant speech-language pathologist providing services to such sites travels extensively, sometimes going to two or more sites per day.

You will have the opportunity to work with several service delivery models practiced in preschools. Preschool children are served individually or in small groups. Children with disorders of articulation, voice, or fluency are usually seen individually. Children with disorders of language are seen individually or in small groups. The trend in preschools is to serve children with language disorders in group settings. Often, language activities may be integrated with other social and educational activities. This will enable a child to experience more natural communicative interactions. Such integrated activities may promote generalization and maintenance.

Types of Clients. Preschool programs serve children who have severe handicaps to those who are nondisabled, so you will have the opportunity to work with a wide spectrum of children. The more severe the physical and sensory disabilities of the children, the greater are their communicative problems. With children who are severely disabled, you will see the entire range of communicative disorders. In some preschools you may work with children using augmentative communication devices. In other preschools you may work with children who primarily have articulation or language delays.

Report Writing and Record Keeping. Some children progress slowly, with others progressing at a rapid rate. In all cases, documentation of treatment and its results is essential. Your clinical supervisor will outline the requirements of documentation and report writing at your practicum site.

Working With Families and Professionals. In preschools, you will learn to provide consultative services for the children's parents and teachers. You will learn to **train preschool teachers and their assistants** on ways to maximize your clients' communication and to reinforce your clients' emerging speech and language skills. Ideally, you also will work closely with the parents of preschool children. Often, initially, it is difficult for parents to accept that their children have communication disorders. In working with parents of preschoolers, you will use the skills you have acquired in previous practicum experiences and in any counselling courses you have taken.

Your work with parents of preschoolers involves training them in conducting **home treatment programs** when necessary. Training parents to work regularly with their child to teach target behaviors and to routinely provide language expansion activities is a major part of your work. Once a parent realizes that a child has a communication disorder and you are there to help the child, the parent may become one of your greatest assets.

Prisons

Prisons are a growing industry in the United States and there are a large number of prisoners with communicative disorders. Speech-language pathology services may be provided in adult prisons and are mandated services in juvenile facilities.

Prerequisites. In addition to a strong background in speech and language disorders, the student preparing to work in a correctional facility will want to have an understanding of criminal behavior and may want to take a class in criminal justice. Before beginning your internship you will be required to pass a security clearance. Also, you may be required to pass a training course that focuses on how to interact with prisoners, how to dress, and how to behave in an emergency.

Supervision. Typically, supervision will be provided by a correctional facility staff speech-language pathologist. In some juvenile facilities, the speech-language pathologist may be an employee of the area school district. Your supervision will be in accordance with all ASHA guidelines and will be coordinated by your university. Although not part of your practicum supervision, you may be observed by correctional authorities as part of their regular monitoring activities.

Prison Schedules. Schedules will vary depending on the facility. Typically, services will be provided between 8 a.m. and 5 p.m., Monday through Friday. At adult facilities, the frequency and duration of services will depend on the needs and availability of your client. For example, you may be seeing a client twice a week for 45 minutes each time. However, there may be times when your client is unavailable because of a personal discipline or **prison lock-down**. Prison lock-down means that all prisoners are locked in their cells because of a security concern.

In a juvenile facility, your services will be regulated by your client's IEP. Refer to the section on public school services and Chapter 5 for more information about IEPs. Also, services will be influenced by your client's personal discipline, facility lock-down, and duration of his or her sentence.

Types of Clients. In correctional institutions, you will see clients with disorders of articulation, voice, fluency, and language. Your clients may have only one disability or may have multiple disabilities. Your clients may have limited education and some may have behavioral disorders. However, prisons have strict rules for earning certain "benefits" and often prisoners are motivated and happy to work with you. If you work in a juvenile facility, you will see clients who have IEPs. For additional information on IEPs, see Chapter 5.

Report Writing and Record Keeping. Accurate and thorough report writing and record keeping are essential components of this setting. Your supervisor will give you complete information on the facility's requirements.

Working With Families and Professionals. Depending on the facility you are working in, you may have little contact with your client's family. However, you may work with the facility's nurse, teachers, or correctional officers. These professionals may assist you in providing effective intervention for your clients. You will find that having to work in a locked facility and relying on each other for your safety helps build a close professional community.

Private Practice

Across the nation, private practices in speech-language pathology are rapidly growing. You might think that private practitioners provide speech-language pathology services only in their office to clients in individual treatment sessions. However, this scenario is only a small part of the picture. Besides working with clients in their offices, private practitioners may **contract** to provide speech-language pathology services for other private agencies. For example, private practitioners may serve skilled nursing facilities, home health care agencies, hospitals without speech and hearing departments, psychiatric facilities, and private preschools. They also may contract to serve children in local public schools.

Some private clinics may **specialize**. For example, one private practice may specialize in pediatric services, with another perhaps serving adults only. Yet another private clinic may have expertise in treating patients with laryngectomy. There also are extensive private practices that hire large numbers of speech-language pathologists who contract to offer services to patients in skilled nursing facilities and home health care agencies.

Prerequisites. Students planning a practicum assignment in a private practice need a broad educational background. Clients may range from infants to elderly individuals. The entire range of communicative disorders may be treated in private settings.

Because the private practitioner is dependent on favorable public relations, you will need to have, or quickly develop, **good interpersonal skills**. You will not only develop your skills in assessing and treating communicative disorders, but also will gain insight into the business aspects of your profession. You will learn about marketing your services to the public and getting reimbursed by insurance companies and such government programs as Medicare.

Supervision. Your opportunities to work with clients in private clinics may be somewhat limited because most expect and request services from an experienced, licensed, and certified professional regardless of the amount of supervision available for a student clinician. Still, there are many opportunities for working under the supervision of a speech-language pathologist providing contractual service to other agencies. Also, a speech-language pathologist with sufficient staff resources may provide additional services through a student clinician for a client who needs more frequent treatment, but cannot afford it. Your supervisor will work closely with you to ensure maintenance of a practice's reputation of quality service. Minimally, all supervision will comply with ASHA's requirements for clinical practicum.

Clinic Schedules. Schedules will vary depending on the type of service delivery in which the private practice is involved. If you are working in a skilled nursing facility, your schedule will resemble that already described. If you are working with clients in the private practice office, your schedule will be influenced by the times clients are available for appointments. Although many practices operate on an 8 a.m. to 5 p.m. schedule, often certain days are reserved for appointments outside of regular business hours (e.g., 6 p.m. to 9 p.m.). Typically, treatment is scheduled for 30-minute sessions 2 to 3 times per week. The duration and frequency of treatment are based on each client's needs and financial resources.

Types of Clients. Clients may range from infants through adults. Disorders can cover the gamut of communication difficulties. Severity may spread across the continuum from very mild to severe. Of course, if you are assigned to a private practice that specializes in a certain area, you will see clients reflecting that area.

Report Writing and Record Keeping. Similar to all practicum assignments, documentation of assessment and treatment is important, and, depending on the private practice, writing and record keeping requirements will vary. Chapter 5 provides general report writing guidelines. In addition to report writing, you may be more directly involved in billing for your services. Your supervisor will assist you in learning the requirements for your practicum site.

Working With Families and Other Professionals. One advantage to working with clients in private practice is that they have sought out your services and are in your office because they want to be. Therefore, it is sometimes easier to maintain family involvement with your clients' treatment. On occasion, however, because of the cost of private speech and language services, some families expect the speech-language pathologist to provide a quick cure for a client. On other occasions, it may be necessary to immediately include family members in a client's treatment because the client's finances or insurance allows only a limited number of appointments for speech-language pathology services.

Regardless of the situation, you will learn to communicate effectively and to work closely with various family members. Communication with other professionals may be written or verbal. Again, depending on the services the private practice you are assigned to provides, you will interact with different professionals. For example, if you are working in a rehabilitation setting or skilled nursing facility, you will collaborate with different members of the facility's staff (e.g., physical therapist, occupation therapist, social worker, nurse, and physician) to maximize your clients' treatment.

Other Clinical Settings

There are many other clinical practicum settings that have not been detailed in this chapter. Among these are the speech-language pathology services provided at adult day health care centers, veterans administration hospitals, and public clinics and private practices. The range of settings in which you might complete your clinical practicum may be limited by demographic factors and your university's resources. More frequently, however, the range is limited only by your own initiative. If you wish to gain practicum experience in a new setting, discuss your interest with your supervisor, clinical director, or academic advisor.

Clinical Internships

Clinical internships may be part-time or full-time. Though a part of clinical practicum, **internships** provide comprehensive, on-the-job experience for more advanced students. Also, an internship typically is completed in an off-campus clinical site. The qualifications of the student clinician and the requirements of the clinical site determine the type of internships available. Students enrolled in **distance learning** programs may have clinical practicum programs designed specifically for that program.

Part-Time Internships

Part-time internships can be divided into two sections, intermittent and daily. **Intermittent part-time internships** allow you to participate in clinical practicum at a given site on a periodic basis. For example, you might receive a practicum assignment at a skilled nursing facility for 2 hours per day, 2 days per week. Other intermittent internships may allow your hours to vary from week to week. **Daily part-time internships** are much closer to the requirements of a full-time internship. You are assigned a clinical site for a specified number of hours and required to participate in practicum each day of the work week.

Part-time internships allow you to schedule your work and academic classes around clinical practicum. Some part-time practicum may be so limited that you will not learn much about the setting and the clients served there. However, in the early stages of clinical practicum, many student clinicians need additional time to assimilate and integrate new information and experiences. For these students, part-time internships are ideal.

Full-Time Internships

Full-time internships require you to participate in a clinical practicum with the number of hours, work days, and holidays parallel to those of the clinical-site staff. If you are participating in a full-time practicum assignment at an elementary school, you might be there from 8 a.m. to 3:30 p.m., Mondays through Fridays for a specific number of weeks or total number of hours. If you were assigned to a hospital practicum site as a full-time intern you probably would be required to arrive at 8 a.m. and work until 5 p.m., Mondays through Fridays for a certain number of weeks or until you earn a specific number of clinical hours.

Full-time internships and even daily part-time internships provide a more comprehensive practicum experience than do intermittent assignments. In full-time internships, you may be able to experience more of the professional and interpersonal aspects of an assigned setting. In addition to direct patient contact, you also may be included in rounds or staffing and be more closely involved with allied professionals. You may attend or even provide staff development (training) inservices. A full-time internship allows you to experience the daily routines and pressures associated with a particular setting and to obtain a better understanding of the personal as well as professional requirements of the work setting. Part-time internships rarely provide you with this opportunity, because you are not on-site long enough.

Because full-time internships are intensive and allow minimal time for class work, they often are reserved for student clinicians in their final term of graduate work or for summer practicum assignments. However, if you wish to take up a full-time internship sooner, discuss it with your advisor.

General Administrative Procedures

A primary goal of speech-language pathology training programs is to provide valuable practicum experience for student clinicians while offering and maintaining clinical services of high quality. Many administrative procedures are necessary to meet this goal.

Facilities and Equipment

The university must ensure that both on-site and off-site **facilities are adequate and appropriate for clinical practicum**. The university speech and hearing clinic should maintain a current inventory of evaluation instruments and supplies, provide a professional and safe environment in which to provide clinical services, and offer adequate supervision and guidance to students from qualified supervisors.

To maintain quality clinical services, the clinic also should use some method of quality review and improvement. This should include measurable goals and outcome indicators. The quality review and improvement process might include such activities as surveys of client satisfaction, review of calibration logs, and review of clinic documentation.

Before placing students in off-campus practicum sites, the university clinic director evaluates the sites for their appropriateness. The clinic director verifies the qualifications and certification status of on-site supervisors, the types and number of clients served at the setting, and the number of clock hours students could obtain. The director may visit the facilities to ensure they are safe and adequately maintained. If you have any concerns about on-campus or off-campus facilities, discuss them with your clinic director.

Supervisor Qualifications

Your academic department verifies supervisors' qualifications to ensure they have met accreditation and university standards. ASHA requires that clinical supervisors hold the ASHA CCC. Supervisors must effectively share information and assist students in developing clinical skills. The university clinic staff maintains and reviews supervisor records as frequently as a clinic assignment is made.

At the end of each clinical assignment, students have the opportunity to **evaluate their supervisors**. These evaluations are usually anonymous. In addition, the university periodically performs peer reviews. Constructive and specific feedback can help the clinical supervisor acquire more effective clinical teaching skills.

Clinic Fees

In conjunction with the university, the department faculty develops a fee scale for clinical services provided at the university speech and hearing clinic, which is often not-for-profit. Funds generated in fees are used to defray the costs of clinic materials, supplies, and equipment. Fees are implemented on a fixed or sliding scale and may be waived for clients unable to afford payment.

You may inform your clients about the clinic's fee schedule; but you have neither the responsibility nor the authority to reduce or waive fees. Clients or parents who ask questions about fees, waivers, payment plans, and so forth should be referred to the clinic office.

Scheduling Practicum Assignments

Scheduling and assignment of practicum experiences are made on the basis of a student's experience, the student's clinical clock hour needs, the student's specific area of interest, availability of practicum sites, the number of clients seeking services, and the availability of clinical supervisors. Because of these and other variables to be considered in making clinical practicum assignments, you may not always get the kind of assignments you desire. However, the better the communication between you and the clinic director (or other individual in charge of scheduling), the greater the likelihood of you having a successful practicum experience. Therefore, follow the format your university uses in registering for practicum each term and for expressing your practicum needs ahead of time.

Student Records

Prior to being admitted into clinical practicum, students' records are reviewed to find out if they meet the academic requirements for clinical practicum. Although ASHA provides minimum guidelines for student performance, individual universities may have additional requirements the students must meet.

The clinic staff maintains records of student clinicians. These records are reviewed periodically to ensure that they meet both the university and ASHA guidelines for clinical practicum, including the types of patients served and number of clinical hours earned. It is important that you accurately communicate through the forms your department uses the clock hours you have earned and the clinical experiences you have completed. Appendix C contains a sample form for recording clinical clock hours earned.

The training director (or the department chair) assures that an evaluation of your performance is written at the end of each clinical assignment. The supervisor discusses your evaluation with you and places a copy of the evaluation in your file. The evaluation of your clinical skills and the corresponding grade will influence your future practicum assignments. If your clinical skills are weak, your continued participation in clinical practicum may be a matter for discussion. If you disagree with an evaluation of your practicum, you should discuss your concerns with your supervisor. If necessary, follow established procedures students must use to protest evaluations.

Clinic Supplies, Materials, and Equipment

While you are in clinical practicum you will use a variety of supplies, materials, and equipment. The university clinic and many off-campus sites provide most of these items. However, you also will be required to purchase some materials, equipment, and supplies you use. You will want to begin building your own inventory of materials and supplies throughout your clinical practicum, regardless of the amount of materials and equipment available to you.

Clinic supplies are consumable items. These include tongue depressors, gauze, cotton swabs, gloves, finger cots, tissue, and disinfectant. Carefully follow your clinic's protocol regarding disposal of these items. Most sites designate specific containers in which to dispose supplies used in oral examinations and materials that have come in contact with saliva or blood during evaluation or treatment sessions.

Clinical materials also are consumable or expendable items. Typically included in this category are tests, test response forms, and such treatment materials as articulation cards, language programs, and books.

Your clinic library or media center may have a wide variety of tests for the evaluation of communicative disorders. Tests are generally arranged by alphabetical order or organized by the type of disorder the test is designed to evaluate. Follow the check-out procedures outlined at your university or clinical site. The same test will be used over and over again by many other individuals, so handle it carefully. Tests are expensive and the less money that has to be spent to replace worn out or lost tests, the more money the clinic will have available to upgrade materials, equipment, and facilities.

As you progress in your clinical practicum you may want or be required to take the opportunity to use many assessment instruments. Instead of continually administering the same test across clients, experiment.

Learn and administer new tests. Find out which tests evaluate what they purport to evaluate, which tests are standardized for specific populations, and which speech and language behaviors might be better evaluated through analysis of speech samples. After you graduate, you will be selecting your own tests. Therefore, take time to learn to objectively evaluate most of the published tests made available to you at a practicum site.

Test response forms also are considered clinic supplies, because they are consumable. Response forms are expensive, especially when they must be supplied to 20 to 40 student clinicians per semester. Use the response forms judiciously. Do not request or take more forms than you need. Some university clinics provide student clinicians with only one response form per semester for each client and require the student to pay for any additional forms needed because of incorrect scoring or response form loss. It is not appropriate to photocopy response forms for clinical use, unless the publisher specifically gives permission to reproduce the forms.

In addition to numerous tests, your clinic will have a supply of **treatment materials**. The type and quantity of materials differ across campuses and clinical sites. Generally available are a selection of articulation cards depicting pictures designed to evoke corresponding phonemes in a variety of word positions. Also, you frequently will have access to picture or photo decks representing many vocabulary and language concepts. Comprehensive language programs and books also may be available. Your clinic may supply different types of toys for use with younger clients. There is an abundance of commercial items available, although often the theoretical basis of the faculty and clinic staff influences the types of materials made available to the student clinician.

Treatment materials are the most individual or personalized of items used in clinical practicum. Therefore, it is not unusual for student clinicians to develop their materials. You can develop your materials by drawing pictures, using computer graphics, using pictures from books or magazines, creating charting forms, accumulating lists of words, phrases, and sentences designed to teach phonemes or language behaviors, and developing an activity file of various treatment techniques and ideas.

Many student clinicians find it functional, as well as beneficial, to allow their clients to create some of their treatment materials. With the assistance of a parent, a young client might be asked to cut pictures out of a magazine and bring them to his or her treatment session to put into a **speech book**. Another client might be asked to bring in newspaper articles to discuss during a treatment session. You may ask clients with good drawing skills to draw picture cards for use in their treatment sessions and home practice assignments.

In the school setting, clinicians increasingly are using **curriculum materials** as treatment materials. Clinicians in other settings may emphasize naturally occurring activities or events to evoke speech and language behaviors. Personalized materials the student clinician creates usually meet a specific need and are, consequently, functional; best of all, they are never checked out by another clinician.

Clinical equipment is nonexpendable. It is something that is used, one would hope, over a long period of time. Clinical equipment generally is much more expensive than supplies and materials. Examples of clinical equipment include audiometers, computers, audio and videotape recorders, sound level meters, auditory trainers, and augmentive communication devices. Less expensive items like flashlights, stethoscopes, dental mirrors, and therapy mirrors also are in this category.

Again, note that the longer the life of the equipment, the more your clinic can invest in new equipment rather than simply replacing lost or broken equipment. Handle the clinic equipment carefully. If you have questions about the appropriate way to utilize an instrument, ask your supervisor for assistance. Be careful when checking out or returning equipment. If equipment is broken or parts missing when you check it out, notify the clinic secretary or your supervisor, so that the equipment can be repaired. When you return equipment, replace it correctly and carefully in its container or storage space.

In this age of rapidly advancing technology, there is an ever-increasing amount of equipment available for the speech-language pathologist. Some of the equipment is priced within the budget of student clinicians, and you may want to purchase a few items to add to your personal inventory. When deciding on the purchase of a piece of equipment, determine if the equipment is something that you will use frequently or if it is something for which there is no substitute. For example, a flashlight is inexpensive, you will use it frequently, and there is not a better substitute for it. An audiometer, however, is expensive, you may or may not use it regularly, but there is not a substitute for it, unless referrals for audiological testing are easily made. On the other hand, an augmentive communication device may be used for a single client, is generally expensive, and, rather than carrying an inventory of augmentative equipment, the client may be referred to a clinic specializing in augmentive communication.

The supplies, materials, and equipment that you need often are dependent on your clinical practicum site. It is to your advantage to work with a variety of materials and equipment in many different clinical settings.

Now that you know some of the different clinical sites and practicum experiences available, you can begin planning your clinical program with your advisor. The clinical practicum portion of your training may be important in choosing the setting in which you want to work after graduation.

3

The Conduct of the Student Clinician

thical behavior and professional demeanor are essential characteristics of the well-respected speech-language pathologist. Training in speech-language pathology includes the acquisition of knowledge about communication and its disorders, together with professional skills in assessing and treating those disorders. However, an equally important part of training is not formally discussed in most textbooks or classes. This part is the acquisition of certain standards of behavior considered professionally appropriate. Professional behavior and the various codes and regulations governing this behavior are discussed in this chapter.

General Professional Behavior

Certain behaviors are traditionally accepted as professionally appropriate and governed by peer influence. Other behaviors are clearly defined and regulated by codes of ethics or other written rules. Throughout your enrollment in clinical practicum, you will have many opportunities to **represent the profession** of speech-language pathology, the university department and its clinic, and the university at large. You will interact with

63

numerous clients, care providers, professionals, and related agencies in the community. You represent speech-language pathologists to people with whom you interact. The profession will be judged by your behavior, and you will begin to establish a reputation that you may build on as your professional career progresses. Therefore, you must demonstrate appropriate and acceptable professional behavior. **Honesty, integrity, respect for others, and a desire to help** are behavioral qualities admired in all people. They are especially important for professional people.

ASHA provides various guidelines to clarify your professional role, behavior, and responsibilities. Equally important, these documents help uphold high standards of service and protect your clients. These guidelines outline certain standards of care and include the ASHA Code of Ethics, ASHA's Preferred Practice Patterns, Scope of Practice, Technical Reports, Guidelines, Position Statements, and the Consumer Bill of Rights.

In addition to specific rules outlined by ASHA in its Code of Ethics and various reports, general rules of professional behavior include **punctuality** in meeting clinical appointments and clinic deadlines, **working cooperatively** with office staff, supervisors, and other student clinicians, **assuming responsibility** for clinic equipment and clinic facilities, **being well prepared** for each clinical session, and maintaining **appropriate dress and demeanor**. Professional demeanor is one of the initial factors on which a student clinician is evaluated. Professional demeanor is a vague term, but refers to such behaviors as appearing confident in your abilities, communicating clearly and appropriately with clients and supervisors, presenting yourself as a mature adult, following prescribed rules, and effectively utilizing clinical time.

Confidence in your ability to help your client is an important characteristic to develop. At the university clinic, you will work with many clients with varied backgrounds. You will probably be nervous when you first talk with your clients, but it is important that you make a good impression. You will often be the first clinic person to contact a client. Your initial meeting with a client sets the stage for future clinical relationships and may influence the client's willingness to pursue treatment. It is important for the client to see you as a **self-confident** and **well-trained person**. The client must believe that you are capable of providing quality clinical services. Also, your clients must believe they are important to you and trust that you will do all you can to help them. A large part of this trust is developed as you initially establish rapport with your clients. There are many significant and insignificant factors that will influence your client's opinion of your abilities. The degrees you have earned probably have the least influence. The way you dress, wear your hair, make eye contact, and shake hands are sometimes overlooked behaviors that will have much influence on your client's desire to work with you. Again, much of the client's initial impressions will be based on your professional demeanor.

Your professional demeanor and clinical ability will also affect other students. At off-campus practicum sites, you are a representative of the university. Administrators, supervisors, medical, health, and allied health professionals may have little knowledge of the university and its training program. Based on your exemplary professional behavior or lack of it, a practicum site may continue to offer or withdraw its offer to provide practicum experiences for other student clinicians. Although student clinicians beginning off-campus practicum should be as well prepared for the assignment as possible, no student is expected to know all of the procedures and regulations of a site. However, each student is expected to **perform appropriately and professionally**. You should meet the deadlines, maintain regular attendance, work cooperatively with the site staff, learn new procedures, and follow the guidelines related to clinical practicum in a particular setting.

Even if you do not have advance knowledge of some of the special rules and regulations of the off-campus site where you will complete your clinical internship, you should know the ASHA Code of Ethics. During your on-campus practicum, you also are expected to know and adhere to the ASHA Code of Ethics and various policies and procedures. Before you begin any clinical practicum assignment, you should reread ASHA's Code of Ethics.

ASHA Code of Ethics

The **ASHA Code of Ethics** (American Speech-Language-Hearing Association, 1994a) gives guidelines of professional behavior for individuals providing clinical services in speech-language pathology or audiology. There is no legal basis for enforcement of the Code of Ethics, except in states that have adopted the code as part of licensure requirements. However, a professional violating the code of ethics may lose his or her ASHA certification, membership in ASHA, or both. As a student clinician and in the future as a speech-language pathologist, you will be faced with many pressures that will demand ethical judgments. Such factors as shortages of speech-language pathologists, increased demands to show profits, and wider scopes of practice can impact your service delivery. Although you are a student, your supervisor will assist you in making the appropriate decision based on ASHA's Code of Ethics and other guidelines. As a professional, you will make your own decisions based on your own judgment and knowledge of ethical practices. Throughout your professional career, you will refer to ASHA's Code of Ethics, guidelines, and position statements to make ethical professional decisions. In addition to learning the various guidelines on professional conduct early on, evaluate your own personal values. If your value system is not consistent with the value system professed by ASHA, you may want to pursue a different career.

The **Ethical Practices Board (EPB)** of ASHA is responsible for interpreting, administering, and enforcing the Code of Ethics. To maintain ASHA certification, you are required to uphold and abide by the Code of Ethics. Also, many employers require that their employees providing speech-language pathology services hold current ASHA certification. Consequently, the Code of Ethics and the EPB have a significant impact on the profession.

All students participating in clinical practicum are required to comply with the ASHA Code of Ethics. The code helps you in developing ethically responsible professional behaviors. The information outlined in the Code of Ethics not only helps you answer questions related to professional and clinical issues, but also to understand the rationale for certain clinic procedures.

The entire code, as well as its revisions, are published periodically in the *Asha* magazine. Also, you may read the code on the ASHA web site. The following discussion emphasizes specific areas of the code; however, you should read and understand the complete Code of Ethics. Appendix D contains the Code of Ethics.

The ASHA Code of Ethics, revised January 1, 1994, is composed of a Preamble, four Principles of Ethics, and numerous Rules of Ethics. The **Preamble** briefly summarizes ASHA's philosophy of service delivery, provides an introduction to components of the Code of Ethics, and lists individuals who are governed by the Code. The **Principles of Ethics** outlines basic ethical behavior. Subdivided under each Principle of Ethics, the **Rules of Ethics** describe more specifically acceptable professional behavior. Obviously, ASHA cannot foresee all instances in which a moral or ethical judgment must be made. Therefore, the Code of Ethics is designed as a guide of minimally acceptable behavior. The four Principles of Ethics are discussed in the following sections.

Principle of Ethics I

> *Individuals shall honor their responsibility to hold paramount the welfare of persons they serve professionally.*

Principle I of the Code of Ethics is straightforward and not easily misinterpreted. Client welfare is foremost. The difficult part for beginning student clinicians, however, is determining what is best for the person being served. If you have a question about the legitimacy, efficacy, or ethics of a particular clinical situation, discuss it with your clinical supervisor. If you have a concern about the safety of a procedure, do not do it until you discuss your concerns with your supervisor. Familiarize yourself with what ASHA considers are some of the factors involved in protecting your clients' welfare.

Preparation. ASHA's Code of Ethics mandates that services be provided competently. In training programs, both the student clinicians and clinical supervisors must be competent. To be competent, one must be well-prepared. At university clinics, student clinicians commonly are required to complete course work in a specific communicative disorder before they are assigned a client with that disorder. Compliance with this policy helps ensure that student clinicians are academically prepared to work with clients with a specific disorder. To be prepared for specific clinical sessions, you should spend time in advance reviewing academic information related to your clients' disorders, your clients' records, and assessment materials including standardized tests you plan to use. Also, you will need to gather treatment materials, forms for charting specific behaviors, and other supplies and equipment. Writing lesson plans, treatment plans, and clinical reports also should be part of this preparation. Assure that you have appropriate knowledge, experience, and supervision before working with a patient with a swallowing disorder, tracheostomy, laryngectomy, or other serious medical complication.

Current ASHA certification is one of the criteria of minimal clinical competence defined by ASHA. Therefore, your clinical supervisors will have the Certificate of Clinical Competence in the areas in which they provide clinical supervision. Your speech-language pathology supervisor will have skills necessary to provide speech therapy for your clients. Minimally, you will have a general background in a specific disorder before you are assigned a client with that disorder. However, you may be required to do additional research to effectively serve your client. During training, your supervisor will refer you to appropriate sources if you are unable to find the information you need. After your formal training and throughout your professional career, you should continue your education and research by being current in your practice and by continuously refining your skills.

ASHA also addresses client welfare and clinical competence by prohibiting service delivery by individuals whose services are hampered by substance abuse, or physical or mental health problems. Obviously, such individuals are not appropriately prepared for effective service delivery. ASHA directs those individuals to seek assistance and to not provide service in the affected area. Whether or not you decide to continue your education in speech-language pathology if you have a substance abuse problem or are concerned about a mental or physical health condition, find someone to help you. Discussions with your clinic supervisors, clinic director, department head, or other faculty will be confidential. They may be able to help you find appropriate services. Acknowledging and addressing certain problems will not necessarily preclude you from clinical practicum. However, as in the case of academic preparation, your supervisor may decide when you are physically and emotionally prepared to work with clients.

Remember, maintaining professional competence is a continuing process. It does not end with the completion of your formal professional education.

Referral. You will not always be able to provide all the services your clients need. Therefore, the requirement that you provide only the services you are qualified to provide means that you should sometimes **refer clients to other professionals**. Some of your clients may need services in addition to those of speech-language pathology. For example, you may have a client recovering from a cerebrovascular accident who appears depressed. It may be appropriate for you to refer the client to a professional who treats depression. Other clients may need the services of a speech-language pathologist who specializes in treating a particular disorder that you cannot treat effectively. For example, a client who has had a laryngectomy may come to see you to learn esophageal speech. If you are not skilled in this area, you would refer the client to a colleague who is. Still other clients may be difficult to schedule because of your case load. Instead of asking them to postpone treatment, you might suggest an equally competent speech-language pathologist. Finally, there may be clients who cannot afford to continue your services. You may know of other speech-language pathology services that are available for free or at a reduced cost. All such clients should be referred to other professionals who can provide more effective or economical services than you can. It is customary to provide several names of qualified professionals when making a referral. You should not refer clients to an individual practicing speech-language pathology or audiology who does not have current ASHA certification. Your practicum site will have a list of qualified professionals for referrals. Your referral list may include other speech-language pathologists, audiologists, psychologists, otolaryngologists, orthodontists, dentists, and physicians.

It is important to refer to individuals who are both qualified and cooperative. If you have had difficulty obtaining necessary information from a professional, you may want to avoid referring to that individual.

As with all other major clinical decisions, you should not make a referral without first discussing the matter with your clinical supervisor. Your clinical supervisor must approve the reason for the referral and to whom the referral will be made.

Discrimination. The code prohibits discrimination. Decisions related to delivery of service must not be based on "race or ethnicity, gender, age, religion, national origin, sexual orientation, or disability." You will provide speech-language pathology services for a wide variety of individuals. Obviously, there will be certain persons you enjoy working with more than others. In fact, as you progress in your training program, you may decide you want to work only with a specific population. For example, you may choose to specialize in treating individuals who stutter. In this case, declining to serve someone with aphasia would not be discrimination. However, discrimination exists if you solely base service delivery decisions on **race, ethnicity, gender, age, religion, national origin, sexual orientation**, or **disability**. It is important to remember that clinical judgments and recommendations must be made on your expertise and clinical data and not on unrelated factors.

Informed Consent. The code covers several rules on providing information to clients. Basically, clients must be given enough information so they can understand all relevant aspects of clinical services that affect them. They can then make a rational decision to seek services or not. Such a decision is **informed consent**. Individuals must be given information related to possible consequences of treatment as well as no treatment.

University clinics do not, as a rule, require individuals refusing treatment to sign written statements verifying such refusal and their understanding of possible consequences of a refusal. Private clinics may ask clients to sign a statement to that effect. However, most clinics require clients to initial or sign a plan of treatment to confirm their knowledge of the proposed services. If clients are not required to submit a written acknowledgment of the treatment plan, you should note in the records when the plan was discussed with the client and the client's apparent understanding of the discussion (Flower, 1984). Each off-campus site will have its guidelines for obtaining client consent that student clinicians should follow.

Clients must be informed fully regarding the nature and possible effects of the service. Also, they must be provided prognostic information. Beginning clinicians sometimes do not know how to reply to clients who ask if a specific treatment will *cure* them or even how a specific procedure will affect their communicative disorder. As you know from reading the Code of Ethics, you are **forbidden from guaranteeing treatment results**. However, you can make an informed, reasonable, prognostic statement. For example, you should not say, "After 6 weeks of treatment, you will no longer stutter." However, you may say, "This type of treatment has been successful with many individuals who had problems similar to yours. Based on the diagnostic information I have and what I think is your level of motivation for change, the chances of improvement in your speech fluency are good." Ethically justified prognostic statements are those that are probabilistic statements based on valid and reliable information about the client and the accumulated scientific evidence in the discipline. There-fore, prognostic statements should not be made without first ensuring that all necessary information has been obtained and is accurate. If there is a gap in our information, you should make it clear to the client. If a satisfac-tory prognostic statement cannot be made, the reasons should be ex-plained to the client. You must discuss your client's prognosis with your clinical supervisor before you report it to the client.

Informed consent also requires that clients be told if the treatment they receive is part of a research program. Your clients must be informed clearly of the nature of research, the procedure to be used, the benefits of partici-pation, and the possible negative effects. The clients must be given a free choice to participate in the treatment research or to opt for other kinds of treatment programs. The clients who agree to participate in an experimen-tal treatment program retain their right to withdraw from it at any time and without prejudice. Potential participants should fully realize this.

Clients also must be fully informed about who is providing the speech-language pathology services and what his or her qualifications are. In the university clinic, as well as at off-campus sites, it is explained clearly to the client that student clinicians provide services under the supervision of a certified professional. You must never misrepresent your status to the pub-lic. In many settings, you will be asked to wear a name tag or identification badge that will give your name and title.

Before providing services, you should check to ensure that your client has signed all **consent forms**. Each site will have different forms. Check with your clinical supervisor, if you are not sure what forms are used at your site.

Treatment Efficacy. The Code of Ethics continues to address treatment efficacy by stating that treatment should not be provided to clients who **may not be expected to benefit from treatment**. The code also prohibits continuation of unnecessary treatment. Again, these are two is-sues that often are difficult for student clinicians to resolve. First, profes-sionals and agencies sometimes disagree about these issues. For example, a speech-language pathologist may judge that a patient with brain injury could benefit from speech-language services. However, the insurance company, judging that the patient would not benefit from treatment, may not approve payment for the services. In this instance, the clinician, who may feel frustrated because the needed service cannot be provided, has not acted unethically in recommending treatment.

Financial factors may adversely affect individuals who are unclear about their values and ethics. Unfortunately, economic factors are impor-tant in maintaining private businesses and the business that holds little re-gard for ethical practice may attempt to put a speech-language pathologist in a compromising position. For example, a speech-language pathologist may be instructed to provide services for a specific number of patients per day. If there are not sufficient numbers of appropriate patients, the clinician may be pressured to increase the caseload by enrolling patients for whom the benefit of treatment is questionable. Clinicians who enroll patients in treatment because of such pressures when they are reasonably sure that a patient would not benefit from treatment (e.g., because of the patient's extremely poor health) will have violated the Code of Ethics and will have acted unethically.

Professionals themselves may disagree on who benefits from treatment and for how long. For example, two speech-language pathologists may not agree on the appropriate chronological age for treatment of a specific communicative disorder. Also, progress of some individuals (for instance, a person with a severe cognitive impairment) may be extremely slow and efficacy of treatment difficult to assess. Clinicians who maintain objective and accurate records of client behaviors will be better able to judge the efficacy of individual treatment than those who rely on subjective judgment and memory to evaluate client progress.

Is it considered unethical to not record every response of a client? No. However, **failure to maintain *adequate* records is unethical.** Adequate records should document changes or lack of changes in the target behaviors over a span of treatment sessions. Continuing the same treatment when repeated measures show no change in client behaviors is certainly unethical. Do you necessarily have to dismiss the client? No. But you certainly should change the treatment procedure.

There is no single formula to determine which individuals can benefit from treatment or when treatment should be discontinued. Social, educational, psychological, and health factors affect your decision. You should evaluate your clients and attempt to make the appropriate determination, but you should never try to enroll or dismiss a client without first discussing the matter with your clinical supervisor.

Confidentiality. Clients' rights to privacy are protected under the Code of Ethics. You are directed to **maintain client confidentiality**, except when you must reveal information to protect your clients' or the community welfare or because you are directed to do so by law. In addition, legal protection of a client's right to privacy is provided by federal and state laws.

Client confidentiality is of ongoing concern at university clinics. There are two reasons for this. First, much of the learning at the university level occurs by individuals sharing information and experiences with each other. Second, persons not directly involved with treatment may observe clients receiving services. Early in your academic career, you will be called on to help ensure client confidentiality. You will observe many clinic sessions, you may present information about clients in certain courses, and you will be involved in student and faculty discussions about clients' evaluations, treatments, and counseling sessions. In all these situations, the clients' rights to privacy must be respected.

Because students frequently discuss their clients with each other, client confidentiality may be violated easily. Observers not directly involved with service delivery may discuss clients in such a way as to violate client confidentiality. You need to be aware of your client's right to confidentiality and monitor both your written and verbal communications to ensure those rights.

Flower (1984) discussed three types of consent related to disclosure of confidential information: implied consent, written consent, and consent inherent in the private interests of the client. **Implied consent** means that individuals seeking services implicitly approve access to their records by staff or support personnel without the need for written authorization. For example, it is not necessary for the clinic secretary to obtain written authorization before accessing a client's record, because reviewing client records is typically a part of a secretary's duties.

Release of information to individuals or agencies outside of a facility requires a written authorization, or **written consent**. The clinic secretary at your university clinic or at an off-campus practicum site can give you information on the consent form required and the procedures for completing it.

Inherent consent that is in the private interests of the client is assumed when release of information is in the best interest of the client. This form of consent generally occurs between the professional and members of the client's family. For example, your client may discuss with you a desire to commit suicide. Of course, you will want to share this information with the client's spouse or other family member. In another instance, you may suspect your client is a victim of child abuse. In this case, you will follow your site's procedures for reporting your concern to the proper authorities. Again, without first discussing a specific situation with a clinical supervisor, you should treat all client information as confidential. This precaution will allow you to avoid the need to justify disclosure of confidential information.

The very nature of university training programs requires some relaxation of the rule of client confidentiality. Students constantly observe assessment and treatment sessions. Consequently, the clinical services offered to individuals through the university training programs are less confidential than those that are offered in private clinics. This is acceptable as long as the client has given informed consent for being observed. The following are guidelines to help ensure client confidentiality.

1. **Do not discuss your client by name, except with your clinical supervisor, clinic staff, or as necessary during clinical meetings**. On-campus, you will be involved in meetings with your supervisor and clinic staff. Off-campus, you may have hospital rounds, student study team meetings, and meetings with your on-site and university supervisors. Obviously in private clinic meetings with your supervisor or affiliated staff, it is perfectly acceptable to identify your clients by name. In fact, you would probably be thought somewhat odd or obtuse if you never mentioned your clients' names.

2. **Do not discuss your client in public areas**. Avoid discussing information about your clients in hallways or waiting areas. If you need to talk about your clients or with your clients, move to a private room. Your discussion will also probably be more profitable if you take the time to find an area where people are not freely moving about and distractions are minimized.

3. **Do not mention your client's name in class presentations or discussions**. As part of class assignments, you may be required to present case histories on various clients you have observed or worked with. You can easily refer to your client as "the client" or give each client an alias.

4. **Do not leave client reports, lesson plans, or other written information unattended**. Promptly file documents in your clients' folders. If you are submitting reports or lesson plans to your supervisor, be sure they are not left on a table or desk that is accessible to the public.

5. **Follow all the office rules regarding checking out and returning client folders and reports**. As a general rule, client files are not to be taken from the clinic area. If files are taken to be used during a clinic session, staffing, or meeting, check-out procedures should be followed, so the clinic secretary can retrieve the files, if necessary.

6. **Do not take client folders home and do not remove information from them**. If you need information from your clients' files, allow time to take the necessary notes. Keep all such notes confidential; do not have client names in your notes. Information must remain in your clients' files to document service delivery.

7. **Do not discuss your client with others**. Unless your client or your supervisor has approved the communication, do not discuss your client with other professionals or persons in other agencies.

8. **Remind your observers that they should respect client confidentiality**. When you are working as a student clinician, other students may want to discuss their observations of your clinic session with you. Help them remember the rules of client confidentiality by modeling appropriate behavior and, if necessary, asking them to not discuss your clients in front of other people.

9. **Obtain written consent to make videotapes or take photographs of clients**. A separate consent should be obtained for any photographs or videotapes used for public viewing, such as at a health fair or community education program. Your clinic secretary should have the necessary forms.

10. **Comply with all clinic rules regarding release of information**. Your clinic will probably have a specific form that must be completed and signed by the client before information is released to another agency. Check with your clinic supervisor or the clinic secretary for additional information. When giving information over the telephone, you also must respect client confidentiality. For example, if you have clients who also are receiving speech-language services in the public schools, their school clinicians may phone you. Be sure you do not reveal confidential information without prior approval from the client. If in doubt as to when you may give information over the telephone, discuss it with your clinic supervisor.

11. **Honor client confidentiality during communications on the Internet**. There are several Internet listserves and chat rooms operating that provide forums for clinical discussions. Students and professionals post questions, concerns, and comments about clients. If you participate in such a listserve or chat room, be careful to respect your clients' rights to privacy. Do not discuss your clients by name or use any information that could identify your client. For example, in certain circumstances your client could be identified by such a statement as, "My client is a 3-year-old female whose mother is a local pediatrician and whose father is a high school principal." It is acceptable to discuss clinical issues, but be cautious and use good judgment.

There are several other rules related to the importance of client welfare. Most of these are self-explanatory, such as not charging for services not provided, maintaining adequate records, and not assessing or treating an individual only by correspondence.

Principle of Ethics II

> *Individuals shall honor their responsibility to achieve and maintain the highest level of professional competence.*

Individuals providing independent speech-language pathology services, or supervising the delivery of those services, **must hold the Certificate of Clinical Competence in Speech-Language Pathology (CCC-SLP)**. Supervision of speech-language pathologists completing their CFY (Clinical Fellowship Year) also must be provided by an individual with a current CCC-SLP. As you know, the CCC is the minimum standard and additional training in specific areas may be necessary to ensure competent service delivery. Your master's degree offers you a foundation on which to build your knowledge. After you graduate, you will be ready to learn and integrate much of the skills that you peripherally touched on in college. As a professional, make it a part of your job to routinely participate in appropriate continuing education activities, read professional journals, and network with other speech-language pathologists.

Scope of Competence.   The field of speech-language pathology is growing rapidly. Service delivery encompasses more and more aspects of client care. Speech-language pathologists work with clients of all ages. Some work with infants, providing early intervention services, sometimes while the infants are still in the hospital. Other clinicians primarily work with school-age children, adults, or geriatric clients. Still others specialize in serving clients with specific problems, for example, clients who stutter, clients with head injuries, or clients needing augmentative communication devices. Obviously, the needs of an infant in the neonatal intensive care unit (NICU) will differ from the 8-year-old child with a language delay, and the needs of a client who recently has had a laryngectomy will differ from the needs of an adult who stutters. Therefore, every certified speech-language pathologist may not be competent to provide services for every client. The Code of Ethics mandates that speech-language pathologists only work in their areas of competence based on their education, training, and experience.

As noted in previous discussions, you may not be expected to know everything needed to serve all your clients, but you should have the basic knowledge and skills to research new information. Your supervisor will always be your resource person, but you should strive constantly to learn on your own and to expand and extend your knowledge.

Continuing Education. As you know, the CCC implies that the minimum educational and clinical qualifications have been met. The Code of Ethics expands on these qualifications by addressing the need for continuing education.

To maintain a high standard of professional competence, speech-language pathologists must **continue their education**, even after they have earned their CCC. Some organizations require members to document a specified number of continuing education units or hours to maintain their affiliation or license. Although not requiring this, ASHA strongly encourages continuing education and awards a certificate of recognition to members who accumulate continuing education units.

You may have already discovered that researchers and clinicians rapidly and constantly produce new information about communicative disorders. Some of what you learned in many undergraduate classes may be outdated by the time you start your clinical practicum. You are busy keeping up with course work, but you must remain current. You can begin the practice of self-study by reading journals and recently published books in speech-language pathology. You also can attend many conferences and workshops to gain current scientific and professional information.

Supervision. The Code of Ethics directs individuals to be well prepared for the services they provide and to require individuals under their supervision to be well prepared. The supervisor is responsible for ensuring that support personnel are appropriately supervised and that other professional staff provide services only within their levels of competence. As a professional you may be assigned a speech assistant to help you provide services. ASHA guidelines require speech assistants to be supervised by speech-language pathologists who have their CCCs, at least 2 years of experience, and some education in supervision. In training programs, the student *uses* the supervisor's license and certification to learn the techniques of the profession. If supervisors determine their student clinicians are not qualified or prepared to work with certain clients, they may assign the clients to other individuals.

You must be well prepared to work with your clients. As part of your preparation, you must acquire and organize information about typical and disordered communication, methods of assessment and treatment, various diagnostic and therapeutic materials, and all clinical procedures including the Code of Ethics.

Principle of Ethics III

> *Individuals shall honor their responsibility to the public by promoting public understanding of the professions, by support-*

ing the development of services designed to fulfill the unmet needs of the public, and by providing accurate information in all communications involving any aspect of the professions.

Accurately represent your services, products, and profession. Principle III instructs that speech-language pathologists must not inaccurately portray their ability, education, credentials, or experience. Statements regarding services or products must be correctly represented. No misrepresentation of services or products dispensed is acceptable. All information provided to the public should be clear and accurate. Advertising is appropriate, as long as it is not misleading, and as long as it complies with contemporary professional standards.

Directly related to accurate representation at the university training program is the need for clients to fully understand that students in the program provide services. This information is given to clients who contact the speech and hearing clinic to inquire about available services. The clients also are told about the clinic schedule and fees. Individuals who want to find other services are referred to qualified speech-language pathologists in the locality.

Principle of Ethics IV

Individuals shall honor their responsibilities to the professions and their relationships with colleagues, students, and members of allied professions. Individuals shall uphold the dignity and autonomy of the professions, maintain harmonious interprofessional and intraprofessional relationships, and accept the professions' self-imposed standards.

Effective professional relationships are important. As a speech-language pathologist you represent the entire profession. In providing optimal client service, you may interact with various professionals. These professionals may be other speech-language pathologists or individuals in allied professions. ASHA recognizes the importance of effective professional relationships by addressing them in the Code of Ethics. In certain instances you will be expected to model appropriate professional behavior, in other instances you may be required to regulate others' professional behavior.

Supervisor Responsibility. The Code of Ethics holds supervisors responsible for individuals working under their direction. In the university training program, your **supervisors are responsible** for ensuring your behavior is professionally appropriate. As you now know, there are many aspects to professionally appropriate behavior including adequately preparing for clinical sessions, protecting client confidentiality, maintaining effective working relationships with other professionals, and so on. In your clinical assignments your supervisors will be evaluating your professionalism as well as your technical and academic skills.

Assigning Credit. The Code of Ethics directs that credit (or recognition) be proportionally given to individuals who have contributed to a written work. Your reports submitted for academic or clinical course work must **contain references and credit other individuals** involved in the work. For example, if you and another student collaborate in evaluating a client and writing the assessment report, both of you should sign the report. (Your supervisor must also sign the report.) If you are reporting information described in a different report, the name of that evaluator and the date of the report should be noted.

Professional Judgment. Regardless of who your supervisor, employer, or referral source is, you must always use your own professional judgment in making **clinical decisions**. For example, as a student clinician, and later as a professional, you routinely will determine which clients need and could benefit from speech-language pathology services. Even though there may be economic issues to consider, your **decision on service delivery must be based on clinical data**. Do not let other individuals' priorities cloud your professional judgment. As you begin your clinical practicum, clearly evaluate not only what your clinical service plan is, but, also, what the rationale behind the plan is. This will help you begin to develop your own problem-solving skills.

Upholding the Standards of the Profession. Individuals must comply freely with the standards of the professions, in this case the standards ASHA suggests in its Code of Ethics and other guidelines. In addition to individually upholding the code, clinicians who believe that another ASHA member has violated the Code of Ethics must report to the Ethical Practice Board (EPB). However, **the student clinician** reports such incidents to the **clinical supervisor**. The clinical supervisor, the clinic director, and the department chair will decide on what action might be taken.

So far, we have highlighted the major sections of the Code of Ethics with which student clinicians may commonly be involved. The code also contains additional rules. Read the Code of Ethics in Appendix D. Then, determine which of the following situations would involve a violation of the Code of Ethics. What would be an ethical way to handle each situation?

1. You were busy studying for midterm exams and "just didn't have enough time" to completely prepare for your clinical session.

2. You are beginning your second year of graduate school. A speech-language pathologist in private practice telephones and asks you to work as an aide. How would you reply? Are there any specific requirements you would need to comply with to be employed as a speech aide? Could you earn clinical clock hours? Could you perform other clinical services?

3. The mother of one of your clients contacts you and asks if you would be available to tutor her child. How would you respond?

4. A clinical supervisor allows students who were continually ill-prepared for their clinical assignments to continue in clinical practicum.

5. You are working with a client who also is receiving speech-language services at another facility. You do not agree with the type of treatment being provided by the other speech-language pathologist. What would you do?

6. Your supervisor suggested that you use certain treatment procedures with one of your clients. You were unsure of how to implement the procedures, but could not get to school during your supervisor's office hours to discuss the procedures. You decided to work with your client anyway, because if you do something wrong, your supervisor will see it and come to help you.

7. A man you have been working with for two months tells you that he just tested positive for HIV (human immunodeficiency virus) infection. He wants to continue treatment, but does not want anyone to know about his medical history except you.

Other Codes and Regulations

Scope of Practice

ASHA has outlined service delivery for professionals in communicative disorders through its scope of practice statement (American Speech-Language-Hearing Association, 1996a) and its preferred practice patterns statement (American Speech-Language-Hearing Association, 1997b). The scope of practice statement describes professional activities and defines which professionals may perform those activities. For example, **speech-language pathologists may not perform audiological evalua-**

tions; however, they may perform pure-tone air conduction hearing screenings as part of a complete evaluation of a client's communicative performance. The scope of practice restricts supervision of specific procedures to those that are defined under that professional's area of certification. More simply, when you complete your clinical practicum in audiology, your primary supervisor will be an audiologist; when you complete your clinical practicum in speech-language pathology, your supervisor will be a speech-language pathologist. Refer to Appendix E for a copy of the Scope of Practice for Speech-Language Pathology.

Preferred Practice Patterns

In addition to identifying what types of services specific professionals may provide, ASHA's preferred practice patterns also outlines **clinical processes, clinical indicators, equipment specifications, expected outcomes, safety and health precautions, documentation, and related references**. As with the Code of Ethics, one of the guiding principles of the preferred practice patterns is the importance of client welfare. Refer to the preferred practice patterns as an introduction to your research when gathering new information about each of your clients.

Reporting Suspected Child Abuse

Although students should first assume that all client information is confidential, there are specific state laws governing disclosure of information to protect the well-being of a client or of the public. A clear example is a clinician's responsibility to report suspected child abuse. Child abuse can include physical, emotional, or sexual abuse. Neglect and child endangerment can also be included in the category of child abuse.

Based on federal laws and regulations, states have established laws regulating the reporting of suspected child abuse. The reporting requirements differ across states. The definition of child abuse, the age range of victims, and the agency to whom the suspected abuse is reported vary also from state to state. Nevertheless, **suspected child abuse must be reported**. In most states, the individual suspecting the abuse must report it. The individual cannot leave the reporting to the agency he or she works for (Flower, 1984).

Child abuse is not always visible or easily identified. Most children are very active, and consequently suffer various accidental scrapes, bruises, and broken bones. You must not jump to conclusions, but you must not disregard signs of possible child abuse. If a child arrives with a bump, bruise, bite, burn, or broken bone, you may want to ask how it happened. If you have a child who repeatedly arrives with various injuries, report it to your clinical supervisor. Again, this may not be a case of child abuse, but your supervisor can investigate further or take other necessary action. Burke (1990) has described the following signs of possible child abuse:

1. **Burns, broken bones, bruises, bites, and cigarette burns**. These are indicators of physical abuse.
2. **Scratches or bruises** on areas of the body other than elbows, knees, or shins. These may be indicators of child abuse, rather than those of an active child.
3. **Bilateral injuries**.
4. **Inadequate or inappropriate clothing**. Examples may include the child who wears sandals in the winter or a warm jacket during hot summer months. Be aware of different cultural influences in evaluating this category. In some cultures, certain items of clothing such as sandals (without socks) are worn throughout the year regardless of the outside temperature.
5. **Unexplained injuries**.
6. **Frequent school absences** when there is no record of a serious illness.
7. **Behavioral difficulties**. These may include lack of trust, depression, hostility, compulsive behavior, lethargy, or withdrawal.
8. **Overly sophisticated sexual knowledge**.
9. **Seductive behaviors with peers and adults**.
10. **Dirty or malnourishment**. These are indicators of neglect and may be accompanied by unmet dental and medical needs.

When you suspect child abuse, inform your supervisor immediately. Each clinical site will have its reporting procedure. You should know these procedures and follow them when necessary.

Dress Code

When people first meet you, they judge you by your appearance and demeanor. With clients, you must quickly establish a degree of trust through both your professional demeanor, attire, and general appearance. A neat appearance and appropriate clothing will positively influence your clients' first impressions of you.

There is not a universal dress code that you must follow in all practicum sites. However, **all clinics have guidelines** for what they consider appropriate professional attire. Contrary to some beliefs, you are not expected to go out and purchase an entirely new wardrobe. Typically, shorts, jeans, sandals, and strapless dresses are not considered appropriate for professional clothing. If you have a question as to whether something is appropriate to wear, do not wear it.

At off-campus practicum sites, dress may be more or less formal than at the university clinic. If no information is offered, ask your off-campus supervisor about the dress code or guidelines at the site. Occasionally, a supervisor will say that, "Anything is okay to wear," while the supervisor and the rest of the staff dress very formally. In this case, it is best to dress as similarly to the staff as possible. In all cases, dressing with a view to appearing professional is desirable.

From being a student during certain times of the day to being a clinician at other times of the day can be a difficult mental transition. Donning professional dress helps you make that transition. It also prompts the client to regard you more as a professional person and less as a student.

Professional Liability

Although you are a student in training, you still provide direct client services when you engage in clinical practicum. You will be expected to provide a certain standard of care and you will be held responsible for your actions. You may be liable for any inappropriate or negligent service that results in damage or harm to a client. ASHA has published a technical report on professional liability and risk management (American Speech-Language-Hearing Association, 1994b). Read this report early in your clinical practicum.

All student clinicians should have **liability insurance** before beginning their clinical practicum. You can obtain information from your clinic office regarding the procedures for obtaining liability insurance. In some locations, students pay for insurance directly to the university. In other locations, students are required to independently purchase insurance and then provide the proof of coverage.

Insurance typically is purchased on an annual basis. A low cost group insurance is available for students and professional practitioners. Information can be obtained at your clinic or by contacting ASHA.

To avoid any suspicion of negligence or malpractice, you must closely follow the ASHA Code of Ethics, comply with all clinic procedures, and maintain appropriate communications with your supervisor. You also should be knowledgeable in current standards of care for the disorders you treat. As you know, periodically ASHA publishes Position Statements and Guidelines. These documents specify ASHA's official position on controversial clinical or scientific issues, recommend appropriate courses of professional actions, and summarize state-of-the-art information on selected issues. You should keep yourself current on these position statements and guidelines.

Health and Safety Precautions

Because you will be working closely with people, you must follow certain health and safety precautions. These precautions help provide protection for you and your clients from various communicable diseases or injuries.

Because you work with many different individuals, you are at a greater risk for **exposure to a communicable disease**, than, for instance, a computer programmer might be. Also, you will work with certain clients who are very susceptible to infection such as patients in the neonatal intensive care unit, elderly patients, and critically ill patients. Many sites follow universal health care precautions. Under universal precautions everyone (patients and professionals) are considered risks for infection (Kemp, Roeser, Pearson, & Ballachanda, 1995). **Materials that require universal precautions include**: blood, semen, vaginal secretions, cerebrospinal fluid, synovial fluid, pleural fluid, any body fluid with visible blood, any unidentifiable body fluid, and saliva from dental fluid.

Each practicum site may have different health and safety regulations. You must follow the regulations of your clinical assignment. Following are some general health procedures.

1. **Get a rubella vaccination**. All individuals should have a rubella vaccination. It is required only one time. Rubella, also known as German measles, is a viral disease often accompanied by a fever and a rash. Although children who contract rubella rarely have any complications, the virus active in a pregnant woman can be a teratogen to a developing fetus, with the possibility of causing intrauterine death, spontaneous abortion, or many types of congenital defects (Benenson, 1990).

2. **Get a mumps vaccination**. Mumps is a viral disease. It is accompanied by fever and tenderness and swelling of one or more of the salivary glands. There is no clear evidence linking mumps during pregnancy with congenital malformations. However, because of the incidence of testicular mumps in the male population, male health care providers often are advised or required to have mumps vaccination. The frequency of mumps has decreased since common early childhood immunization has become available; however, an increase in mumps was reported in the United States in both 1986 and 1987 (Benenson, 1990).

3. **Get a Hepatitis B vaccination**. Like the mumps vaccination, this vaccination is not always required, but is recommended. Hepatitis B is a

form of viral hepatitis and can be transmitted through contaminated blood, needles, or instruments. Onset is rapid and infection can cause severe liver damage (Anderson & Anderson, 1994).

4. **Have a tuberculin skin test** (PPD-purified protein derivative). Tuberculosis is an infectious mycobacterial disease. Generally, it has decreased in occurrence in developed countries, but has stabilized or increased in frequency in the population of persons testing positive for HIV infection. Tuberculosis most often involves the lungs and, if left untreated, can result in death or other serious complications. The initial infection to tuberculosis often is not recognized. This is one of the reasons students, who are in close contact with a variety of individuals in their clinical experiences, are required to have a tuberculin skin test on a regular basis. Clinics may require a skin test annually. Public schools often require the skin test less frequently, because the incidence of tuberculosis is less in children and increases in the aging population (Benenson, 1990).

5. **Protect any wounds or skin lesions**. Use a waterproof dressing, gloves, or both to protect any wounds, sores, or skin abrasions you may have.

6. **Use gloves**. Wear latex gloves when performing oral exams, during any invasive procedure of the oral cavity (such as dysphagia assessment or treatment), or during any contact with blood or bodily fluids with visible blood (ASHA Committee on Quality Assurance, 1990). To protect the client against infection, when wearing gloves do not touch your pencil, furniture, or other unsanitized objects.

7. **Wash your hands after removing latex gloves**. Your hands may become contaminated as you remove your gloves. Therefore, be sure to wash your hands after removing gloves.

8. **Wash your hands before and after working with a client**. Hand washing is considered one of the best ways to prevent the spread of disease. In addition, avoid touching your hands to your mouth, eyes, or nose when working with your clients.

9. **If necessary, wear eye and mouth protection**. If you are working with a client and blood, saliva, or other bodily fluid splashing is possible, you may need to wear eye goggles and a mouth mask (Golper, 1992).

10. **Disinfect or sterilize equipment**. Follow your practicum site's procedures regarding sterilization and disinfection of equipment. Disinfection can be performed using 1:100 solution of household bleach (sodium hypochlorite) to water (ASHA Committee on Quality

Assurance, 1990). Commercial disinfectant also is available. McMillan and Willette (1988) advise that environmental surfaces such as tables, tape recorders, and audiometers be disinfected prior to and following each client contact. However, more recent information suggests that "equipment not contaminated by blood or bodily fluids containing visible signs of blood need not be cleaned after each use" (ASHA Committee on Quality Assurance, 1990).

11. **Use disposable materials**. Whenever possible use disposable materials. After using these materials, follow your clinical practicum site's guidelines regarding disposal of used items.

12. **Stay home if you are ill**. If you are ill, cancel your clinical appointments. You probably will not be very effective as a clinician anyway and may transmit your illness to your client.

13. **Treat the blood of all patients as potentially contagious**. Although it is important to be aware and assess the risk of exposure with each of your patients, you cannot determine the need for infection control based on a patient's case history. Remember, that the use of universal health care precautions protect you and your patient.

14. **Be informed about communicable diseases**. There are many diseases you could be exposed to. However, knowledge about the transmission and prevention of the disease is one of the first steps in defense against the disease. For obvious reasons, the spread of AIDS/HIV infection currently is a major health concern (ASHA Committee on Quality Assurance, 1990; McMillan & Willette, 1988). AIDS (acquired immune deficiency syndrome) is considered the last clinical stage of HIV infection. Present information indicates that transmission is by sexual exposure and exposure to blood or tissue. Although progress is being reported in the drug treatment for HIV infection, there is no known cure for AIDS (Benenson, 1990).

Depending on the work environment, there are other diseases of which the speech-language pathologist should be aware. However, this chapter cannot outline all possible diseases to which one may be exposed. It is hoped that students will seriously consider the potential for exposure to communicable diseases and the potential for exposing others to infections—both the inconvenient types as well as the life-threatening ones—and closely follow all disease control procedures established at clinical practicum sites.

In addition to following health care precautions, you will help decrease the chance of injury to the client by following some basic safety rules. The following is a list of some fundamental rules of safety:

1. **Make sure the clinic area is clean and orderly**. This will help avoid such accidents as tripping over small items left on the floor.

2. **Do not leave children unattended in the clinic**. Children who are left without supervision may cause mischief or injury to themselves and others. They may swallow small objects, play with electrical outlets, pull furniture over, or fall.

3. **Do not let children stand on tables or chairs**. If, for some reason, you want a child to stand on a table or chair, hold him or her with at least one hand.

4. **Check with the parent before giving food**. Occasionally, you may want to use food in your treatment program. Before doing so make sure you have the parent's approval and that the child does not have any food allergies, restricted diet, or swallowing difficulties. If you are working with an adult who is under the care of a spouse or caregiver, check with that person before giving your client food.

5. **Make sure clients who are in wheelchairs lock their brakes**. If they do not do so automatically, advise them to lock their brakes. If they cannot do so independently, lock their brakes for them.

6. **Before pushing clients who are in wheelchairs, make sure their feet are in the footrests or lifted off the ground**.

7. **Do not allow smoking in the clinic area**.

8. **Know where the fire extinguisher is**. In addition, it is important to know how the fire extinguisher works. If there is an emergency, you will not have time to read the instructions on the canister.

9. **Locate the nearest emergency telephone**. Most sites will have a telephone or intercom available for emergency communications.

10. **Adhere to safety procedures at your site**. As you know, each practicum site may have different safety precautions. Do not second guess these. Know and follow all rules established at your practicum setting.

Client Bill of Rights

By now it is obvious that there are many rules governing your behavior for the protection of the profession and your clients. Under these rules, you have certain obligations to your clients and your clients have certain implied rights. However, ASHA thought that implied client rights were not sufficient. ASHA's Task Force on Protection of Clients' Rights (1994) published a technical report in which the **Model Bill of Rights for People Receiving Audiology or Speech-Language Pathology Services** was outlined and discussed. This is a generic document encompassing both children and adults across all service delivery settings. It applies to both speech-language pathology and audiology services and was designed to be easily understandable to the consumer. Many of the principles advocated in the Bill of Rights reflect the rules in the Code of Ethics. For example, one of the rights is "that services be provided without regard to race or ethnicity, gender, age, religion, national origin, sexual orientation, or disability" (p. 61). Before working as a student clinician, read this *Bill of Rights*.

In abiding by the Code of Ethics and state and federal laws, you may occasionally encounter guidelines that could be interpreted in different ways. In all such cases, you must consider the well-being of your clients as the most important basis on which to make decisions. Your supervisor or clinic director will be there to help you make appropriate and ethical decisions. ASHA, your state speech-language-hearing association, and your state licensure agency also are important institutions that help resolve professional questions.

4

The Supervisor and the Student Clinician

An essential component to the success of your clinical practicum as a beneficial learning experience is the interaction between you and your supervisor. As you may expect, your clinical practicum in speech-language pathology is a three-way process involving you, your supervisor, and your client. Your supervisor is your clinical mentor. In many ways, your supervisor helps you acquire the knowledge and skills necessary to become an independent and competent clinician who can provide quality service for clients. The effectiveness of your practicum experience depends, partly, on the relationship developed between you and your supervisor. Each of you has different roles and responsibilities in the development of your clinical skills.

Role of the Clinical Supervisor

Training student clinicians while ensuring quality clinical service to clients is the primary role of the clinical supervisor. In a sense, the student clinicians are the supervisors' clients. It is a supervisor's responsibility to maximize students' learning opportunities. Also, the supervisor must fulfill other managerial or academic obligations. Many university clinics have a staff of full-time supervisors who do little or no classroom teaching. Many other university clinics have academic faculty members supervising clinical practicum. Supervisors also may be assigned a variety of administrative duties.

It is important that a student clinician understand the scope of a supervisor's main responsibilities and some of the limitations to avoid misunderstandings or incorrect expectations. It is equally important that a clinical supervisor be aware of a student clinician's prior experience and clearly defines practicum guidelines and expectations.

What To Expect From Your Clinical Supervisor

The clinical supervisor facilitates your practicum experience. This facilitation includes direct teaching of clinical methods, self-evaluation, clinical analysis, and problem-solving skills. ASHA has developed various regulations and guidelines on supervision. ASHA's Special Interest Division II focuses specifically on administration and supervision and several books have been written on clinical supervision. The ASHA report on supervision in speech-language pathology and audiology identified 13 supervisory tasks (ASHA Committee on Supervision, 1985). These tasks provide guidelines for supervision. Many of them have been integrated into the following sections, providing an overview of what student clinicians can expect from their supervisors.

Develop and Maintain Effective Communication. It is important that you and your clinical supervisor establish a **cooperative working relationship** to enhance your clinical practicum experience and assure the delivery of quality services. Some clinical supervisors are available before, during, and after clinic sessions to discuss issues and questions with you. Other clinical supervisors assign specific conference times. It is the responsibility of the clinical supervisor to provide a forum for appropriate and effective communication between supervisor and student clinician. However, you share in this responsibility. In truth, you may be initially intimidated by your first clinical supervisor. To complicate matters, because of other obligations, the clinical supervisor may not always be readily available to you. Therefore, it is important to remember that (1) your supervisor is available for questions, (2) your supervisor is not a mind reader, and (3) that there may be times when you need to be assertive in seeking advice.

Provide Guidelines of Practicum Requirements. Initially, your clinical supervisor will discuss the **organization of your clinical practicum**

with you. He or she will outline expectations for your performance and requirements of your practicum assignment. For example, your supervisor will explain how and when you will be evaluated and on what basis. In addition to requirements of clinical performance, your supervisor will discuss scheduling, attendance, submission of written reports, and mandatory clinical meetings.

Your supervisor should encourage you to discuss any questions or concerns you may have at the beginning of your clinical assignment or as your practicum progresses. As you continue your practicum, issues related to future practicum assignments or requirements may arise. If your clinical supervisor is unavailable or unable to answer your questions (possibly because the supervisor is a part-time member of the university staff), your clinic director or advisor should be able to assist you.

Provide Consistent Feedback.   Your clinical supervisor will provide consistent feedback on your clinical performance. Of course, different supervisors have different supervisory styles. One supervisor may give **written feedback** at the end of each session. Another supervisor may provide **verbal feedback or modeling** during a session and written feedback after the session. A different supervisor might never interrupt a session unless the well-being of the client is jeopardized. At the beginning of your practicum assignment, your supervisor will discuss the type of feedback he or she will provide.

To maximize learning, your supervisor may arrange **client staffing, role playing**, or other forms of clinical teaching sessions. These sessions may be held on a regular or intermittent basis and before, during, or after clinical practicum sessions. Your supervisor arranges these added learning experiences for your benefit. It is important that you take them seriously by being prepared and an active participant.

Informative feedback may take the form of identifying a behavior that you need to change. For example, beginning clinicians tend to use questions instead of statements: "Can you say /r/?" versus "Say /r/." To give objective feedback, the inappropriate use of questions may be charted by the supervisor. Then your supervisor would share this data with you and ask you to eliminate or decrease the use of such questions by a certain amount. Following up on this communication, your supervisor would again observe a clinical session and chart your use of the question, "Can you say /r/?"

If you think that you are not receiving sufficient feedback or that the feedback is unclear, discuss this with your clinical supervisor. Your supervisor may believe that you understand the feedback that has been given and if you do not make appropriate changes, your supervisor may think you are disregarding his or her recommendations. Remember, feedback does not necessarily imply negative criticism. It is a teaching method that you will frequently use with your own clients.

Assist in Planning Clinical Objectives. Typically, your supervisor will direct you to review your clients' charts or case histories and **develop an assessment or treatment plan** for your first session with your clients. Before your initial meeting with your clients, your supervisor will review these plans with you. The less clinical experience you have had, the more assistance your clinical supervisor will expect you to need.

Your supervisor will help you learn to critically evaluate your clients' speech and language behaviors and learn to develop measurable clinical objectives. Each practicum site will have different ways of writing appropriate objectives. For example in the school setting, you will write objectives related to your students' educational performance. In the hospital setting, you may write objectives related to your patients' ability to successfully complete such daily living activities as stating when they want something to eat. Your supervisor also will help you establish priorities for treatment objectives. Chapter 7 describes some general guidelines for selecting target behaviors. Note, however, that your clinical supervisor must approve all major clinical decisions, including what to teach your clients and how.

Your supervisor also may identify or help you identify **personal objectives** for you to achieve. You may be asked to describe areas of professional growth and how you plan to achieve it. For example, your supervisor may suggest that you need more information related to the nonverbal child or you may identify your own weakness in that area when assigned such a child as a client. To supplement your knowledge in this area, your supervisor might direct you to specific resources or advise you to research the subject area and report your findings to him or her.

Assist in Developing Diagnostic Skills and Assessment Strategies. Your clinical supervisor will observe a minimum of 50% of each evaluation session. You will get feedback on your **selection, administration, and interpretation of tests**. Your supervisor may suggest certain tests or test administration sequences. It is your responsibility to learn each test before you attempt to administer it to a client. To ensure the test is appropriate for your client, you should carefully read the test manual. If possible, practice using the test by administering it to friends. After you have familiarized yourself with a test and practiced administering the test, your supervisor will give you additional help if needed. For example, your supervisor may model both general and specific test administration procedures. Your supervisor also will advise you regarding **informal observation procedures**, client-specific assessment procedures, and assist you in integrating results of standardized tests and nonstandardized observations.

Demonstrate a Variety of Clinical Skills. Beginning student clinicians sometimes are unsure of how to implement the myriad of treatment techniques and principles about which they have read and observed. For example, if you exhibit difficulty with effectively reinforcing a desired behavior, your **supervisor will demonstrate** the appropriate strategy. Some clinical supervisors prefer to actually demonstrate with a specific client during treatment sessions. Other supervisors do not interrupt sessions, but may demonstrate a technique after a session and expect you to implement it the following session. Often, supervisors will inform you in advance if they intend to demonstrate a specific technique during a clinical session. You should request demonstration of certain procedures when you do not clearly understand your supervisor's instructions.

Facilitate Development of Client Management Skills. After you develop your treatment goals, you must determine a progression of treatment. Your supervisor will assist you in **evaluating the needs of your client**, including such variables as determining the initial level of treatment, developing intervention strategies, establishing the performance criteria for each level, and accurately charting treatment results. Your supervisor will encourage you to **evaluate the effectiveness of your clinic sessions** and determine what, if any, changes should be made in your treatment goals or strategies.

In evaluating each of your sessions, it is necessary for you and your supervisor to have accurate information on your clients' performance. You will discover that a set method of charting responses will not be appropriate across all clients and that you may need to experiment with different methods. Your supervisor will suggest different ways to maintain accurate records.

In addition to analyzing client performance, you may expect your supervisor to **require you to analyze your own behaviors** and how they affect client responses. One way your supervisor may assist you in evaluating your performance is by videotaping clinical sessions. You may be required to watch the video independently or jointly with your supervisor. Your supervisor also may chart some of your clinical behaviors (such as your use of positive feedback or method of evoking responses) to show you what you do.

Describe Record-Keeping Requirements. As you know, accountability and documentation are important components of clinical service delivery. Certain record-keeping requirements are common across settings and other requirements may be unique to individual sites. Regardless of the documentation method, closely adhere to the requirements. Whether your client is able to continue treatment or whether your site receives payment for services provided, are only two reasons why appropriate record keeping is essential. Your supervisor will **describe the documentation and record-keeping requirements** specific to your setting. The methods utilized to ensure confidentiality of clinical records also will be outlined and monitored by your clinical supervisor.

Encourage Independent Problem Solving and Self-Analysis.   The importance of the clinical supervisor in providing direct guidance and assistance to student clinicians should not be minimized. Nonetheless, an important role of clinical supervisors is to **teach clinicians independent problem-solving skills** and self-analysis. Regardless of the number of practicum hours completed, you still will encounter clients exhibiting communicative disorders with which you have had little or no experience. Also, although clients with the same diagnoses may exhibit similar communicative performance, each client will have unique problems and behaviors. However, if you have developed the ability to critically analyze both your clients' behaviors as well as your own clinical behaviors, you will be able to make appropriate clinical decisions in a variety of clinical situations. This is not to suggest that each clinician is, or even should be, highly qualified to work with every type of speech and language disorder. Clinicians who specialize can better serve specific clients. However, the clinical decision-making process includes knowing when it is necessary to seek additional information or to refer clients to other speech-language pathologists or different professionals.

Your supervisor will provide guidance based on your level of clinical experience. At each level of your practicum experience, your supervisor will involve you in the problem-solving and analysis process. The supervisor will make suggestions, but will expect you to expand on those suggestions and to generalize ideas across clients and settings. Your supervisor also will expect you to seek information, rather than just waiting to receive instruction or direction. As you progress in your practicum, your supervisor, although continuing to monitor your performance, will provide less and less assistance with decision making and allow you to perform with increasing independence.

Help Develop Verbal and Written Skills.   Your supervisor will facilitate the development of your verbal and written reporting skills by providing you with opportunities for practicing both types of activities. Content requirements and formats of clinical reports vary across supervisors and settings; therefore, your supervisor should provide you with an **outline of professional writing requirements** of your assignment. Also, to help guide you, your supervisor may provide you with **samples of reports**.

Although reporting styles may vary, the need to write clear, concise, and logical reports does not. Your supervisor will **edit your clinical reports** or suggest specific changes. Do not be surprised if you must revise a report more than once. When your supervisor first edits your report, the most obvious problems may be noted. However, after these errors are corrected, more subtle problems may be observed, requiring you to revise your reports further.

Verbal reporting skills will be required at each of your practicum sites. For example at the university clinic, you will need to share information with your clients and their family members. In the medical setting, you may be required to share information with clients' family members and various health professionals. In the educational setting, you will be required to share information with such people as clients' family members, teachers, family physicians, and psychologists. Therefore, your supervisor may require you to **practice your verbal reporting skills** during client staffing, consultation with other professionals, and sharing information with clients and their families. If you have little previous experience with verbal reporting, you might find it beneficial to write out the information you want to cover and practice presenting it out loud. It is also helpful to try to anticipate questions that might arise and prepare answers in advance.

Provide Current Resources. Information is changing rapidly in the field of communicative disorders. Experts continue to suggest new assessment and treatment methods. New instruments and technological devices also are developed frequently. Your supervisor will expect you to use current information, instruments, procedures, and technology and will assist you in locating them. The supervisor will **help you research current information** and use many campus resources including the library, computer laboratories, writing clinics, and so forth. Much information is available on the Internet. For example, ASHA has made many of its Position Papers, Guidelines, and other resources available through its Web site. **Before using material that you found on the Internet, be sure the information is accurate**. Only use information that you obtained from a reliable site (such as ASHA's) or find a second source that validates information you obtained from the Internet. Before you begin clinical practicum, you will have begun to develop a library of various texts and journal articles. Although these texts and articles may be only 1 or 2 years old, by the time you begin clinical practicum, they may already be outdated. It is essential to routinely read your journals and maintain current information on a variety of subjects. ASHA encourages its members to update their clinical information through its continuing education program. Also, some state licensure laws and credential regulations require continuing education units.

Model and Demand Professional Behavior. Your supervisor will **model the behavior expected of you**. For example, your supervisor will be punctual, dress appropriately, protect client confidentiality by not talking about clients in public areas, and so on. Your supervisor will treat you as a professional and will expect to be treated as one. Regardless of your clinical practicum site, your supervisor will expect you to know and comply with ASHA's Code of Ethics. Your supervisor will outline the requirements of your clinical site including the dress code, health regulations, and clinical practicum schedule. If you have any questions about the parameters of professional behavior for your site, ask your supervisor for clarification.

Evaluate Your Clinical Work. Your clinical supervisor also is an instructor who must evaluate your clinical work. Every supervisor must strive to make objective and constructive evaluation of your clinical work. Although there may be times set aside for formal evaluations, every time you receive feedback from your supervisor, you will have received some level of evaluation as well. In conjunction with your clinical practicum, you may receive a letter grade or grade of credit/no credit. Your supervisor will follow your university's guidelines for **evaluation of student clinicians**, but most evaluations include areas such as knowledge of disorders, competence in administering tests and interpreting results, proficiency in developing and implementing treatment plans, readiness to implement and expand on supervisory suggestions, and so on. Many universities are using rating scales that help supervisors assess students' abilities and assists them in improving their clinical skills. Your performance may be compared in terms of accuracy, consistency, and need for supervisory guidance to an optimum clinical behavior called a **clinical competency**. If you have questions about your clinical practicum evaluation, discuss them with your clinical supervisor.

Help, Guide, and Support You. In addition to ensuring quality patient care, a primary responsibility of the clinical supervisor is to **provide appropriate training for the student clinician**. During training, sometimes it may be necessary for your supervisor to give you feedback that seems negative. However, your clinical supervisor's aim is for you to learn, so try not to feel that your supervisor is *picking* on you. As a conscientious student clinician, you can expect your supervisor to be there to help you, guide you, and support you. The supervisor will expect you to have confidence and trust in him or her. Your supervisor is not only **your mentor**, but also **your advocate**.

Off-Campus Clinical Supervision

Often the off-campus clinical supervisor is a professional employee of your practicum site. Off-campus clinical supervisors have their CCCs in audiology or speech-language pathology. Your university training director will have discussed ASHA's requirements for supervision and may have provided a general background of your experience level. However, off-campus clinical supervisors may or may not be fully familiar with your university's training program. Consequently, they may not act or hold the same expectations as the supervisors at the university clinic.

Overview

Your off-campus supervisor will perform many of the same activities identified in the previous section: (1) develop and maintain effective communication, (2) provide guidelines of the practicum requirements, (3) provide ongoing feedback, (4) assist in planning clinical goals, (5) assist in developing diagnostic skills, (6) demonstrate clinical methods, (7) assist in developing client management skills, (8) describe record-keeping requirements, (9) encourage independent problem solving, (10) facilitate development of reporting skills, (11) provide current resources, (12) model and demand professional behavior, (13) evaluate your clinical work, and (14) help you and support you. However, you should not expect off-campus clinical supervisors to be exactly the same as the university clinical supervisor in performing all these and other duties.

Frequency of Supervision. At your off-campus site, the frequency of supervision may be different than you were used to at on-campus clinical sites. The amount of supervision offered at off-campus sites may be more or less. Minimally, the **off-campus supervisors will meet ASHA's guidelines** for the type and frequency of supervision. However, at an off-campus site, you are expected to be able to work relatively independently, but you may be supervised more closely than when you were less experienced. This increased amount of supervision does not mean that the supervisor does not have much confidence in you. The off-campus supervisors may have only a single student clinician to supervise; whereas, university clinic supervisors may supervise up to four clinicians at one time. In addition, in certain cases, you may be working with critically ill patients or providing a therapy, which if done incorrectly, could compromise the client's health. The off-campus site also may have additional supervisory requirements for compliance with insurance requirements.

Unique Aspects of Practicum Sites. Each of your practicum sites will offer you unique learning experiences and have requirements specific to that site. Your off-campus supervisor will let you know about the special components of clinical work in his or her setting. In the beginning, your off-campus supervisor may have to spend extra time in getting you familiarized with the special clinical populations served at the site and the unique clinical and administrative procedures to be followed. Your clinical supervisor may model certain techniques and give you samples of different documentation procedures.

Progress Toward Independence. Expect your supervisor to demand fairly **independent performance** from you. This sounds like a contradiction, based on the probability that you will receive greater one-to-one supervision than at the university clinic; however, it is not. Inherent in an internship placement is the assumption that you are fairly advanced and able to make independent judgments. Because of this, your clinical supervisor certainly will expect you to act relatively independently in planning assessment and treatment sessions, problem solving, researching additional information, and asking necessary questions.

Supervisor Expectations. Your off-campus clinical supervisors may have a general understanding of your clinical experience and academic course work, but probably will not know your specific academic background in detail. They may know what courses you have had, but may not know the scope and orientation of those courses. Consequently, their expectations may be different from those of your supervisors at the university clinic who probably knew the curriculum content and orientation of courses you had and the level of your clinical experience. But the off-campus supervisors may not be familiar with the full details of the university's training program. The supervisors' expectations of you may be based on their general experiences with students of your background. Some supervisors may base expectations on their own educational experiences and the requirements they faced. This is not necessarily a disadvantage, but something of which you should be aware.

Responsibilities of the Student Clinician

Student clinicians must fulfill numerous responsibilities to ensure a successful practicum experience for themselves and to provide effective services to their clients. In essence, though, student clinicians should (a) learn to assess, treat, counsel, and professionally work with their clients and their families; and (b) show systematic progress in their learning of those professional skills.

Throughout your clinical practicum experiences, many of these responsibilities will remain unchanged as you progress in your practicum. However, the expectations of the clinical supervisor change. As you advance and gain experience, you will be expected to fulfill your clinical responsibilities with **less guidance** from your clinical supervisor. Although individual university departments may have additional requirements, the following sections provide a general overview of the student clinician's responsibilities.

Compliance With ASHA's Code of Ethics

As you know from Chapter 3, ASHA's Code of Ethics describes various acceptable professional behaviors. In all clinical practicum settings, **abide by ASHA's Code of Ethics**. It is your responsibility to be aware of the intent of the Code of Ethics and its various principles and rules. You do not want to jeopardize your career as a speech-language pathologist because you have violated the Code of Ethics.

ASHA Preferred Practice Patterns

The ASHA Task Force on Clinical Standards developed an extensive list of speech-language pathology and audiology procedures (American Speech-Language-Hearing Association, 1997b). The **Preferred Practice Patterns** paper was written in generic terms and provides a framework under which service may be provided across various work settings. Intended to be flexible in nature, the *Preferred Practice Patterns* are designed to outline current practices and to be updated as the profession changes. Paramount to the *Preferred Practice Patterns* is the welfare of the client, although many professional issues are covered. The fundamental components of the *Preferred Practice Patterns* include: identification of professionals who perform a procedure, expected outcomes, clinical indications, clinical process, setting and equipment specifications, safety and health precautions, and documentation. In most cases, ASHA policy and related references are also given. Each of these areas is discussed in greater detail in Chapter 3. As you might imagine, knowledge of these preferred practice patterns is important to the student clinician. Referring to the different procedures will provide you with a general guide to a variety of procedures such as speech screening, language screening, augmentative and alternative communication assessment, fluency assessment, and speech-language pathology treatment.

ASHA Scope of Practice Guidelines

American Speech-Language-Hearing Association's (1996a) Scope of Practice guidelines **define the roles** of the speech-language pathologist and the audiologist. You will have both speech-language pathology and audiology clinical practicum experiences. One semester you may participate in speech-language pathology clinical practicum; another semester you may participate in audiology clinical practicum. Because of the diversity of clinical experiences, it is important that you know in which clinical setting what kinds of services are provided. During your audiology clinical practicum, supervised by a qualified audiologist, you would be able to provide various audiological services including, "Activities that identify, assess, diagnose, manage, and interpret test results related to disorders of human hearing, balance, and other neural systems" (American Speech-Language-Hearing Association, 1996a, p. 14). However, when you enroll in speech-language pathology clinical practicum with supervision of a qualified audiologist or speech-language pathologist, your scope of service related to audiology is much more limited and includes only, "Providing aural rehabilitation and related counseling services to hearing impaired individuals and their families"; and "Conducting pure-tone air conduction hearing screening and screening tympanometry for the purpose of the initial identification and/or referral of individuals with other communication disorders of possible middle ear pathology" (American Speech-Language-Hearing Association, 1996b, p. 18). Your scope of practice will also be influenced by your state's licensure laws. As you know, ASHA guidelines are not legal mandates, but licensure laws are.

Clinic Policies and Procedures

The many clinic policies and procedures student clinicians must follow may appear unwarranted to the new clinician. Yet, these policies and procedures enable a clinic to operate effectively and efficiently. Each clinical site will have different policies and procedures you must follow. Typically, the clinic secretary or your clinical supervisor will let you know the policies. Many practicum sites will make **procedural handbooks** available to you.

The following subjects commonly are addressed at the university clinic and any off-campus practicum sites: enrolling in clinical practicum, scheduling clients, ensuring client confidentiality, reserving and checking out materials and equipment, maintaining and working with clients' folders, utilizing the clinic telephone, maintaining clinic records, fulfilling insurance and health requirements, quality improvement, health precautions, and complying with the site's dress code. If you are unsure of a specific procedure or policy at your clinical site, you must get the information from your clinical supervisor.

Client Confidentiality

Because of its importance, the necessity of ensuring client confidentiality has been addressed in several places in this book. Remember that **all information regarding a client is confidential**. Do not discuss a client or a client's family by name in public areas. Public areas include reception areas, work rooms, waiting rooms, and other places outside the clinic. Do not leave clients' records unattended at desks or in workrooms. As a general rule, never remove permanent records from the clinic area. Follow established procedures regarding release of client information to other agencies.

Client Personal and Cultural Belief Consideration

You will work with many clients who have varied cultural and ethnic backgrounds. You are not expected to share each client's values and beliefs, or even to know every culture's traditions; however, your willingness to **accept your clients' diversity** will maximize the effectiveness of your service delivery. You should be aware of assessment, treatment, and counseling considerations in serving a diverse clinical population. Chapter 6 contains specific information about serving multicultural populations.

Clinic Session Preparation

Know the administration and evaluation of diagnostic assessment procedures. Review them before every diagnostic session. Inspect the tests you plan to administer before meeting with your client to make sure the tests are complete, that they contain all required materials, and that the necessary test response forms are available. Although it may be another person's job to stock the treatment rooms, it is your responsibility to have all the necessary materials. In the middle of an oral-peripheral examination, you cannot blame someone for not providing the needed supplies. To avoid wasting assessment or treatment time, **prepare and organize all materials** and **forms** in advance of each session.

In advance, **check any equipment** that you plan to use in your clinical sessions to ensure it is working properly. Make sure you know how to operate equipment you plan to use. Some distressing problems can occur with common tape recorders. They may be broken or the batteries may be dead. Not infrequently, student clinicians have recorded an entire clinical session only to find that the pause button was depressed instead of the record button.

Carefully **review data** obtained in previous sessions to determine appropriate beginning levels and possible sequences of treatment for the sessions for which you are preparing. Make sure the materials you have selected are the most appropriate for the target behaviors you plan to teach. The best organized and most creative materials are ineffective if the target behaviors are inappropriate or unrealistic. If you are working with a new client or in a medical setting where others place information in your client's chart, **review the chart** before beginning each treatment session.

Diagnostic Instrument Choice

Select and use evaluation procedures and instruments that are appropriate to the client. Select procedures and instruments that are **valid, reliable, nonbiased, and comprehensive**. The evaluation procedures must sample behaviors adequately. Report with caution the results of tests administered to clients outside the standardization population. Use informal or naturalistic observation of a client's communicative skills as a part of each evaluation. This type of assessment is used to provide a more comprehensive analysis of a client's spontaneous speech and to provide a basis for evaluation when standardized instruments are not appropriate. Standardized tests can supplement information obtained from analysis of a client's conversational speech.

Develop Measurable Treatment Objectives. Develop measurable treatment objectives based on diagnostic results or reassessment of a client's **current communicative skills**. You may continue to work on objectives established the previous semester, if they still are appropriate for the client. Do not believe erroneously that you are always required to develop "original" objectives—even though the previous semester's objectives may still be applicable.

Submit Written Assignments Promptly. Your clinical supervisor will notify you of timelines and due dates for written assignments. Each practicum site will have **different writing requirements**. University clinics typically require an initial written summary, daily lesson plans or a semester treatment plan, and a final summary or progress report. Submit written assignments on time, because it is important for many reasons. First, completing assignments on time suggests that you are dependable and that your practicum assignment is a high priority to you. Second, your written work reflects your knowledge of your clients, their communicative disorders, and of assessment and treatment procedures you plan to implement. A promptly submitted report will help the supervisor give you timely feedback. Third, your reports may suggest to the supervisor the level of supervision you need to work effectively with your client. To understand the formats and to practice writing various kinds of professional reports before or during your clinical practicum assignment, see Hegde (1998a).

Treatment Plan Development

An effective treatment program may fail if it is not properly sequenced for each individual client. For example, if the initial target behavior is defined as the correct production of a phoneme in sentences, you may never get started at all. Therefore, **plan and sequence treatment** using the initial and continuous assessment data. Plan realistically for the time available within each session. Design maintenance procedures early in the treatment sequence. Include the family in the treatment process. Use clinical procedures based on replicated research and technology. Finally, include the client as an active participant in the intervention process. Read the second part of this textbook and other books for details on treatment procedures (Hegde, 1998b).

Accurate Clinical Record Maintenance

Maintain an accurate and comprehensive record of your clients' clinical histories and related information in their permanent files. **Maintain clinic files** in the order established by the clinical site.

Continuous measurement of target responses throughout the treatment sessions and charting them in the form of line or bar graphs will make it easier to see client progress or lack of it. Such graphic and other quantitative measures enable you to find out quickly if treatment is appropriate or if modifications are needed. Graphs also allow you to provide the client (or parent) with a visual representation of progress. Therefore, record and analyze your clients' responses during all assessment and treatment sessions. Learn efficient and accurate charting skills to record the client responses.

Maintain an **accurate and complete chronological log** of clinical activity. This log is a necessary part of the documentation and analysis process. A review of a client's file should show the client's progress. Record keeping requirements are discussed in more detail in Chapter 5.

Apply Information Learned in Academic Courses

In planning for evaluation and treatment sessions, **draw from the information you learned** in your academic courses. This seems like a fundamental assumption that should go without mentioning, but occasionally there are students who differentiate between material learned in academic courses and material learned in practicum assignments. Some students fail to see the relevance of what they have learned in the classroom to clinical work. The more you are able to integrate academic and clinical assignments, the greater is the value of both. You also will find that information learned in one class that focused on a particular disorder can be expanded and generalized to other communicative disorders. The information you acquire in your academic studies is the foundation on which you build your independent professional skills and clinical experience.

Research Information. Research information will be needed to fulfill your clinical assignments. Your clinical supervisor may provide you with **resources** or you may **independently locate materials**. Know the library resources, including current and past periodicals, latest books, and computerized information search programs that are available for finding research information. If you are unsuccessful at resolving a particular clinical question independently, request assistance from your clinical supervisor.

Ask Questions. Although expected to work increasingly independently, you must learn to **seek assistance** when you have questions. You should not continue an aspect of your practicum when you are not sure of something. If you are unclear about clinic policies and procedures, if you are not certain about implementing a specific treatment plan, if you are not sure about directions given by your supervisor, or if you just forget something that was said, ask for clarification.

Your clinical supervisor does not always immediately know when you need help. If you think you are not getting enough assistance from your supervisor, evaluate your own behavior before assuming that your supervisor "doesn't have time" or "doesn't care." Some clinical supervisors will be very structured in scheduling times for questions, meetings, and staffing. Others will be less structured and expect student clinicians to approach them with questions as they arise.

Clinic Session Self-Evaluation

Do not expect your clinical supervisor to evaluate all your sessions. To make independent clinical judgments, **learn to self-evaluate** your clinical work. You will learn to analyze objectively your clients' behavior and your behavior. This self-analysis is an essential part of clinical practicum. The skill will enable you to successfully modify evaluation and treatment plans and to continue to use and expand on information that you acquire throughout your professional career.

There is an ever-increasing number of assessment instruments in communicative disorders. To further confuse students, there are many contradictory theories and treatment strategies. If you can objectively evaluate your clinical behaviors and those of your clients, you can establish the most effective treatment for your clients. Also, you will be better able to find out what academic areas or clinical skills you should target for personal improvement.

You are not expected to know automatically how to evaluate your clinical sessions. Your supervisor is responsible for helping you acquire this skill. In helping you acquire self-evaluation skills, your supervisor may respond to your questions with additional questions. Your supervisor may suggest areas of research rather than giving you a specific manual or reference. Also, when you are having trouble working with a client, your supervisor may not immediately step in, but allow you time to analyze and resolve whatever problem you are having.

Attendance Maintenance

Attend all scheduled clinical sessions promptly. If you are ill or have a personal emergency, **notify your clinical supervisor** and, if part of your clinic's protocol, your clients. Studying for examinations, leaving for a vacation, or simply being unprepared are not acceptable reasons for canceling a clinical appointment. Also, begin and end your clinical sessions on time.

Professional Behavior

Sometimes it is difficult to be a student on the one hand and a professional on the other. But remember that although you are in training, **you are a professional** helping people with communicative disorders.

Know how to make others view you as a professional. Do some of your fellow students generate more of an aura of professionalism than others? If you look at their behaviors, you probably will find individuals who have spent much time becoming knowledgeable about their clients' communicative disorders. They will have prepared thoroughly and organized their clinical sessions. They also will have given thought to how they speak and dress.

Student clinicians who present themselves as professionals also treat their clients, supervisor, clinical staff, and other professionals with respect. In turn, the student clinicians are treated as professionals.

Clinical Clock Hour Log Maintenance

You are responsible for maintaining a log of the clinical clock hours you have earned. Maintain both a **daily** and a **semester log**. University speech and hearing clinics have formats for recording clock hours. Carefully follow the format established at your clinic, because you may not get credit for incorrectly recorded clock hours. Appendix C contains sample clinic hour recording forms you may reproduce and use for your records.

Clinical Supervisor Relationship

You will work with many supervisors. Each may have a different supervisory style. Regardless of your practicum site or the supervisor you have, it is important to **maintain contact** with your supervisor. If you have any questions or concerns about your assignment, contact your supervisor. If you had a great experience in the clinic, let your supervisor know. Do not expect your supervisor to know everything that happens in each of your sessions. Also, do not expect your supervisor to always know when you need help. Work cooperatively with your supervisor and assume some of the responsibility for maintaining effective communication with him or her.

The interaction between the clinical supervisor and student clinician is the basis for learning in the practicum setting. To ensure optimal training for the student clinician and quality service for the client, the supervisor and the student clinician should diligently fulfill their respective responsibilities.

Enjoy Practicum Experience

All this work and all this responsibility, and now you have to enjoy yourself! Yes. At least, as you gain knowledge and clinical independence you should feel some personal fulfillment. Often, your clients will know if you dislike what you are doing. More importantly, if you never find joy or satisfaction in your clinical practicum, you should re-evaluate your professional objectives, because you may have chosen to pursue the wrong career.

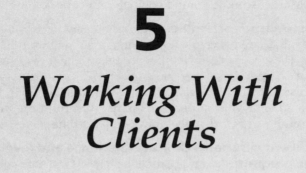

5

Working With Clients

n your academic course work, you were responsible for memorizing and assimilating new information. As a student clinician your major task is to learn professional skills in working with clients who have communicative disorders. These skills include scheduling clients, evaluating their communicative skills, developing and implementing treatment plans, writing a variety of reports, maintaining adequate records, working with families, and coordinating services with other professionals.

Scheduling Clients

Scheduling clients is one of the initial steps in beginning clinical work. Depending on your clinic's policy, either you or the clinic secretary may schedule your clients. It is your responsibility to confirm appointments with the secretary, regardless of who is responsible for the initial scheduling. Several factors influence the scheduling of clients. Such factors include:

1. **The student clinician's schedule.** Your clients will need to be scheduled around your class schedule, your work, and other obligations. Remember, that your clinical practicum is viewed as a professional responsibility and your outside employment may not take precedence over

your clinical practicum. You may be asked to change your employment schedule, if scheduling around your job cannot be accomplished.

2. **The supervisor's schedule.** Supervisors may have obligations such as teaching academic courses, advising, or serving on university committees. These variables will influence the availability of certain supervisors. Also, part-time supervisors may be hired. In these cases, the supervisors may only be available after their full-time job is over. For example, one of your supervisors may work full-time in the public school setting and work at the university part-time.

3. **The student clinician's clinical experience and level in the academic program.** As a rule, student clinicians are not assigned clients with disorders in which the students have had no academic training. Therefore, if you have not had any course on stuttering, you will not be assigned a client who stutters. Client family issues, behavioral issues, or complexity of a disorder will also influence scheduling. As much as possible, beginning student clinicians will be assigned clients with less complex needs.

4. **The type, frequency, and duration of service needed.** The needs of each client will influence the type, frequency, and duration of service provided. Many variables are involved. For example, certain clients may need individual treatment, with other clients benefiting from interaction in a group setting. In other instances, clients with more severe disorders may be seen more frequently (e.g., 4 to 5 times per week), whereas, clients who are close to being dismissed may be seen as few times as 1 or 2 times per month. The severity of the disorder, as well as client health and ability to attend to task, influence the duration of appointments. Sometimes clients with more severe disorders need to be seen frequently, but for shorter periods of time. Certain clients fatigue easily because of health problems. Other clients' optimal attention to tasks may be 20 to 30 minutes.

5. **The population served.** For the convenience of working adults, the clinic hours may include many evening appointments. Your clinic may have both day and evening hours to accommodate a variety of schedules.

6. **The clients' cultures.** Cultural and religious factors also can affect scheduling. Religious holidays must be considered. While it is rare for services to be provided on Sunday, certain individuals may not be available for service on a Friday or Saturday. Also, clients with certain cultural backgrounds may prefer not to be grouped with members of the opposite gender. Other cultural and religious factors must be considered.

7. **The clinical site.** Each clinical site has different priorities regarding client scheduling. At a university clinic, clients must often be sched-

uled around the needs of the students and supervising faculty. At a hospital, the client's health care and the schedules of allied professionals must be considered. In private practice, the convenience to the client is paramount.

8. **Financial resources.** The policy for payment of services will vary at each clinical site. In some cases, the client's ability to pay for services will determine the length and duration of the treatment. For example, a client may have insurance that pays for 10 hours of speech therapy and the client can afford to pay for 5 more hours. Unless the site is willing (and able) to waive any remaining fees, the client's treatment would be restricted to 15 hours.

University Clinic Schedules

University clinics schedule clinical sessions based on the availability of clinical supervision, convenience of clients, the schedule of student clinicians, and the operating times of the clinic. Because of the number of variables involved, university clinic schedules may change from semester to semester.

Most university clinics usually operate during regular business hours, Monday through Friday, with some evening sessions available for clients who cannot attend during the day. Clients typically are scheduled for two to three sessions per week. Sessions range from 30 to 60 minutes. Diagnostic sessions may be scheduled for 1 to 2 hours. Clients are scheduled for individual or group treatment sessions.

Initial Client Contact. At the beginning of the term, you will receive your clinical assignment. You will be given your clinic schedule and your supervisor or clinic director will assign you appropriate clients. Beginning clinicians are assigned 1 or 2 clients, with the more advanced clinicians possibly working with 3 to 4 clients.

At many schools, student clinicians are responsible for telephoning their clients to schedule them. If one of your clients cannot attend at the proposed time, notify your supervisor and the clinic secretary. You will be assigned another client to contact.

The initial contact with your clients is an important step. You should plan what you want to tell the clients or their families. Use the following general guidelines to make your initial telephone contact with your client:

1. **Introduce yourself, your credentials and the purpose of your call.** For example, "Hello, this is Jennifer Jones, a graduate student cli-

nician at the University Speech and Hearing Clinic. I'm calling to schedule speech services for your daughter, Lisa." If the client has not been seen previously at your clinic, be prepared to answer questions about the clinic's policies and procedures. New clients will have questions about fees, clinic schedules, parking, the type of supervision provided, the frequency of supervision, qualifications of the supervisors, length of the semester, qualifications of the student clinicians providing services, and related services available (e.g., audiology).

2. **Discuss the client's schedule.** Tell the client when his or her appointment is. Some clinics also may send written appointment cards to clients. If you contact your clients more than 5 or 6 days in advance, telephone them again the day before their first appointments to remind them of the date and time. This will help reduce the number of missed appointments.

3. **Clarify ambiguous information and request additional information.** For instance, parents sometimes complete a line incorrectly on the case history; they may write the current date on the line requesting their child's date of birth. In addition, you may want to review information that seems too brief. Also, request clients or parents to bring all reports from other speech-language pathologists or related specialists they have seen. As appropriate, verify the primary language of the parents and of the client. Discuss the need for an interpreter.

4. **Give information about parking permits and clinic fees.** Tell clients where they can park. If a free parking permit is possible, tell them how they can acquire one. If clients state they are unable to afford the clinic fee, ask them to see your clinic director (or follow the policy already established at your clinic). You do not have the authority to make decisions about fee reduction or to set up a payment schedule.

5. **Give directions to the clinic.** New clients may not know where the university clinic is. You are familiar with the campus and may not think in terms of how to get to the clinic from other areas of the community. Therefore, have a map of the campus and city available when you first contact your clients. With the help of the map, give accurate directions. Redundant information is usually helpful to an individual unfamiliar with the campus. For example, you might say, "then turn left on Lakeview, you'll be going east. Go to the third stoplight which is Trout Avenue, and turn right, then you'll be heading north."

6. **Give directions to the clinic waiting room.** Tell your clients that you will meet them in the waiting room after they have completed any business at the clinic office. Each clinic has its procedures for the first meeting with clients. Follow the procedures at your university.

7. **Ensure that the client has the correct appointment date and time before ending the phone call.** After you have answered the client's questions and given directions, tell them you will see them at the appointed date, time, and place. "O.K., I'll see you on Monday, September 2nd at 9 a.m. at the clinic waiting room."

Hospital Schedules

Your hospital schedule will coincide with the typical business day, usually from 8 a.m. to 5 p.m. Because many hospitals provide speech-language pathology services 6 days a week, you may be asked to schedule practicum on some weekends. There will be many variables to consider in your hospital schedule and one of the keys to success is flexibility. The following are some factors to consider:

1. **Determine the frequency and duration ordered for speech therapy.** In medical settings, inpatients often are scheduled for speech services 5 to 6 days a week, for 1 hour each day.

2. **Determine the optimum schedule for your patient.** Attempts are made to schedule services at times that are most beneficial to patients. Patients may be seen one or two times a day. One factor influencing their treatment schedule is the length of time they are able to effectively participate in evaluation or treatment. For example, clients may have been prescribed speech-language services five times per week for an hour each day. However, if they are unable to attend for a full hour, they may be seen for 30 minutes during the morning and again for 30 minutes during the afternoon. Another factor influencing the schedule is the type of treatment provided. For example, if you are working with a client who has dysphagia, you may coordinate his or her treatment with the meal schedules. Sometimes, you may go in early to work with the patient before or during breakfast or you may stay late to work with the patient at dinner time.

3. **Coordinate your schedule with the nursing staff.** Though your hospital assignment may require you to begin at 8 a.m., you may not immediately begin direct patient contact. Much of the nursing patient care occurs early in the morning. This care may include such activities as administering medications, providing breakfast, toileting, and bathing. Therefore, you must coordinate your schedule with the nursing staff.

4. **Coordinate your schedule with other patient rehabilitation services.** Besides speech services, a patient may be receiving other rehabilitative services, such as physical and occupational therapies. To

determine your schedule, you will need to check with other professionals providing services to your patients.

5. **Allow time for meetings and conferences.** In the hospital setting, conferences are scheduled to discuss patient care and progress. These conferences are called rounds and are attended by the physician and other members of the medical team. The rounds may be specific to patient rehabilitation, in which case members of the rehabilitation team attend. Rounds are often scheduled between 8 a.m. and 9 a.m.

6. **Adjust your schedule around a regular family visit.** Often, you need to train certain family members to work with your patient in the hospital and at home after the discharge from the hospital. In such cases, find out when it is most convenient for the family member to attend the treatment sessions. Although you want to involve the family in your patient's treatment, there also should be times when the family can be with the patient to just visit. There is the occasional family member who can be at the hospital only at a certain time because of transportation, work, or school obligations. Schedule your sessions so your patients will have some private moments with their families.

7. **Adhere to your schedule.** After you have consulted with other staff and determined a schedule of therapy for a medical patient, remain with the same schedule as much as possible. As patients are discharged and new patients enrolled, some schedule changes will be necessary.

8. **Be punctual.** Your patients' schedule may be full. Many specialists may schedule their services. The doctors, nurses, physical therapists, occupational therapists, and family members all want to have time with your patients. To ensure your patients receive the total amount of therapy they are entitled to, begin and end your treatment sessions on time.

9. **Schedule time for indirect services.** Schedule time for report writing, consultation with other professionals, and family consultation. Also, schedule time for your own breaks and lunches.

10. **Verify your appointments with the secretary.** If you are working in an outpatient setting, the receptionist or secretary may schedule your clients. As much as possible, clients are scheduled for a regular time during their entire enrollment. For example, one of your clients may be scheduled for speech services every Monday, Wednesday, and Friday from 10:00 to 10:45 a.m. Your schedule will change as clients are discharged and new clients are added.

School Schedules

In the educational setting, caseloads may be large and several service delivery models may be used. (Refer to Chapter 2 for additional information on different service delivery models.) Because of this, scheduling may seem overwhelming to the beginning clinician. To begin the scheduling process, use the following guidelines:

1. **Determine the type of schedule.** The two common types of schedules are block (intensive cycle) and intermittent. In **block scheduling**, specific students (or schools) receive services 4 to 5 days a week for a certain number of weeks (for example, 6 weeks). After the predetermined length of time, service is rotated to the next group of students (or schools). In **intermittent scheduling**, all students and schools are served each week. For example, the speech-language pathologist assigned to serve two schools might provide services on Mondays and Wednesdays at one school, and Tuesdays, Thursdays, and Fridays at the other school.

2. **Determine what types of service delivery models you will use.** Your schedule will be influenced by the service delivery model used. Many school clinicians provide a combination of the traditional pull-out model, consultation model, and classroom-collaboration model. Each model requires different amounts of time and considerable coordination with the other professionals involved. For more information on these models, refer to Chapter 2.

3. **Determine how often each student on your caseload will receive service.** Certain students may require more intensive service than others. Generally, students who are close to attaining their objectives and being dismissed are seen less frequently than students who are just beginning to learn new behaviors. Students with more severe disorders may be seen more frequently than students with less severe disorders. You must provide services for the amount of time specified in the student's IEP.

4. **Determine if students will receive treatment individually or in a group.** Certain students require individual treatment and other students may benefit from treatment in a group setting. Although students receiving individual treatment receive more of your individual attention, group treatment also has advantages. The group setting may better reflect students' school environment than does a student's interaction with only the speech-language pathologist. To aid generalization and maintenance in a private practice, you can ask family members and

the client's friends to attend and participate in your client's treatment. However, in the public school setting this is rarely possible. So, effective use of the classroom setting or group setting can aid in generalization and maintenance by better reflecting students' school environment by enlisting other students to assist with your clients' treatment. In addition to becoming discriminative stimuli (see Chapter 9) for the target behaviors trained, other children can act as models for the target behaviors.

5. **Consider school and class schedules.** You must find out the times of recess, lunch, class dismissal, school assemblies, and so on. Several of your students may be receiving services from other professionals, including the school psychologist, resource specialist, adaptive physical education specialist, or physical therapist. There also will be certain periods of the class that the teacher does not want the student to miss on a regular basis.

6. **Allow time for consulting with teachers, testing, writing reports, and meeting with parents.** Consultation and collaboration with the classroom teacher is essential to your effectivness in the school setting. Be careful to allow sufficient time to work with the classroom teacher. Generally, this time will have to be scheduled before or after school or during the teacher's breaks. Also, testing students, writing reports, and meeting with parents are important components to your school service delivery. To avoid canceling treatment sessions, schedule blocks of time for these activities in advance.

There are many factors to consider in developing your schedule for service delivery in the schools. The preceding items provide a brief overview of issues faced in school scheduling. Appropriate implementation of any type of schedule requires effective communication with the classroom teachers and other specialists serving the students on your caseload. When you participate in your school internship, your supervisory clinician or the university supervisor will provide you with practice in scheduling and decision making regarding scheduling options.

Scheduling Guidelines Summary

Because of the number of factors involved, scheduling a client (or patient, or student) can become an art form of its own. Although frequency of service and procedures for scheduling clients will differ across settings, the following are common factors to include in implementing your schedule at any practicum site.

1. **Schedule sessions to optimize the effectiveness of treatment.** Make decisions about time of day, length of session, frequency of treatment, group or individual treatment, and direct or indirect (e.g., consultative) service delivery. In making your decisions, follow the clinic guidelines on these matters.

2. **Coordinate speech-language pathology service with other services.** Avoid conflicts with other professionals by developing effective communication with them. Make sure you know what other professionals your client is receiving services from, when the services are provided, and what the treatment objectives are.

3. **Follow your schedule.** Be punctual in beginning and ending sessions. Alter your schedule as little as possible and communicate any changes in your schedule to all individuals affected by the change.

4. **Allow time for indirect services.** Schedule time for paperwork, evaluations, conferences, and breaks.

Assessment of Clients

Prior to being enrolled for treatment of communicative disorders, individuals must have a complete speech-language assessment. The assessment allows you to determine if a communicative disorder exists, and, if it does, the nature and extent of that disorder. In addition, the evaluation allows you to gather enough information to include recommendations on possible treatment objectives, treatment procedures, and timelines for treatment.

Many university training programs have a "diagnostic clinic" designed for the sole purpose of evaluation. Other clinical settings may have clinicians who perform only assessments and are not involved in treatment. However, most speech-language pathologists are involved in both assessment and treatment.

It is not the purpose of this section to provide a comprehensive assessment guide, but to give an overview of the components of evaluation, with emphasis on the university clinic setting. Read one of the many excellent books on evaluation and diagnosis (Emerick & Haynes, 1986; Peterson & Marquardt, 1990; Tomblin, Morris, & Spriestersbach, 1994).

University Clinic Assessment

At the university clinic, the initial assessment procedure begins after an individual has contacted the clinic regarding a communication problem. Under your clinical supervisor's direction, you will assess individuals with a variety of communicative disorders. Assessment procedures vary, depending on disorders, clients, and clinicians. However, the following procedures are common to all assessments.

1. **Discuss your assessment plans with your clinical supervisor before meeting with your clients.** Also, notify your supervisor of the time of the scheduled evaluation.

2. **Obtain a case history.** A completed case history form is required prior to scheduling an individual for an evaluation. Occasionally, the clinician and client may complete the case history during the initial interview. The case history can be very extensive and often includes prenatal, birth, and developmental information; medical, social, educational, and occupational history; and, previous related evaluation and treatment results. Following receipt of the necessary information in the clinic office, an evaluation is scheduled.

3. **Interview the client (or parent).** The interview allows you to clarify information reported on the case history and obtain additional information either omitted or inferred from the case history. Information obtained during the interview suggests the types of testing that you will need to perform. Also, the interview is an information-giving process in which you explain the assessment procedures and results to the client, parents, or both.

   • **Each interview will vary** depending on the type of disorder, related problems, and so on. Some interviews will be relatively short and others may be lengthy. Typically, the more complicated the medical history, the longer the interview. You also may be involved in a lengthy interview with clients who have received treatment from other agencies. When an interpreter is required, the interview time must be extended. Interviews also may have different formats. To assess the communication skills of a child, you will interview the parent. You may or may not include the child in the interview. You may want to include the child with a fluency disorder in the interview; whereas, a child with a language disorder may not be able to participate in the interview, because of limited expressive vocabulary.

   Two problems are commonly experienced by beginning clinicians in the interview. Both are usually due to the reliance on a preset interview format.

   • First, it is not uncommon for beginning student clinicians to have some **difficulty establishing rapport** with their clients during the interview. This is sometimes from the inappropriate use of closed-ended questions (only answerable by "yes" or "no") and the use of the case history form as an interview guide. Following the case history line-by-line, beginning clinicians sometimes question the client on matters the person has already responded to on the case history. For example, you might ask, "Has Josh had ear infections? Has he had any seizures? Has Josh had mumps?" and so on. Generally, it is more effective to summarize information on the case history and request verification. For example, "You noted on the case history that Josh was sick for several weeks as an infant. Tell me a little bit more about that." This is not to imply that you should not ensure that all necessary information is accurately supplied, but, in most cases, redundant questions should be avoided. If you observe that the informant has difficulty giving information clearly, to clarify information, you may want to ask redundant questions. In this case, try and rephrase the questions so that they are better understood by the informant. Sometimes vague or confusing responses are the result of misunderstanding the question, rather than not wanting to answer the question. In cases where the informant does not want to answer the question, you may need to use other interviewing techniques.

- Second, **ignoring or bypassing, important information** is another problem related to relying on an interview "script." For example, you may ask a question about educational history, "What grade is Josh in?" By waiting only for the response to the question in order to pursue the next question, you may miss important information that the parent reports. It is important to direct the interview, but it is equally important to listen and respond to all that is said in the interview. Appendix F contains a sample of an interview.

4. **Perform an oral-peripheral examination.** An oral-peripheral examination is performed to investigate the structural and functional integrity of the speech mechanism. Consider integrating the following procedures in your oral-peripheral examination:

- Systematically evaluate the oral-peripheral mechanism during each examination to avoid overlooking any areas. That is, always evaluate structures in a certain sequence. For example, some clinicians begin with general facial features, then progress to examination of lips, teeth, tongue, hard palate, and so on. Other clinicians begin examining the oral cavity first and then examine peripheral areas.
- Verbally describe your observations while audiotaping. It is helpful to orally record the evaluation. This step will allow you to continue the examination without having to stop and write notes.
- Observe the speech mechanism during activities such as laughing, speaking, and eating, if the client refuses to allow invasive procedures during the oral examination. Perform the examination later in the evaluation session or in a treatment session, if the client is enrolled for speech services.

5. **Screen the client's hearing.** ASHA guidelines require an audiometric screening as part of a complete speech and language assessment. University clinics routinely screen the hearing of clients as part of a speech and language assessment. In other practicum settings, an audiometer may not be available to the speech-language pathologist. Therefore, the clients are referred to an audiologist. In the public school setting, the school nurse, licensed as an audiometrist, often performs hearing screenings. Before evaluating individuals wearing hearing aids, it is important to find out when the person last had an audiological evaluation. Also, perform a hearing aid check to determine if the hearing aid is functioning.

6. **Obtain speech-language samples.** The speech sample is sometimes referred to as an "informal" assessment procedure, which seems to diminish the importance of analysis of the sample. However, the conversational speech sample is one of the most important assessment instruments available to you. It allows you to evaluate your client's communicative abilities in a natural context. It is essential to the assessment of a client's actual speech and language performance. When obtaining and analyzing a speech and language sample include the following:

   - To ensure the reliability of the speech sample, obtain more than one sample.
   - Direct conversation to provide clients with opportunities to produce a variety of language structures (e.g., declaratives, interrogatives, different verb tenses, and so forth).
   - If possible, sample conversation in a variety of environments. In adult evaluations, the interview commonly is used to obtain at least a portion of the conversational sample. At the university clinic, other environments can be sampled easily. Sample clients' speech while they are speaking on the telephone, speaking with the clinic receptionist, or speaking with a bookstore salesperson.
   - Assess more than just the client's mean length of utterance. In your analysis of the speech sample, include information about the client's semantic, morphologic, syntactic, and pragmatic productions.
   - Use the speech samples to examine articulation skills.
   - Compute overall speech intelligibility.
   - Analyze production of phonemes. Note specific erred phonemes, types of errors (e.g., omissions, substitutions, distortions), frequency of errors, and percentage of occurrence. You also may describe specific error patterns (e.g., syllable reduction, cluster reduction, fronting).
   - Observe voice characteristics: quality, pitch, intensity. Note such behaviors as the number of pitch breaks in a 5-min speech sample, or the absence of adequate breath support.

- Measure the types and frequency of dysfluencies in the sample and calculate the dysfluency rate. Refer to Appendix G for a discussion on types of dysfluencies and how to calculate them.
- Use effective and appropriate stimuli to evoke conversational speech. Clinicians evaluating children often use pictures, books, and toys to evoke speech. The recurring problem with pictures is that they often evoke single-word responses. Using books typically does not result in an adequate conversation sample. Children often prefer to look at the pictures than to talk to the clinician. You can use toys to gather a speech sample; however, again, some children become involved in playing with the toys and do not engage in conversation. Before bringing out pictures and books for children to describe, try to involve them in conversation. If a child is school aged, ask about most and least favorite school activities, favorite teachers, what happens to students who get in trouble in the cafeteria, best friends, school bully, and so on. The preschool child may respond to similar questions about preschool or siblings, educational programs on television, cartoon shows, and so forth. Sometimes, you can tell the child something about yourself first to stimulate speech. For example, "I have a puppy that is so silly. Yesterday he ran through the sprinklers and then came and jumped all over me! I bet you have a silly puppy, too. Tell me about your puppy."

If you have a difficult time obtaining a valid sample or if you need a second sample, you may want to use one of the following methods.

- **Record a short conversational sample between a parent and the child.** The two should be alone in the room. Use audio or video recording. Tell parents why and what you are doing. Ask them to talk (or play) with their children as they normally would.
- **Ask parents to maintain a daily log of their children's speech for one week.** Help parents take this request seriously and organize their note taking by providing them with a small notebook with their child's name written on it. You even may want to attach a pen or pencil to the notebook. This is one way to get a more complete view of the language of a young child who is reluctant to participate in activities in the clinic. Although the information may not be fully accurate, it will give you a better idea of the child's language performance as well as an idea of the parent's perception of the child's communication skills. A parent may report that his or her child uses only single words. However, while recording the child's speech for a week, the parent may find that the child is using some two-word phrases. Another parent might report that his or her child has a large vocabulary. The record of verbal productions may confirm or con-

tradict this report. Refer to Appendix H for information on obtaining and analyzing speech samples.

7. **Administer standardized tests.** There are a number of standardized tests designed to evaluate communicative disorders. They should adequately sample behaviors. Review tests before administering them. You must know the administration and scoring procedures. If you have to concentrate on remembering administration or scoring procedures to the exclusion of observing your client, you may miss important behaviors exhibited by the client. For example, if you are unfamiliar with the *Peabody Picture Vocabulary Test*, you may be busy figuring out basals and ceilings and miss the child's preservative responses or uncooperative behaviors. It is important to remember that the information obtained from a standardized test is only as good as the examiner. Standardized tests can be used to substantiate your clinical observations, but should not be used to replace those observations.

8. **Use reliable, valid, and culturally nonbiased tests.** Test selection must be appropriate for the client. Read and evaluate the information provided in the test manual. Determine if the test meets reliability and validity standards. Review the normative demographics to assure your client's ethnicity is adequately represented in the sample. Look at the test stimuli to determine if there are pictures or vocabulary that are culturally biased. In California public schools, certain tests have been prohibited for use with African American students because of potential biased results. Be sure that you follow the guidelines for test use at your site.

9. **Use other evaluation instruments.** Technology is providing speech-language pathologists with an array of computerized equipment to quantify data that were previously evaluated subjectively. If equipment such as the Visi-Pitch, Nasometer, or Computerized Speech Lab are available at your university clinic or practicum setting, take the time to learn and use them.

10. **Conduct disorder-specific evaluation.** Depending on the type of disorder you evaluate, other types of testing and sampling may be performed. Most of these will be disorder-specific. For example, you will assess stimulability of misarticulated sounds in evaluation of articulation disorders. You may analyze reading samples in your assessments of fluency disorders.

11. **Discuss impressions and recommendations.** At the end of the assessment, discuss your initial impressions of the child or the client with the family or the client. Let them know that a more detailed analysis and report will be given in the future. Communicate every-

thing in simple and direct language. After discussion with your supervisor, give your recommendation.

12. **Analyze the results and write the report.** Find out what the combined test scores, the oral-peripheral examination, and speech sample results mean. It is not sufficient to report only test scores without also making both objective and subjective clinical observations. Based on your analysis of the client's speech and language skills, make recommendations for or against treatment. If treatment is recommended, report client specific objectives, prognosis for obtaining the objectives, and possible duration of treatment. If treatment is not recommended, state clearly the rationale for not recommending treatment. Discuss your assessment plans with your clinical supervisor before meeting with your clients. Also, notify your supervisor of the time of the scheduled evaluation.

Reassessment of Clients

Clients returning to the university clinic for a new term of treatment should be reassessed before continuing treatment. A reassessment of all areas of speech and language typically is unnecessary. For example, it is not necessary to readminister a battery of language tests to a client diagnosed with a fluency disorder who had no previous indications of a language problem. Important reassessment data needed for the continuing client may be the results of a speech sample, hearing screening, oral examination, course of the disorder in the absence of treatment, and baselines of target behaviors. See Chapter 8 for procedures for establishing baselines.

Reassessment is important to establish the progress or improvement in the client's communicative behaviors. Accurate record keeping, probes, and self-evaluations also are necessary. Specific tests may be administered at the clinician's (or supervisor's) discretion.

Additional procedures and timelines for assessment and reassessment of clients are mandated by insurance companies and the public schools. Find out about these procedures and timelines from your supervisor.

Establishing a Working Relationship With Client and Family

To treat clients effectively, you should establish a good working relationship with the client and the family. Individuals with communicative disorders and their families initially may feel uncomfortable with the treatment process. They may not know much about the treatment, its duration, and its effects. Clients and their families may not begin treatment with the same level of knowledge or enthusiasm that student clinicians do. Therefore, you should educate clients and their families about their responsibilities, the treatment procedures, and their effects. To this end, you must establish good communication between yourself, your client, and your client's family. Because you are learning to do this, you also should maintain constant communication with your clinical supervisor. When working with clients and their families, consider the following guidelines.

1. **Before you discuss important issues with your clients, obtain your supervisor's approval.** Also, when you do not know the answer to you clients' or their families' questions, tell them that you will find out from your supervisor. Then, discuss the questions with your supervisor and find out how to answer them. On occasions, because of the complexity of the information to be presented, your supervisor may decide that he or she needs to talk with the family. In such cases, the supervisor will probably include you in the discussion, so you will learn to handle such issues.

2. **At the beginning, give an overview of the planned services.** Briefly describe to the clients or families the reassessment results, the planned treatment, expected results, and what the family members should do at home, along with follow-up and booster treatment procedures. In talking with clients and their parents, use simple, direct language. Do not give obscure answers that are couched in incomprehensible speech-language jargon. When you need to use technical terms, describe them, define them, and give everyday examples. However, do not talk down to people. For example, when the father of a child with a language delay is a professor of English, do not try to explain prepositions that you want to teach the child. Similarly, if the mother of a child is a physician, do not try to describe the velopharyngeal mechanism in everyday language (Hegde, 1998b).

3. **Repeat important information.** Your clients may be hearing a lot of new information at one time. Do not be afraid to repeat important information several times. For example, you may explain something at the beginning of a discussion and ask if the client understands your description. Later using different words or putting it in a different context, you may give the same information. At the next meeting, you may repeat the information again. It is not unusual for clients to report that they, ". . . were never told that." It's not because they are trying to be

difficult, but because they were hearing so much new information at once, that they did not assimilate (or learn) all of what you said.

4. **Always give accurate information.** Do not bluff. An often asked question is: what caused the speech or language problem? Why does my son stutter? Why can't my youngest child talk, while two older children are doing fine? The parents assume that research will have provided answers. But the research information may not provide a clear-cut answer that satisfies clients or their family.

5. **Tell parents and clients that it is difficult to point out the cause of a disorder in a given client.** Our knowledge of disorders and their potential causes are applied to groups of persons, not to specific individuals. For example, you can say that we know many potential causes of stuttering including hereditary predisposition, faulty learning, environmental stress, instability in the nervous system, and many others. But clinicians cannot say why a given child or adult stutters, because several factors may come together to produce a problem and most of the factors may be obscure.

6. **Discuss the sequence of treatment with your clients.** Explain that treatment will begin at a simple level and progress gradually to more complex levels. For example, "I will begin training the /s/ sound in single words. First, I will teach the sound at the beginning of words. After Jason masters the sound in words, he will learn to use them in phrases and sentences. Finally, Jason will learn to produce the sounds correctly in conversation—here at the clinic and at home and school." Explain too that, although a target behavior may be established quickly in the clinical setting, it takes additional work to establish that behavior in everyday communicative situations.

7. **Allow sufficient time to ask questions.** Any time you give technical information, make sure the clients and their families understand by inviting questions and comments.

8. **Answer questions on treatment outcome in probabilistic terms.** You may tell the parents that they may see some improvements in their child's fluency after 3 months of treatment, but you may not say that "John will be speaking fluently in 6 months." Point out to parents that the effect of treatment will depend on many factors, including the motivation of the client, the amount of family support, duration of treatment, and so forth. Recall that ASHA Code of Ethics specifies that you not guarantee treatment outcome.

9. **Ask family members to observe treatment sessions.** This helps the family to understand the treatment process and the abilities of the

client. Schedule time to discuss what they see with you. Answer questions that the family may have and give information to begin integrating the family into the therapeutic process. Be sure to tell the client and family that their questions and input are always welcome.

10. **Empower family members to be active participants in the client's treatment.** Let family members know the importance of their involvement in the treatment process. Early on, give family members responsibility for working with the client during therapy sessions and when at home. To help formalize the family's involvement, provide charting forms or other written material. Routinely, ask for feedback regarding the family's and the client's progress when working at home. Give positive feedback and supportive instructions. Make any necessary changes in the client's and family's homework. With a client reluctant to comply with family members' instructions, give the home assignment and explain that it is you, not the family member, who is expecting it be completed.

11. **Regularly review your clients' progress with their families.** Give periodic progress reports to parents of child clients. Invite parents into the treatment room. Allow sufficient time for you to share information and answer questions. You may obtain valuable information related to your clients' treatment if you periodically schedule 10- to 15-minute sessions with parents. Discuss their child's progress only in the treatment room. Avoid discussions in the hallway, waiting room, and such other places, because they compromise client confidentiality. Also, such discussions usually are hurried and noncommunicative. Again, repeat important information. Use redundancy to help clients and their families remember.

The ultimate goal of treatment is to integrate the behaviors trained in the clinical setting into a client's everyday communicative environment. To do this, it is necessary for you to work closely with the client's family so that they support the newly established communicative behaviors at home and in other nonclinical settings. Remember, families are an integral part of the treatment process. Family members can provide important information regarding not only your clients' disorders, but also the family dynamics. Also, family members can be invaluable in assisting with generalization and maintenance of target behaviors. In medical settings, other health care providers can also be used to assist with generalization and maintenance of target behaviors. In school settings, teachers are invaluable members of the intervention team and can provide help with generalization and maintenance. Maintenance strategies are described in Chapter 10.

The Internet's Role

The use of technology has expanded rapidly in the last decade. Twenty years ago, only a few people envisioned the future of the personal computer. Students understand better than many people the opportunities use of technology and the Internet presents. Because of electronic mail (e-mail), students can readily communicate with professors and other students. **They can discuss theoretical and clinical issues with experts and other students** thousands of miles from their home. Also, the Internet offers **easy access to libraries, papers, electronic journals, and support groups**. However, students are only a handful of the individuals using the Internet for communication and research.

Before parents or family members bring clients in for an evaluation, it is not unusual for them to have made inquiries related to their concern about the client. For example, prior to the inexpensive availability of the Internet, if parents suspected their child had autism, they may have discussed their concern with their pediatrician and their child's preschool teacher. Also, they may have read an article or two in a popular magazine. Now, parents and family members who have Internet access often have spent some time researching their concerns. In their Internet research, they may have accessed journals published by different professional associations, support groups composed of parents with similar concerns, professional discussion groups, articles from popular magazines, and advertisements for materials, treatment techniques, speakers, and other people and materials that offer all the answers and "cures."

Parents, family members, and clients who have taken the time to research on the Internet before meeting with a speech-language pathologist may be very knowledgeable about a disorder. Some people may be motivated and willing to apply their knowledge to assist with treatment. Occasionally, their understanding of a particular disorder may be helpful in completing the evaluation and may decrease the amount of treatment time needed. Unfortunately, other people may be very misinformed. As you know, there is much misinformation published on the Internet. Also, it is easy to take information out of context or without understanding the background or related information. You can re-educate many people by explaining what is known and what has been proven to be effective in working with specific disorders. In addition, you will encounter people who resist learning the facts. They may insist that you provide a certain therapy that they read about on the Internet. In this case, you and your supervisor may choose to not work with the client.

Regardless of the type of client or family member you encounter, it is important that you be well-informed. Know as much as you can about the disorders your clients have. In addition, know what information and misinformation is published on the Internet. Know the latest "fads" and be able to explain why these treatments are or are not appropriate.

Report Writing

Speech-language pathologists write different types of reports on clients they serve. **Diagnostic reports** provide comprehensive information on a client's pretreatment status. **Treatment plans** describe short- and long-term goals and the procedures used to obtain those goals. **Lesson plans** describe treatment planned for one or a few sessions. Client performance is described in different formats, including **progress reports, final summaries**, and **discharge reports**. For a variety of clinical reports and opportunities to practice them, see Hegde (1998a).

In addition to generic reports, public agencies have specific reporting requirements. **Individualized education programs (IEPs)** are required in the public schools for individuals with disabilities, 3 through 21 years of age. The **individual family service plan (IFSP)** is required for individuals with disabilities, birth through 2 years of age, and their families.

In medical and rehabilitation settings, assessment of functional skills are often the focus. Occasionally, a checklist may be used in lieu of a written report.

The general format and content of a variety of reports are discussed in the following sections. Written report requirements will vary from practicum site to practicum site. At each practicum site, you should find out what specific reporting procedures must be followed.

General Guidelines on Report Writing

Written reports satisfy many needs and there are several reasons why clear, comprehensive reports are essential. Written reports document the status of a client and thus provide a basis for future comparisons. Also, they provide an efficient form of communication with other individuals. In clinical training programs, supervisors judge a student's knowledge and writing skills by his or her written reports. Also, insurance companies and other third-party-agencies use reports as a basis from which to determine if payment will be made for speech-language pathology services. Besides, many different individuals including allied health professionals, educators, clients, and the clients' family members also read the reports. Each person who reads a clinical report is likely to make certain assumptions regarding the clinician's training and professional skills. Sometimes, families judge if the clinician fairly represents their family member's abilities and concludes if the clinician "likes" the client.

Although content is the most important element of your report, clear, concise presentation, neatness, and accurate use of vocabulary, grammar, spelling, and punctuation also are important. In fact, probably the first impression formed of your report is based on how the report looks, which may or may not have anything to do with your clinical abilities. As a general rule, consider the following in writing reports.

- Write in complete sentences.
- Spell all words correctly.
- Use correct punctuation.
- Present information in a logical sequence.
- Do not use nebulous or ambiguous statements.
- Provide as much detail as necessary to clearly describe the client's communicative abilities.
- Avoid making inferential judgments without substantiating data or qualifying statements.
- Avoid the use of jargon.
- Avoid the use of such qualifiers as like, very, rather, and so on.
- Do not use sexist or culturally biased statements or make assumptions based on stereotypes.
- Use correct margins and line spacing. Follow the format requested by your supervisor.
- Use the required type of paper. Most clinics require you to use nonerasable white bond paper. However, initial drafts of reports may be typed or printed on lower-grade paper.
- Proofread your reports before submitting them.
- Submit only high quality computer print-outs or typed reports.
- Do not submit anything without page numbers.
- Always keep a copy of your report.

Some beginning student clinicians may not know where or how to begin their first reports. Find out if your university provides report writing guidelines or samples of reports as references. If neither of these are available, refer to past reports for a writing format. The university clinic often requires more detailed reports than are typically required (or necessary) at other practicum sites. The rationale behind the overly detailed reports is that if information is not included in the report, then possibly, you did not observe or consider it. Also, if you know how to write a detailed report well, you can always write brief reports equally well. See Hegde (1998a) for multiple exemplars on general, technical, and professional writing.

The following sections offer guidelines for you to write different kinds of reports. Follow the requirements on the format, style, and content of reports specified at each of your practicum sites.

Treatment Plans

After the assessment is completed, write treatment plans that describe short- and long-term objectives and the procedures for achieving those objectives. A well-written treatment plan and accurate progress notes will allow another clinician to review the client's records and begin treatment based on the supplied information. ASHA's Professional Services Board (1984) requires written treatment plans that are reviewed and changed as the client's needs change. Dr. Paul-Brown (1994), director of ASHA's speech-language pathology division, recommends that the discussion of the treatment plan with the client and the client's family be noted on the treatment record. ASHA states that the following information should be contained in a treatment plan.

- Prognostic statements.
- Written long- and short-term objectives based on conclusions and recommendations of an evaluation.
- Statements regarding type, frequency, and duration of treatment.

In addition to this information, treatment plans include descriptions of target behaviors, stimuli to evoke responses, topographical aspects of responses, performance criteria, response consequences, probes to measure generalization, maintenance training, dismissal criteria, and follow-up treatment (Hegde, 1998a, 1998b). This information is detailed in the following section.

The preparation and writing of treatment plans will vary from setting to setting. Public schools, clinics, and insurance companies have their own formats. In the following section, common components of treatment plans are presented, along with examples specific to certain clinical settings. You are likely to receive additional instructions at individual practicum sites.

Writing a Treatment Plan. The comprehensive treatment plan describes treatment from the beginning of treatment to maintenance of trained behaviors in natural environments. It details both the client's performance and the clinician's performance, as well as the interaction between the two. The treatment plan does not have to be lengthy, but it should be comprehensive (Hegde, 1998a, 1998b). When you write a treatment plan, do:

1. **Briefly summarize identification data.** Describe background information, current performance levels, and purpose of treatment.

2. **Describe target behaviors.** Include both long- and short-term objectives in your description. Write objectives that are client-specific (that is, appropriate and useful to the client), valid, and measurable. Ideally, you will have established baselines of target behaviors before preparing a treatment plan. Chapter 7 provides information on the selection of target behaviors.

3. **Describe stimuli to evoke responses.** You must determine if pictures, objects, conversation, or orthographic symbols will be used to obtain a specific response. You also must decide if visual, auditory, or tactile stimulation will be used. You must identify the setting in which training will be performed (e.g., in the clinical setting, in the client's home, and so on). It is not uncommon for training to begin at a single word level with the presentation of pictures in the clinical setting and advance to the spontaneous speech level with conversational interaction in extraclinical environments.

4. **Describe topographical aspects of responses.** Response topography identifies the level at which training is initiated (e.g., at the syllable level) and the levels of progression. Response topography is not disorder specific, but is used in treatment across all communication disorders. For example, a client with a voice disorder initially may sustain an appropriate pitch only during single-word productions. A client with an articulation disorder may only produce or imitate the target phoneme accurately only at the single-word level.

5. **Specify performance criteria.** Describe the rate of accuracy that will be accepted as the criterion for moving through the training hierarchy. Distinguish between modeled and evoked responses.

6. **Describe response consequences.** Describe how you increase desirable behaviors and decrease undesirable behaviors. Specify any treatment modifications in the progress report or final summary. Response consequences that increase or decrease behaviors are discussed in Chapters 8 and 9, respectively.

7. **Describe probes for generalization.** Probes measure generalized production of trained behaviors. However, they frequently are absent from treatment plans, perhaps because some clinicians think they are implied within the training sequence. To ensure that probes are not omitted, describe their use in the treatment plan. Answer the following questions in describing probes: When will probes be administered? What type of probe will be utilized? What is the criterion? What hap-

pens if the criterion is or is not met? See Chapter 8 for details on probe procedures. Appendix I has a sample probe procedure and recording sheet. Also, a reproducible form is provided for your use.

8. **Describe the maintenance program.** Describe how you program maintenance of target behaviors. Include in the description how you plan to train other individuals in the client's environment.

9. **Describe the dismissal criterion.** This criterion typically reflects production of the target behaviors in conversational speech in both clinical and extraclinical settings. Written dismissal criterion helps ensure accountability. See Chapter 7 for recommended criterion.

10. **Describe follow-up or booster treatment.** After clients have met a certain performance criteria, they are dismissed from frequently scheduled treatment sessions. However, many clients require "booster" or "follow-up" sessions to maintain a certain proficiency level. For example, a fluency client who has established 98% fluent speech in clinical and extraclinical settings may be dismissed from twice-a-week treatment sessions. However, he or she should be scheduled for periodic follow-up sessions to assist in maintenance of fluency skills. You should specify the intervals for follow-up sessions in your initial treatment plan. Refer to Appendix J for a sample treatment plan.

Lesson Plans

Writing Lesson Plans. Although you have written a comprehensive treatment plan, you also may be required to write session-by-session or weekly lesson plans so the supervisor knows what you are doing in a given session. As part of your planning and preparation for clinical sessions, you will write lesson plans for each of your clients. At the university clinic, lesson plans commonly are developed on a weekly basis and submitted to the clinical supervisor in advance for approval. The lesson plan typically contains the following information:

- **Treatment objectives.** Write the treatment objectives for your client. For example: *The production of /s/ in word initial positions at the evoked level, with 90% accuracy.*
- **Procedures and materials for obtaining the objectives.** Describe how you will implement the treatment objectives, include materials and treatment procedures. For example: *The /s/ picture cards and /s/ objects will be presented to the client. The client will be required to name each picture. All correct /s/ productions will be verbally reinforced. All incorrect /s/ productions will be interrupted by a verbal "No" or "Stop."*

Information contained in the lesson plan may be similar to items identified in the treatment plan (e.g., response typography, criterion levels, management of consequences). However, the lesson plan does not always allow for a complete view of the client's treatment. The lesson plan describes what is done in a session or two, whereas the treatment plan describes the total sequence of treatment for a given period. Refer to Appendix K for a sample lesson plan and Hegde (1998a) for additional examples.

Individualized Education Plans

Writing Individualized Educational Programs. Public Law 94–142 (and its many amendments) mandates a free, appropriate public education and related services for all children and youth who have a disability. Speech-language pathology is a part of **designated instructional services (DIS)** under special education services. A written **individualized educational program (IEP)** is required for each child, ages 3 through 21 years, who receives special education services.

IEPs originally were formulated to provide for management, communication, and accountability in special education services. The IEP is more of a management plan than a treatment plan. Also, it is a contract between the school and the family. The IEP describes what will be trained, but not the specific training procedures. Specific rules regulate the development, writing, and implementation of IEPs. There are many legal requirements regarding the timelines for services, identification, referral, assessment, enrollment and dismissal of students, the rights of parents, and due process. The following section gives you guidelines on writing the speech-language IEP.

Content of the IEP. A speech-language pathologist writes an IEP for each student he or she serves. The parents are important members of the IEP team and provide input regarding the delivery of special education services for their children. An IEP must be developed before a student can receive services. An annual meeting to review the IEP is required, although meetings may be held more frequently. **IDEA 1997** (Individuals with Disabilities Education Act, revised in 1997) is the recent revision of P.L. 94–142. In addition to annual review of students' progress, IDEA 1997 requires periodic progress reports. Many IEP forms are used, but the basic content is the same. To provide a comprehensive management plan, the following information must be included on an IEP (California State Department of Education, 1989; Dublinske & Healey, 1978; Individuals with Disabilities Education Act, 1997):

1. **Give the identifying information.** Write the child's name, address, phone number, birthdate, and parent's name(s) on the IEP. Also, write the student identification or folder number on the IEP. Note the child's grade, primary language, and English language proficiency on the IEP.

2. **Describe the child's present level of performance.** State current communicative performance, including both receptive and expressive speech and language skills, behavioral problems noted or reported, related educational strengths or weaknesses, and contributing history or current developmental or health information. Also, report learning styles. Present levels of performance must be based on at least two assessment procedures. Report test scores as standard scores or percentiles. Both standardized tests and speech samples typically are utilized to describe communicative skills. Sometimes you may refer the reader to a separate diagnostic report rather than repeating the information. For example, you might write: *For additional information, see diagnostic report 4–10–98*. Report sufficient information to develop appropriate objectives. Information about the student's strengths should be noted. Include relevant information obtained from interviews with parents and teachers.

3. **Describe how the disability affects the student's educational performance.** Indicate how the disability affects the student's involvement, progress, and participation in the typical curriculum. You must report the child's present levels of performance as compared to educational performance. For instance, report how the 6-year-old child's speech intelligibility of 50% affects his or her educational performance. For example:

> *Sandy's speech in the classroom is 50% intelligible and does not allow her to successfully participate in oral presentations. Also, her teacher is not able to understand many of the questions and responses Sandy produces in class.*

4. **Describe objectives.** List long-term goals to describe the child's expected performance for an entire school year. Objectives (or short-term goals) reflect steps necessary to obtain the long-term goal. In some cases these objectives are referred to as **benchmarks**. Write measurable objectives (or benchmarks) that have a completion date, and performance criteria. For example:

> **Goal:** *Increased sentence length in classroom conversation and oral presentations to a minimum mean length of utterance of 4.0 words by_____(specify a date).*
> *Objective: By_____(specify a date), following picture presentation, Jennie is expected to produce 10 sentences, containing a minimum of 4 words, with 90% accuracy at the evoked level over three sessions. Progress will be measured by response charting.*

Base the long-term goals and the objectives on information reported in the present levels of performance. The goals and objectives should help meet the student's needs that were reflected in the description of the present levels of performance. Develop objectives that demonstrate incremental steps toward the goal. As much as possible develop goals that relate to educational benchmarks (or goals). Other IEP team members, especially the parents, provide input regarding the development of the student's IEP goals and objectives. The speech-language pathologist will guide the selection of treatment goals that are appropriate to the student's current abilities. At the annual review meeting, note the status of the goals and objectives. Some of these may have been met, others may not. Work on some goals or objectives may not have begun yet. There is no required number of goals or objectives.

5. **Describe special education services required.** Specify the type of service that will be provided, the frequency of the service, the duration of each session, and the location of the service on the IEP. For example, speech services may be provided as follows:

> *Group therapy/2x per week/40 minutes each session in the speech-language pathologist's office.*
>   or
> *Teacher consult/1x per month/30 minutes each session in student's classroom.*

6. **Describe the amount of time the child will spend in the regular educational program.** Note the child's participation in regular education on the IEP. For the speech IEP, you may abbreviate the amount of time the child will spend in regular education as a percentage (e. g., *95% per week*). You also may list it as an exclusion (i.e., all the time

except the time the child spends in speech): *all but 2x per week/40 minutes each session.*

7. **Describe when the services will begin and end.** Write the beginning and ending dates of service on the IEP. Services should begin with minimal delay. Initiation of service often begins the next school day or week after the IEP meeting. If an IEP meeting is held at the end of the school year, services begin as soon as school resumes. Because an annual review is required of each student enrolled in special education services, you must write the duration of service for one year or less. Note this in month/day/year format (e.g., 11/10/99).

8. **Describe how progress will be reported.** In addition to the annual review of the IEP, you must report the child's progress to parents regularly. On the IEP, note if you will periodically report progress by sending a report card, progress report, or other type of communication.

9. **Specify the rationale for special education services.** The rationale or justification for service is based on an established criteria for enrollment. In an IEP, indicate if the child is to be enrolled in, continued, or dismissed from special education services.

   The criteria for speech-language pathology services are based on legal requirements and are not always consistent with common practices in the community. As noted before, a 5-year-old child with a frontal lisp may receive speech-language pathology services through a private agency, but may not be eligible for speech services in the school until he or she has reached the age of 8 years. Your school district will provide you with a summary of their eligibility criteria for speech-language pathology services.

   The justification for service can be brief or lengthy, because:

> *Language needs cannot be met in the regular education setting. Standardized test scores reflected performance 1.5 standard deviations below the mean in all language areas. Analysis of a conversation sample revealed errors in syntax and morphology and limited semantic abilities.*

> *Conversational speech is 15% dysfluent. Speech needs cannot be met in the regular education classroom.*

10. **Describe all professionals providing services.** The child receiving speech-language pathology services also may be receiving other special education services. Include related services that are educationally necessarily. Give the names of all services and all service providers on the IEP. Following is an example of a list of services and the individuals responsible for providing them:

    - Counseling: School psychologist
    - Medication follow up: School nurse
    - Speech services: School speech-language pathologist
    - Special reading lessons: Reading specialist
    - Hearing services: Educational audiologist

11. **Get the signature of all individuals attending the IEP meeting.** The names, positions, signatures, and dates of participation of all the individuals attending the IEP meeting must appear on the IEP. Regular education teachers have a place to sign, as does the special education teacher. Other specialists such as the school psychologist and the school nurse may sign the IEP. Get the parents' signatures on the IEP, indicating consent with the IEP for their child's placement in special education. Parents dissenting with the recommended IEP may be provided a separate line to sign or box to check, but a signature may still be required to indicate attendance at the meeting. The child also may attend and be a member of the IEP team. If appropriate, have the child sign the IEP form. If an interpreter is used at the IEP meeting, get the interpreter's signature and write his or her title on the IEP.

12. **Note additional IEP information.** Write (or check) the following information on the IEP:

    - Date of annual review.
    - Date of 3-year evaluation.
    - Eligibility for extended school year.
    - Recommendations for specific materials, methods, or equipment needed to accomplish the goals.

    To reduce paperwork, many school districts use computerized forms or checklists for their IEPs. Computer-generated and checklist formats should be diverse enough to allow the development of an individualized program. This is not a problem with most programs. If none of the already written objectives are appropriate, there usually is a space for other objectives to be written. Your school site will supply you with IEP forms.

Individual Family Service Plans

As an amendment to P.L. 94–142, Public Law 99–457 -Part H (now revised to Part C) established an early intervention program for infants and toddlers and their families. This program requires that an **individual family service plan** (IFSP) be written for children with disabilities, ages birth through 2 years. The IFSP must be developed by a multidisciplinary team of professionals and the child's parent(s). The IFSP contains the following information.

- Present levels of performance (physical, cognitive, communicative, and self-help).
- Family needs and strengths related to assisting the child.
- Intervention goals and the way progress will be measured.
- Types of services the child will receive.
- Initiation and duration of services.
- The name of the case manager.

The IEP and IFSP are similar in that they both describe clinical and educational objectives, types of services to be provided, and the beginning and ending dates of services. The IFSP differs from the IEP because of its emphasis on family involvement. The IFSP targets not only the needs of the child, but the strengths and weaknesses of the family and how these influence the child's development. Emphasized in the 1997 revision of IDEA is the location of services. According to this revision, services should be provided in the natural environment. For young children, this often translates to providing services in their homes. The IFSP incorporates public school services and the services of other public agencies (e.g., families may need respite care services or social welfare services, as well as educational and rehabilitation services). The case manager is selected based on the needs of the child and the family. Basically, the case manager is responsible for identifying, coordinating, and monitoring services. The case manager may be a speech-language pathologist, audiologist, special education teacher, psychologist, social worker, or other professional. A review of the IFSP is required every 6 months, compared with the IEP's annual review.

Diagnostic Reports

Diagnostic reports are written following the evaluation of a client. A diagnostic report is a summary of case history, assessment data, clinical impressions, conclusions, and recommendations. It provides a clear, written statement of the client's communicative abilities at the time of the evaluation. It also provides a forum for communicating with other professionals. At times, the diagnostic report may be used to help obtain payment from an insurance company for the services provided. At other times, it may be used for research; therefore, it is important to clearly document information and differentiate between subjective statements and objective data.

Each client's file must contain a diagnostic evaluation. A copy of an evaluation performed at another facility may be included in a case file (ASHA Professional Services Board, 1984). When you are assigned a client who has been evaluated by another clinician, obtain a copy of the diagnostic report for the client's file.

There are several formats for writing diagnostic reports (Emerick & Haynes, 1986; Flower, 1984; Hegde, 1998a; Knepflar & May, 1989). In addition, reporting requirements vary at each practicum site. To write a diagnostic report, use the following outline, or modify it for different practicum settings.

1. **Give identification information.** Give this information at the beginning of the report. Include the following: the client's name, file number, address, phone number, date of birth, age, diagnosis, date of evaluation, name of the evaluator, and the name of the individual who referred the client. If applicable, also note the client's occupation or school level and parents' names.

2. **Write a statement of the problem.** Describe briefly the client's presenting complaint. To be explicit, write the client's comments verbatim and identify them as such in the text. For example: (1) *Mrs. Applegate stated her voice was "scratchy and old sounding."* (2) *Mr. Thomas reported that he stuttered. He said that his "blocked speech" occurred most frequently when he spoke on the telephone.* Note the client's words by using quotation marks. If someone other than the client was the informant, indicate it: *Mr. John Jones, who accompanied Johnny to the clinic, was the informant during the interview.*

3. **Write the diagnostic report in the past tense.** You are writing about performance that you observed during the assessment. For example, write: *Joan omitted final consonants in her spontaneous speech.* Your observation of the client is limited to a specific time and your statements must be limited to those observations.

4. **Give background information.** Describe the client's background. Obtain this information from the client's case history, client interview, and reports by other professionals. Detail relevant information in this section. Do not report unrelated provided information. Include the client's developmental history, medical history, social and family history, and educational history in this section. For some clients, it will be

necessary to report only certain areas, for other clients, all areas will need to be documented. For example, for a child with language problems, educational background must be described in some detail; but for an adult man with a hoarse voice, detailed educational history may not be necessary. If the reported medical history was unremarkable for speech and language development just say that: *The reported medical history was unremarkable*. However, if a number of illnesses were reported, or if many medications were or were continued to be prescribed, then carefully document this in the report. Note in this section any previous speech-language pathology services the client has received. Report previous diagnoses. If you summarize information from another professional's report (another speech-language pathologist, a physician, a teacher), always give the professional's name, credentials, and date of report.

5. **Summarize assessment information.** Describe results of the pure-tone audiometric screening, oral peripheral examination, and speech and language assessments.

6. **Include statements regarding the client's general behavior.** Include in your behavioral observations such information as the client's attending behavior and cooperativeness. For example: *The client was cooperative and attended to all tasks with minimal verbal prompting throughout the 1-hour evaluation session. Results were considered representative of the client's abilities.*

7. **Perform an audiometric screening.** This is a part of all speech-language evaluations. If it is impossible to perform the screening, note this in the diagnostic report and refer the client for an audiological examination. If a client is wearing hearing aids, perform a hearing aid check before the speech and language assessment to ensure that the hearing aids are functioning.

8. **Perform an oral peripheral examination.** This is a standard part of diagnostic evaluation. The amount of information that must be written in the report will depend on the results of this examination. If no abnormalities were observed, then briefly describe the results. Write in detail any structural or motorical deviations observed.

9. **Describe in detail the speech and language assessment.** Include information about the client's articulation, voice, fluency, receptive language, and expressive language. You should report results of standardized testing, language sampling, and informal clinical observations of communicative abilities. Do not just list test scores, say what they mean. For example, the statement that *"The client scored a raw score of 9 on the auditory comprehension subtest of the* Preschool Language Scale–3" means little to your readers, unless they have memorized the test or have the test administration booklet in front of them.

10. **Quantify results of your client's speech sample.** Report the total number of words in the sample. When reporting certain behaviors (e.g., correct use of plural /s/), give the percentage of occurrence or the specific number of times its production was evoked. For example: *The client produced the plural /s/ correctly 75% of 27 obligatory contexts in which it was evoked.* This statement is more meaningful than: *The client three times produced the plural /s/ correctly.* If the client omitted specific speech or language structures, give the total number of opportunities (or obligatory contexts) he or she had to produce them. For example: *The client did not produce the plural /s/ in 10 phrases that should have contained the plural /s/.*

11. **Present the information in a logical and organized sequence.** Describe observations relevant to speech, language, voice, fluency, and other aspects in separate paragraphs. Do not confuse the reader by writing about articulation performance in sections describing fluency and voice.

12. **Write a statement about each parameter of speech.** This will suggest that all aspects of the client's speech and language were evaluated, even if no disorder or deviation was exhibited in some areas. For example, if you made no mention of fluency in your report on a child with an articulation disorder because you found no problem with it, the reader cannot be sure of this. Therefore, such a statement as, *Analysis of a 200-utterance speech sample revealed 97% fluent speech*, is necessary.

13. **Do not cross professional boundaries.** When you present assessment information, limit yourself to speech-language functions. A common problem occurs when guessing at cognitive levels. The speech-language pathologist cannot report IQ scores. Neither can you diagnose psychological disorders (depression, mental retardation, etc.). However, you can report behavior that you have observed. For example, you might write: *The boy appeared withdrawn throughout the evaluation.* That is, he sat with his arms crossed through most of the evaluation and was never observed to make eye contact with the examiner.

14. **Summarize your impressions.** This section is a summary and interpretation of all the information gathered in your assessment. Report the type and severity of any communicative disorder in this section. Also report if no communicative disorder was exhibited. If a cause for a found disorder is known, you may report it in this section. You may make a statement about the prognosis here or report it in the recommendations section.

15. **Write recommendations.** In this section include the type and amount of service needed, further assessment required, and/or referral to other professionals. Although specific areas of need should be identified, do not report exact objectives. As you know, additional evaluation, including baselines, may need to be performed before starting treatment. You must confer with your clinical supervisor before making specific recommendations.

16. **Sign the report.** Conclude the report with your name, title, and signature. Your clinical supervisor also must sign the report. Therefore, type his or her name and title. Refer to Appendix L for a sample diagnostic report and to Hegde (1998a) for a variety of examples.

Progress Reports

Progress reports provide information about treatment procedures, a client's performance, and further recommendations. There are several types of progress reports. Two types of commonly used progress reports are described in this section. The first type of progress report is written daily or for every session to document the client's performance. Because they are brief, daily progress reports often are called **progress notes**. The second type of report is written periodically to summarize a client's progress for a specific treatment period. At the university clinic, the periodic report may be called a **Final Summary** or **Progress Report** written at the end of a semester or quarter. Both types of reporting document necessary clinical information.

Daily Progress Notes. You should chart your client's performance in each session. Your practicum site may provide you with a recording form or you may develop your own. This recording form will include spaces for the client's name, the date of the session, the objective(s), stimuli, client responses, response consequences, and remarks. If you are using unique materials or equipment, you may want to note that on the recording form. A sample treatment recording form is illustrated in Appendix M.

Record the results of each clinical session on a chronological log as soon after the session as possible. This enables you and your supervisor to review the treatment session and make necessary modifications. It also provides a means of communication among professionals. It gives enough information for another clinician to serve your client if you are unable to do so.

One form of charting and reporting client progress is referred to as SOAP notes (Flower, 1984; Golper, 1998). **SOAP** stands for subjective, objective, assessment, plan. Use the following guidelines in writing SOAP notes.

1. **Describe your impressions of the client in the subjective section.** For example: The client appeared very alert and cooperative. He stated, *"I'm ready to work hard today."*

2. **Write measurable information in the objective section.** For instance: *The client produced four syllable phrases with 80% accuracy in 40 out of 50 trials (40/50).*

3. **Describe your analysis of the session in the assessment section.** You also may compare the client's performance across sessions in this section. For example: (a) *Production of /r/ increased from 65% accuracy during the last session to 90% accuracy during today's session.* (b) *Withdrawal of visual models resulted in a decrease in accurate production of single syllable words from 90% to 65%.*

4. **Outline the course of treatment in the plan section.** You might simply state: (a) *Continue current treatment activities.* (b) *Continue training production of functional CVC words at the imitative level.*

SOAP notes are more commonly used in the medical setting, but also may be used at other practicum sites. If a lesson plan has been prepared in advance of each session, you may sometimes write the results of the session directly on the lesson plan. Because the lesson plan has already detailed the activities, you may just specify a percentage after an activity. For example: *Initial /s/: 90% at the word level. Medial /l/: 30% at the phrase level.*

Regardless of the form of recording, the data should be accurate and recorded during each session. At the end of the sessions, you may write additional notes. You may make subjective statements, but do not confuse them for observed facts. Also, support your statements with observable data. In writing progress notes remember:

- Write legibly.
- Date entries.
- If required, use a pen, preferably black ink (black ink photocopies more reliably than blue).
- Initial or sign your name on all progress notes. At certain clinical practicum sites your supervisor will cosign your progress notes.
- Be accurate.
- Report objective data.
- Avoid qualifiers such as "seems to" or "appeared," unless you report specific behaviors to support your assumptions.
- Record progress notes immediately following your clinic session.
- Only use abbreviations or jargon that others will understand. Obviously, these usages may change depending on the site.

Several abbreviations are used in writing progress notes. Refer to Appendix B for some of the commonly used abbreviations. Appendix N contains a sample of progress notes.

Periodic Progress Reports. In medical and private clinics, periodic progress reports are written to summarize a client's treatment and its results. Procedures and their effects on the client's communicative behaviors are described. Again, depending on your practicum assignment, there will be different requirements for writing progress reports. Following is a list of information you will include in most progress reports.

1. **Give client identification information.** List the client's name, age, address, phone number, occupation or school status, and birthdate. If applicable, give the name of the parent or spouse.

2. **Describe the period covered by the report.** Note the dates that the treatment period began and ended. Also note when treatment was originally initiated, if different from the beginning period of the report.

3. **List the number of sessions the client attended.** You will want to carefully document how many sessions your client actually attended. You may be reporting on a treatment period covering 3 months in which your client only attended six sessions.

4. **List the length of the treatment sessions.** You will see clients for differing lengths of time. Some clients may attend 60-minute sessions and others only 30-minute sessions. Include the length of time you spend with your client in each progress report.

5. **Briefly summarize the client's status at the beginning of the treatment period.** State briefly the client's status before the reporting period. Also, do not write as detailed a description of the client's status at the beginning of the treatment period as you did in your diagnostic report. Give only a brief overview of his or her communicative abilities at the beginning of the treatment period. For example, you might state that: *An analysis of conversational speech in the clinic setting revealed 85% fluency. Analysis of an audiotaped sample of the client's conversational speech at home revealed 82% fluency.*

6. **Summarize the treatment plan.** Describe the treatment objectives and procedures. Include enough information for the reader to know what your progression of treatment was and what stimuli and response consequences were used. If the procedure described in the treatment plan was modified, describe the changes and justify them.

7. **Describe the client's performance.** Describe how the client's target behaviors changed during the course of the treatment. Make such objective statements as, *"At the beginning of treatment, Tom's voice was judged hoarse on 90% of his utterances. At the end of the semester, he was judged hoarse on 10% of his utterances."* Include tables and graphs that summarize quantitative data and show changes over the course of treatment.

8. **Summarize your conclusions and recommendations.** Include in this section your overall impressions of treatment effectiveness. Make a prognostic statement and recommendations based on that prognosis. Did your client make progress? Do you expect your client to continue to make progress? What type of intervention will enable the client to continue to progress? For example: *John demonstrated progress throughout this treatment period. Based on his performance over the past 3 months, prognosis for continued progress is good. It is recommended that John continue to receive treatment for his voice disorder. To be most effective, treatment should be given two times per week for a minimum of 30 minutes each session.*

9. **End your report with your name, title, and signature.** Also include your supervisor's name, title, and signature. Refer to Appendix O for a sample progress report and to Hegde (1998a) for multiple exemplars.

Final Summaries. At the end of each semester, you must prepare a report for each of the clients you served at the university clinic. This is a report of the client's treatment. The final summary is sometimes interchangeable with a progress report. It contains information similar to a progress report, but often provides more detailed information. As in a progress report, include the following in a final summary:

- Give client identification information.
- Identify the period covered by the report.
- Give the number of sessions attended by the client and the length of the sessions.
- Summarize the client's status at the beginning of the treatment period.
- Summarize the treatment plan.
- Describe the client's performance and improvement.
- Discuss your conclusions and recommendations.
- Identify yourself and your supervisor.

See Appendix P for a sample final summary and Hegde (1998a) for multiple exemplars.

Discharge Reports

A discharge report is written at the time clients are dismissed from treatment. Clients are dismissed because they no longer need treatment or do not benefit from it. Others may be dismissed because they do not attend treatment sessions regularly or have stopped coming to the sessions. Some clients may be dismissed or may dismiss themselves from treatment because they cannot afford it.

The discharge report follows a format similar to that of the final summary. It covers the treatment period from the beginning of treatment to the discharge date. Regardless of the title of the report, a final report is always prepared when a client leaves treatment at any facility. In this case, the discharge report and final summary may be the same.

Record-Keeping Procedures

Besides writing various kinds of reports, student clinicians are responsible for maintaining the client files and an accurate log of their clinical practicum hours. Therefore, you should know the general procedures of maintaining the client records and your practicum records.

Client Files

Because they are confidential, clinic files are kept in a secured area such as a locked room or in a locked file cabinet. As noted previously, (a) you should never leave clinic files unattended; (b) never release copies of reports to other professionals or agencies without prior written approval from the client; and (c) you should not take clients' files home.

You are responsible for maintaining your clients' files in a complete and orderly fashion. Follow the procedure established at your clinic for filing documents, recording phone calls, and so on.

To ensure that all necessary information is in their files and is current, review your clients' files periodically. Ask your clients if the phone numbers and addresses in their files are correct. Note all changes in the clients' folders and report them to your clinic secretary.

The following information should be included in client records (Paul-Brown, 1994):

- Client identification information. Telephone number, address, file number, and so forth.
- The name of the individual or agency that referred the client.
- Client history including any related information from other agencies, such as copies of medical reports, IEPs, psychological evaluations, and so on.
- The name of the speech-language pathologist (and student clinician) responsible for service delivery to the client.
- A diagnostic report. This report may have been performed at another facility.

- A current treatment plan, including specific objectives and prognosis.
- Indication of when the treatment plan was discussed with the client or the responsible member of the client's family.
- Notations regarding conferences held with other professionals.
- Treatment reports, progress reports, and final summaries.
- A chronological log of all services provided for the client.
- Daily progress notes reflecting current status of treatment objectives.
- A signed and dated consent for release of information.

At the university clinic, client files should also contain a signed and dated consent to be observed. All records must be signed by an individual holding current ASHA certification.

Practicum Hours

Student clinicians are responsible for maintaining a log of their clock hours earned in clinical practicum. Your university probably will provide you with a form for reporting these hours. Because you will not always be seeing clients for an entire hour, often you may need to report fractions of hours. Use a consistent system for recording clock hours earned. For example, do not report a 30-minute session one time as ½ hour, another time as 30 minutes, and still another time as .5 hr. At the end of the term, totaling your hours will be much easier if your reporting is consistent and systematic. Use the following guidelines for reporting clock hours and fractions of hours.

60 minutes = 1.0 hour

55 minutes = .9

50 minutes = .8

45 minutes = .75

40 minutes = .7

35 minutes = .6

30 minutes = .5

25 minutes = .4

20 minutes = .3

15 minutes = .25

10 minutes = .2

5 minutes = .1

All clock hours must be verified by a signature of the supervising speech-language pathologist. Chapter 1 describes the activities that may be counted as practicum hours.

Working With Other Professionals

To provide effective services to their clients, speech-language pathologists frequently must work with other specialists. You often will see clients who receive services from such professionals as a physician, physical therapist, psychologist, or special education teacher. You may need to coordinate your services with the service delivered by these professionals. You also must refer clients to other specialists for services. For example, you probably will refer an individual who comes to see you about a voice problem to an otolaryngologist for a laryngeal evaluation. You will refer the individual who does not pass his or her hearing screening to an audiologist for an audiological examination. (Refer to Appendix Q for a sample referral letter.) You will consult with professionals in allied health and education professions. To enhance services to clients, speech-language pathologists must develop a working relationship with these professionals.

To work effectively with other professionals, you should know about their services. Following is a summary of the services provided by different specialists with whom you may work.

Health and Allied Health Professionals

To work effectively with other professionals, you must know something about their roles. Following is a summary of the services provided by different specialists.

1. **Audiologist.** The **audiologist is a specialist in the identification, measurement, and rehabilitation of hearing impairments.** Whether you work in a medical setting, private practice, or educational setting, you will work closely with audiologists in many instances. For example, you will refer clients who do not pass their hearing screenings to audiologists. Also, you may find that some of your clients have hearing aids that are not functioning correctly. The audiologist may recommend repair, modification, or replacement of the hearing aids. You may work closely with the audiologist in developing a rehabilitation program for a child with a hearing impairment or in developing a program for community access to assistive listening devices. Audiolo-

gists and speech-language pathologists collaborate in treating an individual who has had a cochlear implant. Also, the audiologist is trained to screen for the presence of a speech or language disorder and may refer individuals to you for speech or language services.

2. **Cardiologist.** The **cardiologist is a physician with specialized training in cardiovascular diseases** (heart and circulatory disease). Because of the nature of their specialty, cardiologists most frequently work with adults, but there are children who also require their services. You may not work frequently with cardiologists, but occasionally you will work with children or adults who have some form of cardiovascular disorder. For example, some of your clients may have a genetic syndrome. Many such syndromes are associated with a high incidence of cardiovascular disorders. Some of the prematurely born infants and children you work with also may have cardiovascular problems. The cardiologist may refer individuals to you who have voice problems because of their reduced lung capacity. You need to find out from the cardiologist what physical abilities you reasonably can expect from your clients. You also need to know if medications your clients are taking may affect speech or behavior (e.g., lethargy, attention span, memory).

3. **Dietitian.** The **dietitian is a professional with training in nutrition and diet.** The dietitian is responsible for planning and managing the food service in health care settings. In certain settings, you may work closely with the dietitian in treating patients with swallowing disorders. You will need the dietitian's assistance in providing appropriate foods for your patient's treatment and meals.

4. **Neurologist.** The **neurologist is a physician with specialized training in function and disorders of the nervous system.** Within neurology, there are subspecialties such as pediatric neurology. It is not unusual for the neurologist to work with individuals who also have speech or language disorders. The neurologist may work with individuals recovering from a cerebrovascular accident (CVA), head trauma, or a variety of other neurological disorders.

The neurologist may request a speech and language assessment of a client recovering from a CVA or head trauma. You must provide detailed information, including prognosis for speech and language rehabilitation and treatment recommendations.

Your clients with aphasia, Parkinson disease, or Alzheimer disease may be seeing a neurologist or will have seen one. The neurologist can provide information about the extent and location of brain involvement, affect of current medications, and prognosis.

Neurologists also work with individuals with behavior disorders. For example, you may be working with a child who begins receiving medication for aggressive behavior. You may need to document any change in speech or language performance after the child takes the medication.

If you work with a client with a seizure disorder, he or she likely will be receiving services from a neurologist. If you suspect a client of having undiagnosed seizures, you may refer the client to a neurologist. You will want to know from all your clients if they are taking medication that may affect their speech, attention span, or alertness.

5. **Occupational Therapist.** The registered **occupational therapist (OT or OTR), provides evaluation and treatment of daily living skills for individuals with disabilities.** This includes assessing and retraining such skills as dressing, cooking, and bathing. The OT also may be involved in training clients in the use of adaptive living devices. Adaptive living devices help individuals live more independently. They include such equipment as modified eating utensils, modified cooking equipment, adaptive equipment for self-dressing, and so on. In some settings, the OT provides "cognitive therapy." Basically, cognitive therapy involves the same activities you provide in language therapy that involve comprehension, memory, judgment, and reasoning. Your most common interaction with the OT will be in working with patients with dysphagia. Depending on the setting, either the OT or the speech-language pathologist heads the dysphagia team. There has been much discussion between speech-language pathology associations and occupational therapy associations regarding which profession should be responsible for treating dysphagia and providing "cognitive therapy." Follow the guidelines provided at your clinical site.

Because of the overlap in services, it is essential that you regularly communicate with the OT. You want to provide maximum clinical service without duplicating efforts. To provide effective clinical service, the OT will need to know your role in treatment of dysphagia and communication. Also, the OT will need to know the patients' communicative abilities. You will provide them with information on the patients' receptive and expressive language. You also will give suggestions on how the OT can help enhance the patients' communicative skills.

6. **Orthodontist.** The **orthodontist is a specialist in dental occlusion.** You will work closely with the orthodontist providing services for a client with cleft palate, other craniofacial anomaly, or myofunctional disorder. The orthodontist may request a detailed speech evaluation from you. In some instances, your reports will be critical in helping the orthodontist determine the course of treatment for the client. As always, you will want to provide accurate, detailed information.

7. **Otolaryngologist.** The **otolaryngologist (commonly called an ENT) is a physician specializing in evaluation and treatment**

of disorders of the ear, nose, and throat. The speech-language pathologist often has a close working relationship with the ENT. You and the otolaryngologist may share such clients as individuals with voice disorders, chronic otitis media, hearing loss, or laryngeal cancer. A few instances in which you might work with an otolaryngologist are described in the following paragraphs.

If you are working with a child who has a history of chronic otitis media, you should find out what types of medical treatment the child is receiving from the otolaryngologist. You should closely monitor the child's hearing and refer to the physician if there is a decrease in hearing abilities.

If you have a client who has been diagnosed with vocal nodules, the otolaryngologist may consult with you regarding treatment. The otolaryngologist may suggest a trial period of voice treatment before recommending surgical intervention. You carefully will document progress in voice treatment and refer your client back to the otolaryngologist.

You may work with the otolaryngologist in educating the individual facing laryngectomy. After you receive a referral from the otolaryngologist, you will educate the client about communication options following laryngectomy. The laryngologist will inform you of the surgery schedule, and you will meet with the client soon after the surgery to provide an immediate method of communication. You also may arrange for a person who already has had a laryngectomy to meet with your client before and after surgery.

8. **Pediatrician.** The **pediatrician is a physician specializing in the medical care of children.** You may refer children to their pediatricians because of suspected hearing or vision problems, chronic health problems (allergies, colds, and so on), or unusual behaviors such as poor attention span.

   You will encounter some pediatricians who are knowledgeable about communicative disorders and many who are not. Unfortunately, a few pediatricians continue to erroneously advise parents that their children will outgrow a communication problem. One of your responsibilities is to educate pediatricians about early intervention for speech and language disorders. One way to do this is to provide regular progress reports regarding any of their patients for whom you may be providing services.

9. **Physiatrist.** The **physiatrist is a physician with specialized training in rehabilitative medicine.** The physiatrist directs the rehabilitation of a patient who is disabled. Although there are many reasons for the disabilities experienced by the physiatrist's patients, often the disability is caused from CVA or head trauma.

In the medical setting, you may work closely with the physiatrist who may refer patients to you. He or she may request you to give a detailed report on patients' communicative skills, speech and language prognoses, and recommendations. Too, you may offer suggestions to assist in patients' re-entry into their school, work, or home.

10. **Physical Therapist.** The **registered physical therapist (RPT or PT) provides assessment and treatment for disorders related to physical and musculoskeletal injuries.** In the hospital and rehabilitation setting, the speech-language pathologist and physical therapist often provide services for many of the same patients.

   The physical therapist provides you with information about patients' motor abilities and optimum positioning and posture for a patient. This information can be essential in developing an appropriate eating program or successful implementation of an augmentative communication device.

   You will provide the PT with information about patients' communication skills. The PT may want to know what types of instructions (e.g., single-word commands) a patient can understand.

11. **Prosthodontist.** The **prosthodontist is a dentist with specialized training in the development and use of prosthetic appliances.** The speech-language pathologist and prosthodontist may consult regarding a client with insufficient velopharyngeal closure. You may refer a client with velopharyngeal incompetence (VPI) to a prosthodontist. A prosthodontist may ask you to help assess velopharyngeal adequacy in a patient before and after a prosthetic appliance is used. You also may be asked for suggestions regarding choice of appliances.

12. **Radiologist.** The **radiologist is a physician specializing in the evaluation and treatment of disease with radioactive substances (X ray).** The radiologist also may perform brain imaging with patients such as those with aphasia. You and the radiologist also may share such patients as those with laryngeal cancer and swallowing disorders.

   Your most frequent contact with the radiologist may involve patients with swallowing disorders. The radiologist may perform videofluoroscopy for patients with dysphagia. You may give suggestions regarding positioning of the patient and textures and types of foods to use during the evaluation. You will work closely with the radiologist in evaluating results of the videofluoroscopic examination.

13. **Registered Nurse.** The **registered nurse (RN) is responsible for most medical care prescribed by the physician for the patient.**

Because registered nurses work closely with patients, it is important for the speech-language pathologist and nurse to develop effective communication. The RN can provide information on a patient's daily communicative skills. Another part of patient care is provided by the **licensed vocational nurse (LVN)** or licensed professional nurse (LPN). The LVN is frequently identified as a nurse's aide, has less medical training than the RN and delivers such care as bathing and feeding patients and taking vital signs.

The nursing staff will request information from you on the patient's receptive and expressive abilities. The staff may give you information about communicative attempts of patients. They also may help identify patients needing your services. Because the nursing staff typically has the most contact with the patients and their families, it is critical for you to develop a good working relationship with them.

14. **Social Worker.** The **social worker is often a member of the hospital's rehabilitation team working closely with the patient's family.** You can obtain information about community services that your clients may need from the social worker. You also may ask the social worker to intercede with your patients' families who are having difficulty. For example, if you are serving an elderly patient in his or her home, you may observe that neither the spouse nor the patient is able to prepare meals adequately. The social worker may be able to obtain part-time help for the couple or arrange for delivery of meals through social service agencies that provide such services as prepared meals delivered to the home.

Educational Specialists

1. **Adaptive Physical Education Specialist.** The **adaptive physical education specialist has specialized training in physical education.** Such specialists have been trained to work with individuals with disabilities. Their services often include providing physical education programs for individuals with disabilities. For certain students, they may also provide gross and fine motor activities. You probably will not work closely with the adaptive physical education specialist; however, they often are members of the IEP team.

2. **Educational Audiologist.** The **educational audiologist specializes in working with children in the public schools.** The educational audiologist provides assessment and management of hearing disorders for children in the public schools. As a school-based speech-language pathologist, you may frequently interact with the educational

audiologist. You may have children on your caseload who are deaf or have limited hearing. Also, you may have children you suspect may have hearing problems or you may be working with a child who has had a cochlear implant. In all these cases you will want to consult with the educational audiologist to ensure optimal service delivery.

3. **Principal.** The **school principal is responsible for the day-to-day operations of the school, including the education and well-being of all students.** The principal can influence a school staff's behaviors and dispositions toward the speech-language pathology program. It is important for you to discuss your program's goals with the principal. Keep the principal informed about such matters as the caseload size and types of disorders. Help principals realize the importance of your role in the educational community by regularly communicating with them, maintaining highly visible and effective service delivery, documenting and communicating results of service delivery, and participating in certain school committees.

4. **School Nurse.** The **school nurse is a registered nurse with additional training in laws related to public schools.** The school nurse often is responsible for screening students' hearing and vision. The school nurse maintains a health history for each student and often acts as a liaison between the educational staff and other health professionals. Often, the school nurse is knowledgeable about your students' family history and may provide important background information.

You will consult regularly with the school nurse about students with hearing loss, voice disorders, and chronic health problems. You may refer students to the school nurse who have poor dentition (such as unrepaired dental caries). You also may refer children with suspected hearing or vision problems to the school nurse.

5. **School Psychologist.** The **school psychologist is trained and credentialed to work in the public school setting.** The main duties of the school psychologist include testing students to determine their educational strengths and weaknesses. They also determine appropriate educational placement and recommend intervention techniques. The school psychologist may provide some family and student counseling.

The school psychologist may request you to perform speech and language assessments with some of the students he or she is also evaluating. The school psychologist will ask your opinion regarding how a child's communicative skills may affect educational performance.

You may need information from the school psychologist about a student's cognitive abilities. You also may ask for help from the school psychologist on managing a child's behavior problems during your treatment sessions.

It is important for you to establish an effective relationship with school psychologists because they are often the leaders of the IEP team. They can provide support for your program by making appropriate referrals and abiding by your speech and language recommendations.

6. **Special Education Teacher.** The **special education teacher is a credentialed teacher with additional training in specific disabilities or disorders.** Many students receiving services from a special education teacher also need the services of the speech-language pathologist. Teachers of special education include the following: teacher of the hearing impaired (HI); teacher of the learning handicapped (LH); teacher of the severely emotionally disturbed (SED); teacher of the orthopedically handicapped (OH); teacher of the severely handicapped (SH); teacher of the visually impaired (VI); and, resource specialist (RS).

You may work with many of these educational specialists. You should develop good communication with them so you can coordinate your services with their services. For example, if the SH teacher is training a child to sit in his or her chair for 5 minutes by using a token reinforcement system, you may follow through with this procedure when you work with the child individually. Conversely, you may be teaching the use of present progressive with a child. You may ask the LH teacher to instruct the child to correctly use the present progressive in the classroom setting and reinforce the correct responses.

7. **Teacher.** The **regular education teacher is one of the most important professionals with whom you will work.** The classroom teacher is responsible for assuring an appropriate education for each child in his or her class. Regular education teachers are involved in many school activities and work closely with other teachers and parents.

Unless you are assigned such a select caseload as only children with severe disabilities, many of your children will be in typical education classrooms. These children spend the large majority of their day with the classroom teacher and a small fraction of the day with you. In addition, many of your children with severe disabilities may be in regular education. Many schools have adopted a policy of **including** all children in the regular education class. In *inclusive* schools, instead of being in a special education program most of the day and sharing only such activities as recess with their peers without disability, children with disabilities are educated in the typical classroom. Special education teachers and other specialists may visit the classroom to support the student and the teacher.

The effectiveness of your treatment may be assisted or hampered by your relationship with the classroom teacher. It is important that you maintain ongoing communication with the regular education teacher. To maximize a child's education and speech therapy, you should understand what and how a teacher is teaching. You may incorporate the curriculum into your treatment. In other cases, you may provide services in the classroom or help the teacher modify his or her method of teaching to increase your student's comprehension and success. Chapter 2 contains additional information about the different types of service delivery models in the schools.

Guidelines on Establishing Collaborative Relationships With Other Professionals

Regardless of your professional setting, you should be able to communicate effectively with other professionals and obtain all needed services for your client. You should show other professionals that the services you provide are valuable and that the client needs your services as much as theirs. The following are some guidelines that help you accomplish these important goals.

1. **Provide high quality service.** This will help develop a reputation for excellence. Be well prepared for each clinical session.

2. **Develop good communication with other professionals.** Provide clear, concise, and relevant information. In your reports, describe the effects of your services in direct and measurable terms. Minimize the use of jargon that other professionals may not understand. Provide charts, graphs, and tables when they seem to show the progress of your clients more clearly than just the written narrative.

3. **Be courteous.** Occasionally, you may be angry with another professional or just in a bad mood. Regardless, of how you are feeling, when you communicate with another person, it is important to be courteous. If you offer an inappropriate or unexpected display of temper, that is how you will be remembered. Also, the other professional may not listen to the content of the message you are trying to convey. As you know, you can disagree and present you viewpoint in a gracious manner.

4. **Understand the services provided by other professionals.** To effectively collaborate with other professionals, it is essential you understand their roles. Learn not only the definitions of their duties, but try and understand how their responsibilities to your clients affect their job. For example, teachers who must demonstrate that their class is at a certain academic level, may become disheartened when a child with special needs enrolls in their class. It is not because of the child, but because of the other pressures from the administrators, the community,

or both. Rather than judging that these teachers do not like children with special needs, work with them to help the student and the class perform optimally.

5. **Respect the services offered by others.** It is important that you understand and demonstrate respect for the role other professionals play in the treatment of your clients. As a student clinician, you are focusing on speech-language pathology. Therefore, you may sometimes feel that your services are the most important. They are important, but others offer equally important service. The amount of training or prestige an individual has does not ensure the importance of their contributions. Remember, the assistant who drives your client to the grocery store and the neurosurgeon who removed a tumor from your client's brain, both are important in helping your client live successfully.

6. **Respond promptly.** Reply readily and accurately to inquiries from clients and professionals. When you delay responding to a client, parent, or professional, they may feel you think they are not important enough for you to make time for them. Too, they may have urgent information, concerns, or questions.

7. **Acknowledge referrals.** Send a thank-you letter to all professionals who refer a client to you. He or she may follow up with additional helpful information or provide you with more referrals. Also, acknowledging referrals is a chance to educate others about your services.

8. **Send reports promptly.** Send out assessment and progress reports to those professionals who have referred the client to you. If necessary, talk to the referring professionals during the course of the term to keep them informed about your services.

9. **Educate other professionals about communicative disorders.** Any time you discuss a client or your services with other professionals is an opportunity to educate them about speech-language pathology. Offer accurate information about your services and the needs of particular clients. Be a resource person for other professionals.

10. **Respect professional boundaries.** Give information only about speech-language pathology. Do not give information, advice, or treatment that is not within the realm of speech-language pathology. Refer the clients to other professionals for needed services.

11. **Talk to your supervisor before you contact another professional.** Remember that when there is a need to contact another professional, student clinicians must first discuss this with their clinical supervisors to get their advice and approval.

The Internet's Role

The Internet is just one of the many innovations in technology that is impacting speech-language pathologists. However, second only to the personal computer, it may be the one that has been of most assistance to many speech-language pathologists and other professionals. Communication between professionals has increased because of the Internet. For example, on the Internet you will find many **subscriber e-mail lists** and **electronic bulletin boards** that function as communication networking tools for professionals with similar concerns. There is an e-mail list for people involved in the treatment of dysphagia. You may find occupational therapists, physical therapists, radiologists, and neurologists, as well as speech-language pathologists posting questions, answers, and comments to this forum.

In addition, there are many journals that can be accessed via the Internet. You are no longer restricted to the journals offered by ASHA or available through your local library. You can read articles published by other professions. This may give you a more thorough understanding of certain disorders and help you understand the concerns of other professionals.

Telemedicine is an application that has not been used by speech-language pathology, but may have future uses. In telemedicine, a patient may be several thousand miles from a specialist providing the service, but they are linked by the Internet or other technology. The provider may offer information directly to the patient or to another specialist who is directly treating the patient.

You will want to maintain current skills in the rapidly expanding area of technology. E-mail, lists, electronic publishing, and telemedicine are only a glimmer of our technological future.

So far, you have learned about various structural and organizational aspects of clinical practicum. You know that you will have opportunities to learn the skills of the profession in a variety of clinical settings. In completing your clinical practicum or internship, you must follow many administrative and ethical rules, regulations, and guidelines.

Once you understand the structures and procedures of clinical practicum, you may concentrate on the clinical methods of speech-language pathology. You will have learned about these methods in various courses taken prior to enrolling in clinical practicum. In the second part of the book, we give you an overview of these methods that help you treat clients with communicative disorders.

6

Multicultural Issues in Clinical Practicum

Because of the rapidly changing composition of society in the United States, the issues of diversity and multiculturalism are currently in the forefront of government, business, and education. Historically, ASHA has had policies regarding nondiscrimination based on gender, race, linguistic background, and other factors. In 1998 ASHA published a position statement and technical report extending this nondiscrimination policy to students and professionals who speak English with nonstandard dialects or accents (ASHA Joint Subcommittee of the Executive Board on English Language Proficiency, 1998). Over the past several years, ASHA has developed various other guidelines and position statements on effective and appropriate delivery of clinical services to people with diverse linguistic and cultural background. ASHA also has sponsored numerous workshops and conferences on multicultural concerns to educate the professionals. Furthermore, to coordinate its activities relative to minority populations, ASHA has an Office of Multicultural Affairs.

To effectively serve the growing culturally and linguistically diverse population of the United States, ASHA considers recruitment of individuals from diverse cultural, racial, ethnic, and linguistic backgrounds a priority in professional education. In 1992 ASHA published its **Multicultural Action Agenda 2000**, which includes increased efforts to recruit individuals with multicultural backgrounds to the professions of speech-language pathology and audiology (Cole, 1992). ASHA continues to emphasize the importance of diversity through various avenues, including recruitment and retention of minorities (Goldberg, 1994). However, recruitment of minority students with diverse linguistic backgrounds has created some professional training issues.

Student Clinicians With Multicultural Backgrounds

Students from diverse cultural and linguistic backgrounds may face several challenges at the university level. These challenges include the possibility of having a weak academic background and dealing with an educational system dominated by white middle-class values and training structures, along with limited financial support. These are universal problems across disciplines and educational programs in the country. However, because of the obvious emphasis on speech and language proficiency in the field of communication sciences and disorders, nonnative English speakers or speakers who employ an English dialect other than standard American English (SAE) sometimes are dissuaded from majoring in communicative disorders. It is important to remember that individuals should not be discriminated against because of race, ethnicity, language, dialects, or cultural differences. In fact, ASHA's Code of Ethics prohibits such practice. To emphasize its stand on this issue, ASHA published in a position statement and technical report regarding students and professionals who use a nonstandard English dialect or accent (ASHA Joint Subcommittee of the Executive Board on English Language Proficiency, 1998). This paper addresses people who: were not born in the United States and learned another language before they learned English; who were born in the United States and learned another language before they learned to speak English; and who were born in the United States and speak only English. It does not discuss the issue of students or professionals who have not yet become proficient in English as their second language.

As noted in this paper, student clinicians need not necessarily speak standard American English (SAE). However, to succeed in clinical practicum and later in professional practice, all student clinicians should possess a certain standard of SAE linguistic competence. Campbell (1994) suggested that in the United States student clinicians in communicative disorders may speak one of the dialectal varieties of English. More importantly, the student clinicians should possess proficiency in English or an English dialect to achieve above average academic performance. For admission and matriculation to most graduate programs, students must earn a minimum grade-point average of B.

ASHA has not yet developed a standard for English language proficiency for the practice of speech-language pathology in the United States

(Campbell, 1994). ASHA's position statement refers primarily to students' knowledge of communication and its disorders, their skills in evaluating and treating these disorders, and the students' ability to model the speech or language target. In addition to ASHA's position, some training programs have found it essential for students' intelligibility to be evaluated. Most universities have established certain speech and language proficiency standards for all student clinicians, regardless of their language history. Some training programs may require all students majoring in communicative disorders to have their speech, language, and hearing screened. Following the screening, certain students may be referred for additional evaluation. Diagnostic testing may reveal the need for intervention and some individuals may seek elective clinical services. In general, as a student clinician you should:

1. Develop a thorough knowledge of normal and disordered communication and communication development.
2. Acquire effective diagnostic and intervention skills.
3. Learn to effectively communicate with clients from a variety of cultural, ethnic, racial, and linguistic backgrounds.
4. Develop the skill to model all target behaviors required of your clients. For example, for articulation therapy, you will need to be able to model each of the English phonemes or allophones.
5. Learn to write clearly and concisely, using correct grammar.

An issue that has not received much attention is that clinicians with multicultural backgrounds may or may not possess cultural sensitivity. They still may need to study the cultural and linguistic differences of other groups. Therefore, the recommendation that clinicians should study and understand the cultural and linguistic background of clients they serve applies to *all clinicians*.

If you have concerns regarding your oral or written communication skills, discuss them with your advisor. If you are a student clinician with a diverse cultural or linguistic background, you may encounter certain obstacles, but you also will encounter many rewards: excellent employment opportunities, many research questions to be investigated, and colleagues who are eager to share your unique knowledge and experiences.

ASHA Position Statements

Numerous articles about multicultural issues have been published in the various ASHA journals. In addition, ASHA has published several position statements. These position statements reflect ASHA's philosophy regarding multicultural and bilingual issues and help guide today's service delivery to these populations. All student clinicians should have a basic knowledge of the various position statements. The following section gives an overview of several of them.

Bilingual Speech-Language Pathologists and Audiologists

ASHA does not certify an individual as a bilingual speech-language pathologist or audiologist. However, ASHA (American Speech-Language-Hearing Association, 1989) defines certain competencies necessary for being identified as bilingual for the purpose of clinical service delivery. A bilingual speech-language pathologist is one who speaks his or her own language proficiently and speaks (or signs) at least one other language with native or near-native proficiency. Communication skills should encompass all parameters of oral or manual language including the appropriate grammar, meaning, and social use.

In many geographic areas of the United States, there is an immense need for bilingual speech-language pathologists. ASHA strongly supports efforts of universities in recruiting bilingual students. There are many student clinicians who are bilingual. Before identifying yourself as a bilingual student clinician, be sure to examine ASHA's definition of a **bilingual speech-language pathologist** and your own language skills. Some people who have grown up speaking two languages often use one language predominantly and, hence, the other language is forgotten or no longer used proficiently. A person may speak two languages well enough to engage in such communication as social exchanges, but may not be proficient enough to provide clinical service in both languages. Some of the competencies ASHA suggests the bilingual clinician should have include the following:

1. The ability to describe the development of speech and oral (or manual) and written language for both bilingual and monolingual individuals.
2. The skill to differentiate communication differences from communication disorders in oral (or manual) and written language through the use of both formal and informal evaluation.
3. The ability to provide treatment in the client's primary language.
4. Knowledge of various cultural factors related to service delivery (American Speech-Language-Hearing Association, 1989).

Review these standards. You may already have proficient language skills in two or more languages or you may want to upgrade certain language skills. If you are bilingual, find out from your advisor if you may be certified as a bilingual speech-language pathologist in your state. This may be a part of the licensure or credential process in your state. If you are not bilingual, you may want to take classes in a second language to enhance your knowledge of a different language and to gain some insight into what it is like to be a speaker of a minority language who is required to learn a new language in which to communicate. Besides, employment opportunities for bilingual speech-language pathologists are excellent.

Clinical Management of Minority Language Populations

Depending on your work setting and geographical area, you may be one of the almost 50% of ASHA members providing service to individuals who do not speak English as a native language (American Speech-Language-Hearing Association, 1993). In response to the needs of its members and as part of its service to minority populations, ASHA published a position paper entitled "Clinical Management of Communicatively Handicapped Minority Language Populations" (American Speech-Language-Hearing Association, 1985). The paper discusses competencies you should have for evaluation and treatment of individuals with communicative disorders who are minority language speakers. These competencies include those listed in ASHA's other position paper entitled "Definitions: Bilingual Speech-Language Pathologists and Audiologists" (American Speech-Language-Hearing Association, 1989).

The position paper on "Clinical Management of Communicatively Handicapped Minority Language Populations" (American Speech-Language-Hearing Association, 1985) suggests methods that can be used when a competent bilingual specialist is not available. If you are a monolingual student intern at a clinical practicum site serving individuals who are bilingual or monolingual in a language other than yours, you may implement some of ASHA's (1985) suggestions for serving minority language populations. These include:

- Contracting with a bilingual speech-language pathologist or audiologist to serve as a consultant;
- Employing an itinerant bilingual speech-language pathologist or audiologist to provide services for a specific language population;
- Collaborating with university bilingual speech-language pathology and audiology programs;
- Developing an interdisciplinary team that consists of at least one bilingual professional who also is proficient in language development and nonbiased assessment procedures;
- Creating CFY and practicum sites for individuals from bilingual speech-language pathology and audiology programs (American Speech-Language-Hearing Association, 1985).

The paper (American Speech-Language-Hearing Association, 1985) also discusses the **use of interpreters** or **translators**. In working with multicultural populations, you may have to rely on interpreters or translators. Interpreters may be trained professionals, the client's friend, or one of the client's family members. Guidelines for the use of interpreters include training the interpreter, planning assessment sessions, use of the same interpreter, and use of natural assessment measures. For more specific information, refer to the "Clinical Management" position paper and to the section in this chapter, "Guidelines for Working With an Interpreter."

Social Dialects

The American Speech-Language-Hearing Association's (1983) position paper entitled "Social Dialects" clears some of the confusion regarding the role of speech-language pathologists serving individuals who speak in dialects other than standard American English. Historically, some speech-language pathologists have considered dialectal variations as disorders to be treated. Some lay persons tend to make negative judgments about people who speak dialects that are influenced by a second language. ASHA's position on this matter is unequivocal: The dialectical varieties of standard English are not disorders. To appropriately evaluate a communicative disorder, the clinician should differentiate between linguistic variation because of a dialectical difference and linguistic variation because of a speech, language, or hearing disorder.

You may work with individuals with linguistic variation because of dialectical differences when those individuals have **chosen** to receive treatment. For example, you may work with clients who wish to change or reduce their specific accents. Also, you may work with individuals who speak a dialectical variation of English (e.g., Black English) who wish to learn standard American English. In this case, your clients may want to retain their native dialects, but, in certain situations, be able to code switch to standard American English. For example, many clients are happy with and are proud of their dialects, which reflect their cultural heritage. However, they may find the acquisition of the standard dialect to have social or occupational advantage. Remember, except in the case of elective services, you can only recommend speech therapy for those individuals who exhibit a language disorder and not a language difference.

Provision of English-as-a-Second-Language Instruction by Speech-Language Pathologists in School Settings

The effectiveness of school-based speech-language pathologists is partially dependent on their ability to work collaboratively with teachers and other educational specialists. Speech-language pathologists include curriculum in the context of their treatment, teach sections of classes, and work with individual students in the classroom. Teachers provide opportunities for students to generalize skills learned in speech-language therapy and rely on the speech-language pathologist to help students who are having difficulty with comprehension or written and oral language. Because of the increasing demands on educators, the roles of the different personnel sometimes become blurred. The increasing diversity of the school population has added to the confusion of professional roles. According to ASHA (ASHA Joint Subcommittee of the Executive Board on English Language Proficiency, 1998), speech-language pathologists with appropriate training in instructing students who have English as a second language may provide this service. Speech-language pathologists who have not received the necessary linguistic, theoretical, and methodological training should not provide direct instruction in English as a second language (ESL), but may collaborate with ESL instructors for assessment and treatment of appropriate students. As with other areas of professional practice, if you are not trained or prepared to provide a specific service, do not do it.

Some of ASHA's (1998) suggestions for collaborating in ESL instruction include the following:

- Before an assessment, discuss with the ESL teacher such issues as language development and code switching during second language acquisition, socialization, and language use in the classroom and community.
- As part of an assessment, discuss with the ESL teacher such issues as the student's test performance, specific test results, and methods and strategies for maximizing the student's learning.
- During intervention, continue to collaborate with the ESL teacher, discussing ideas and resources, and coordinating goals, objectives, and activities related to the communicative disorder connected to those of developing proficiency in English.

If there is not an appropriate ESL program available, ASHA suggests that the speech-language pathologist act as a consultant to the teachers and other professionals and advocate for the child. In all cases, the speech-language pathologist should be aware of cultural and linguistic factors that affect a student's education and progress in speech therapy. Also, the speech-language pathologist should be sensitive to a student's and his or her family's cultural and linguistic differences. In the educational setting, it is important that a communicative disorder not be misinterpreted as acquisition of a second language and that second language acquisition is not diagnosed as a communicative disorder.

Available Resources

There are many excellent resources available for second-language students as well as for professional clinicians. ASHA is a major source of information. As a member of the National Student Speech-Language-Hearing Association (NSSLHA), you will have access to ASHA's various publications. *Asha,* the monthly publication, typically contains information on professional issues, including those that affect multicultural clinical services.

An excellent source is a bibliography of publications on multicultural issues maintained and updated by ASHA's Office of Multicultural Affairs. The bibliography contains publications on almost all aspects of speech-language disorders that address multicultural issues. Your clinic director or supervisor may have access to the bibliography.

There are now several books and book chapters on multicultural speech-language pathology, special education, and general education (Adler, 1993; Battle, 1998; Cheng, 1991, 1995; Hamayan & Damico, 1991; Kayser, 1995; Khami, Pollock, & Harris, 1996; Langdon & Cheng, 1992; Mattes & Omark, 1991; Payan, 1984; Payne, 1997; Roseberry-McKibbin, 1995; Screen & Anderson, 1994; Seymour & Nober, 1998; Taylor, 1986a, 1986b; Trueba, Cheng, & Ima, 1993; Trueba, Jacobs, & Kirton, 1990; Van Keulen, Weddington, & DeBose, 1998; Westby, 1994; Yavas, 1994). Make use of these and other resources in understanding clients of diverse cultural backgrounds and in planning clinical and educational programs for them.

Assessment Issues

Evaluation, or **assessment**, is a multifaceted process that involves interactions between the examiner, the client, the client's family, and various educators, physicians, and allied professionals. To make comprehensive and accurate evaluations, the speech-language pathologist should possess knowledge of normal and abnormal communication development, knowledge of standardized tests, effective test administration skills, good observation skills, and interviewing skills. In addition, to make nonbiased assessment of nonnative speakers or speakers who use dialectical variations, the clinician should have a knowledge of linguistic standards of the client's community, the client's culture and values, and sensitivity to cultural variations. The clinician should also be aware of any prejudices he or she may have that may contribute to biased assessment results.

In ASHA's 1993 Omnibus Survey (American Speech-Language-Hearing Association, 1993), 15.5% of the respondents reported specific graduate coursework related to communication disorders among multicultural populations and 10.6% of the respondents reported specific graduate coursework related to limited-English-speaking population. Avenues for obtaining information included on-the-job education, self-study, and continuing education. However, 49.8% of the respondents reported that they provided services for individuals who did not speak English as a native language. This means that practical exigencies demand that clinicians who do not have adequate training in multicultural speech-language pathology provide services, anyway. Obviously, there is a need to have training at the university level for working with multicultural populations.

Because of the complexity of evaluations in general and evaluation of culturally diverse populations, this section does not attempt to give all the information you will need to evaluate each type of client you may encounter. Your university may offer a specialized class on multicultural issues or offer culturally relevant information in each of your classes. Nonetheless, you may have to independently gather additional information for specific clients. The following information provides a framework you can build and expand on, depending on your clients and their backgrounds.

Before the Evaluation

Culturally sensitive planning is needed to conduct assessment that is appropriate for all clients, especially for clients of cultural diversity. Take the following steps in planning your assessment sessions:

1. **Know the cultural background of your clients.** Try to understand the client's dispositions, values, and expectations regarding communication and its disorders. This will assist you in establishing rapport with your clients and their families, which, in turn, will help you more efficiently and accurately evaluate your clients. Your interview will be more productive because you will know to whom to address your questions, what types of questions will be most effective, what types of questions should be avoided (or carefully worded), and what types of responses to expect. A knowledge of the cultural background of your clients also may influence the way you structure your assessment, your selection of tests, and your choice of materials for language sampling. Also, to work most effectively with your clients, you should know the dispositions and practices regarding such nonverbal communication modes as eye contact, smiling, handshake, and touching. Many miscommunications and misinterpretations can be avoided, if you are aware of the meaning of these and other behaviors in specific cultural groups. Remember, what is desirable or acceptable in one culture may not be desirable or acceptable in another culture.

2. **Understand how your life experiences may influence your attitude toward a client.** It is almost impossible for one to be totally without prejudice. You have grown up in a community and culture that held certain values. When you encounter individuals who challenge those values through their own beliefs and lifestyles, you may react in a prejudicial manner. Because you view yourself as a person without prejudice, you may attempt to rationalize behavior that is unacceptable, but which you do not want to judge. In other cases, you may find yourself disliking a client for no apparent reason. You may hold such prejudicial beliefs as "people who wear white shoes after Labor day have no class" or "people of color have less intelligence than white people." Regardless of the extent of your prejudicial beliefs, the more you can acknowledge them, the more you will be able to change them, and the less influence they will have on your evaluations. Try to use the self-analysis as an exercise in being nonjudgmental.

3. **Know the beliefs and behavioral dispositions toward communicative disorders.** It is important to understand your client's belief regarding the origin of a communicative disorder. For example, Harris (1993) reported that in some Native American groups a child's disability may be considered a gift from the "Creator." In such Southeast Asian communities as the Hmong, only disabilities that are physical or obviously mental are taken seriously. Knowing an individual's beliefs will affect the structure of your questions, evaluation tasks, counseling, and family involvement in treatment. Your treatment procedure for a disorder in a culturally diverse child may be the same as the one you use with other clients because of the demonstrated effectiveness of the procedure. Nonetheless, you may provide different types of counseling or activities for family involvement in treatment.

4. **Know phonological and linguistic differences.** You may not always know your client's primary language before the evaluation, but you may have some clues based on information in the case history or previous evaluations. As much as possible in advance of the assessment session, study the phonological and linguistic characteristics of your client's native language or dialectal variation. During the assessment session, you should be able to judge if certain behaviors are related to a difference or a disorder and whether in-depth evaluation is in order. For example, in the Hmong language the only final consonant is /ng/ (Cheng, 1991), therefore, evaluation of English morphological skills of the Hmong child learning English as a second language may need to place most emphasis on receptive morphological skills. This would be done with the understanding that expressive skills may be slow to emerge but because of transition from a sound system very different from English and not because there is a language disorder.

5. **Know health statistics.** The prevalence of certain diseases varies across race and culture. Therefore, you need to know health statistics that are relevant to an understanding of a particular client. For example, if you are working with children who are from a population that historically has a high incidence of otitis media, you may explore your clients' hearing history and health care treatment in greater detail than you would otherwise.

6. **Select standardized tests that are appropriate to the client.** Review each test's normative data before choosing tests for your assessment. Many tests do not have norms for various cultural groups. Therefore, to avoid biased test results, do not use tests that are not standardized on the particular group to which your client belongs. Also, avoid tests that sample only a small number of people representing the culture of the person you will be testing. Do not attempt to modify an existing test to use with your client. Instead, rely on spontaneous speech samples, observation of behaviors, and interview information.

7. **Choose material that is culturally appropriate.** Use materials that are culturally appropriate for such activities as vocabulary sampling and spontaneous speech sampling. Avoid materials that depict stereotypes of cultures. If possible, use materials that accurately reflect the client's culture. To obtain the best speech sample, attempt to select materials that the client relates to and feels comfortable with.

8. **Determine if you will need to use the services of an interpreter.** Before the evaluation session, judge the need for an interpreter. You may judge this through information from the client's case history form, from the clinic secretary, or by telephoning the client. If you are unsure of the need for an interpreter, plan to use an interpreter. It is easier to excuse an unneeded interpreter than to locate one at the last minute or to have to postpone a session because an interpreter cannot be found.

9. **Train your interpreter.** After you have selected an interpreter, discuss the evaluation session with him or her. Review the format of the session, discuss specific interview questions and provide training for any tests to be administered. Also, discuss your expectations regarding the interpreter's behavior during and after the evaluation session. Include in your discussion such professional issues as maintaining client confidentiality, not guaranteeing treatment outcome, and so on. If possible, use an interpreter with whom you have worked before whose skills you know and who knows what you expect. If you are working with a new interpreter, find out what the interpreter's experience is and what type of additional training he or she needs. Role play different testing situations in training your interpreter. For additional infor-

mation, refer to the section in this chapter entitled "Working With an Interpreter."

During the Evaluation

In evaluating multicultural clients, you need to take such special steps as:

1. **Be sensitive to cultural issues.** Before your session, you will have reviewed information related to your client's culture. During the session, be aware of and respect cultural communication practices. For example, in the client's culture it may not be acceptable to touch the top of an individual's head. Know what behaviors are considered rude and which are considered polite. For instance, in Asian cultures, maintaining a constant eye contact with a teacher or an authority figure is considered rude. Also, students are encouraged to listen more and talk less. Therefore, silence and lack of eye contact on the part of an Asian child may not suggest a pragmatic language disorder. Such understanding not only will help you establish better rapport with your clients, but it will help you evaluate your client's communicative performance more accurately.

2. **Talk to the client, not the interpreter.** At the beginning of the session, through the interpreter, introduce yourself and the interpreter to the client. Explain what the interpreter's role is and what your role is. For example, "I am Julie Smith, and I will be evaluating your son's speech and language today. This is Mr. Yang, and he will be interpreting for us during this session." Although it is important to acknowledge the interpreter's presence, you always should look at the client or family members when you are talking to them.

3. **Explain why you will be asking questions.** Certain ethnic and cultural groups may not be used to responding to direct questions. It may be considered threatening or rude. At the beginning of the evaluation, explain that you will be asking some questions and why. When you ask specific questions, explain why they are necessary. Often, you will be able to tell from clients' and family members' body language if continued use of such questions are necessary.

4. **Use the appropriate title of the cultural group.** In advance, find out what the acceptable title is for the individual's cultural group and use the title appropriately during the evaluation session (Battle, 1998). Also, determine how different family members and significant individuals are referred to. For instance, in Asian cultures, it is not common to address older relatives by their name. They typically are addressed in

terms of the relation. If an Asian boy is accompanied to the clinic by his uncle and you are talking to the child, it is preferable to use the phrase "Your uncle" and not "Mr. Kapoor." If possible, find out how the family hierarchy affects interaction. For example, are there certain titles for the maternal grandmother and the paternal grandmother? Does one have more interaction or influence with the family? If you are unsure of an appropriate title, ask your client. You may feel slightly embarrassed to ask, but it will make your client more comfortable to know you are concerned about using correct terms, and it is much better than finding out at the end of an hour-long session that you have used certain names and titles inappropriately or incorrectly.

5. **Find out the client's primary language.** During the course of your interview you will find out what the primary language used is. Remember to determine whether different languages are used at home, school, or work. Also, if clients have acquired disorders (e.g., aphasia) find out what language they used premorbidly and what language is now used.

6. **Conduct an ethnographic interview.** An ethnographic interview is one that focuses on the client and his or her interactions within the family. The ethnographic interview is directed by the responses a family member provides to such questions as: Who is the primary person whom children talk to in your family? What do the boys talk about? What do the girls talk about? How do they learn to speak? (Tomblin, Morris, & Spriestersbach, 1994). There are many other questions that would be appropriate for the ethnographic interview. Basically, you are trying to learn about the dynamics of the culture and of the particular family, and how your client fits within that culture and family. This will help you idenify if there is a disorder and assist you with future intervention.

7. **In a naturalistic context, obtain an adequate sample of your client's speech.** If possible, obtain more than one speech sample, in different settings, and with different individuals. Obtain samples from home and work or school. For many of your clients the speech sample will be your best source of information. From an adequate sample, you can judge various parameters of language, articulation, voice, and fluency. Also, you can gain an understanding of which antecedents enhance linguistic performance, which diminish performance, or which seem to have no impact. You may obtain a speech sample with your client talking with different members of the family. This will give you additional diagnostic information and possibly give you information for future treatment sessions. For example, you may determine which family member seems most appropriate for working with the client at home.

8. **Sample social and cognitively demanding language.** In both simple and complex language, people discuss familiar events, share personal experiences, and answer simple questions about stories to which they have listened. To succeed in educational programs and in many businesses, individuals must learn to use complex and technical language. The skills needed to succeed include such abilities as telling or writing imaginary stories, making persuasive arguments, describing complex ideas or events, and following directions (Tomblin et al., 1994).

9. **Use standardized tests that are culturally relevant and contain appropriate norms.** Even then, understand the limitations of standardized tests. Review each individual test item to ensure it is appropriate for the individual's culture (Mattes & Omark, 1991). For example, in certain rural agricultural areas of California, some children of migrant farm workers may never have seen an elevator or an escalator. A child's inability to identify one of these on a test might lead you to an inaccurate conclusion regarding the child's vocabulary. However, the same child may have an excellent vocabulary for various farm implements. Even though most tests are normed for a particular culture or age group, some clinicians choose to adapt and use tests with clients of different cultures or ages. This is not recommended. However, if you think you have no alternative to a certain test, you should alter the testing procedures. Changes might include increasing response time, repeating or rewording instructions, recording the response verbatim (versus marking correct versus incorrect judgments), or altering test vocabulary to reflect the cultural background of the client (Erickson & Iglesias, 1986). Remember, that you will not be able to use normative data when attempting to interpret the results of a test you have altered.

10. **Administer a test in one language at a time.** Do not present one test item in one language and another test item in a different language. If you are administering a test that has been normed for two different languages, completely administer the test in one language before administering the test in a second language.

11. **Be aware of individual differences within each culture.** Do not stereotype your client based on information you have about his or her background. Regardless of the client's ethnicity, culture, age, or gender, each client and his or her family are unique.

12. **Use a variety of methods to evaluate performance.** Do not rely on standardized test scores as the only method of assessing a client's communicative performance. Obtain information about performance in the home through interviewing family members, speech samples

audiotaped in the home, or home visits. If possible, determine how the client communicates with different individuals including various family members, friends, or colleagues. With school-age children, obtain information about their communicative and academic performance in school.

13. **Obtain case history information orally.** You may obtain some preliminary case history information in writing. However, review and verify this information with the client (Terrell & Terrell, 1993). Also, allow the client to expand on the information during the interview. Some clients may not have the reading and writing skills necessary to respond to written questions through writing. In some cases, clients may avoid writing information that they think is sensitive, but may report the same information verbally. Therefore, during the interview, give your clients and their family members the opportunity to discuss the client's medical history, developmental history, and so on.

14. **When assessing a child, ask parents to compare performance of that child with other children who are at home.** It may be difficult to find developmental or normative data for certain clients. Also, if the child has limited English skills and potential for evaluation in the native language is limited, sometimes comparing communicative development with like children yields useful information. Parents often can describe how older or younger siblings communicate. They know generally how much language their children use, what sounds they do and do not produce, what kinds of directions they follow, and what types of communicative interaction they engage in.

15. **When assessing a school-age child, ask teachers to compare performance of that child with other children in the same classroom.** Classroom teachers are an excellent source of information on children's pattern of communication. For example, you may have a 5-year-old client who is from a linguistic population for which there is little normative data on speech and language development. However, the child's teacher may have in her or his classroom several other children from the same linguistic and cultural background. The teacher can report observed speech and language behaviors of your client and how those behaviors compare to the children of similar age and culture in the class.

16. **If necessary, train test-taking skills.** Most tests provide opportunities to practice required responses (e.g., pointing to a picture or naming a picture). Individuals from certain cultural and linguistic backgrounds may need additional time and opportunities to learn the

required response. For example, some individuals may be reluctant to point, others may not be used to responding to direct questions from strangers. When you have gathered background information on your client's typical communicative behaviors prior to the assessment session, you will have an idea of what types of responses will be easier to evoke and which will require additional time and practice.

17. **If necessary, complete the evaluation during subsequent visit or visits.** As with all your clients, familiarity with the clinician and the clinical setting will help evoke more valid communicative behaviors. In addition, some cultures do not view time as a perimeter in which a task must be completed (Tomblin et al., 1994). Also, multiple samples of your client's speech and language will increase the reliability of your assessment results. During your initial evaluation session, your client may be hesitant to speak and respond to questions with only short answers, giving the impression of a limited mean length of utterance or restricted vocabulary. A sample obtained in the client's home, on a second occasion in the clinic setting, or during interaction with another family member might yield different information. Other activities, such as the initial interview and administration of standardized tests, may take more time with certain populations. As they meet with you on repeated occasions, your clients begin to feel more comfortable with you. They then are more likely to accept such intrusive activities as the oral examination.

18. **Find out what the home and school environments are like.** If possible, schedule a visit to the client's home. If your client is in school or day care, schedule a visit to that setting. Observe the client in the extraclinical settings. Find out how the client interacts with different individuals. If appropriate and practical, interview key people in your client's life. Try to understand the types of activities your client enjoys during the course of a day. If your client is a child, observe what types of toys are available at home and what types of play activities are attractive to your client. Because of time and supervisory constraints and distance from the clinic, home or school observation is not always possible. If direct observation in natural settings is not possible, seek detailed information on verbal, nonverbal, and recreational activities in which the client engages at home, school, work, and other nonclinical settings.

19. **Conduct trial speech therapy.** After you have gathered information about your client's strengths and weaknesses, conduct some trial speech therapy. This type of dynamic assessment helps you understand the client's learning strategies. This can give you information about how quickly your client learns new tasks or information and what modifications need to be made in treatment targets and procedures.

After the Evaluation

Multicultural factors affect how you analyze and interpret your assessment data. Therefore, after the evaluation is completed, take the following steps to make appropriate analyses and recommendations:

1. **Talk with your interpreter.** Let your interpreter give his or her impressions of the session. The interpreter from the same cultural background as the client's may have certain insights or knowledge that you do not. If a sample was obtained in the client's native language, analyze the results with the interpreter. Although you may not be able to obtain a complete analysis of all language structures, you should be able to obtain information regarding speech intelligibility, general vocabulary use, and basic pragmatic skills. Make as complete an analysis of language structures as practical. Review any information in need of clarification. Discuss modifications you would like the interpreter to make in future sessions.

2. **Analyze your results.** Determine if your client exhibits a language disorder in his or her primary language. Remember, a speech or language difference because of second language acquisition or dialectical variation is not a disorder. Treatment in such cases is purely elective.

3. **Schedule a follow-up session.** Find out if the client's status has changed since the last session. If it has, make a reassessment of the child's communicative performance. Review the assessment or reassessment results with the client and his or her family. If the client needs help understanding what you are saying, rephrase it. Invite the client to ask questions and allow sufficient time for the client to respond. Pay attention to the client's body language and the questions the client asks to help determine if the client appears to understand what you are saying. Vocabulary and concepts you take for granted may be new to someone outside the field of speech-language pathology and especially to someone not familiar with your communication patterns.

4. **Understand how what you are saying may be interpreted by your clients and their family members.** Remember, the importance of understanding the values of a particular culture. Your clients may be members of a group that does not believe that humans should intervene when there is a disability. Therefore, they may accept your diagnosis, but be unwilling to follow up with treatment. Other clients may believe a disability is a disgrace and not want to acknowledge its existence. Still others, may believe the disability is caused by the client's lack of trying. In all these instances, you will encounter roadblocks that you must deal with in providing effective treatment.

In essence, **flexibility**, **knowledge**, and **sensitivity** are the key concepts in assessing clients of multicultural backgrounds. Standard and standardized procedures often are not suitable with such clients. As noted, although some modification in existing procedures may be appropriate, too much departure from standardized procedures may mean that you have devised a different method of assessment. In such cases, you cannot interpret the results in the prescribed manner. For these and other reasons considered so far, you may need to devise your own assessment procedures to suit your clients. When you see a need to devise client-specific procedures, consult with your supervisor to assure reliability and validity of your procedures.

Treatment Issues

There is very little research on treatment efficacy for multicultural populations. Most clinicians use treatment procedures that are known to be effective or are based on their personal experiences. When research has not specified unique procedures needed to treat clients of specific cultural backgrounds, you only can use the standard procedures that are known to be effective. However, you should use such techniques with a great deal of caution. You should modify treatment procedures based on known cultural factors. You also should keep detailed records to document the effects of such procedures and their modifications. In planning your treatment sessions for culturally diverse clients, consider the following suggestions and consult other sources (Adler, 1993; Battle, 1998; Cheng, 1991, 1995; Hamayan & Damico, 1991; Kahmi, Pollock & Harris, 1996; Kayser, 1995; Langdon & Cheng, 1992; Mattes & Omark, 1991; Payan, 1984; Payne, 1997; Roseberry-McKibbin, 1995; Screen & Anderson, 1994; Seymour & Nober, 1998; Taylor, 1986a, 1986b; Trueba, Cheng, & Ima, 1993; Trueba, Jacobs, & Kirton, 1990; Van Keulen, Weddington, & DeBose, 1998; Westby, 1994; Yavas, 1994).

1. **Use culturally appropriate stimulus materials** "Kayser, 1995". Review stimulus items you have selected to ensure they are not offensive to your clients. For example, if your client is a vegetarian Hindu, you may want to omit stimulus pictures that show individuals eating meat, especially beef. If your client is a Muslim, you may want to avoid pictures that depict the consumption of pork. As much as possible, pictures of people should include a sample of people from your clients' culture or ethnic background. For example, if you are working with African American clients, you will want to have pictures depicting that ethnic background. However, do not use materials that depict stereotypes of the culture.

2. **Use activities that reflect your client's environment.** Because treatment sessions that are relevant to the client's culture may best hold his or her interest, use activities that are culturally relevant. For instance, if you plan to use certain kinds of games as back-up reinforcers in treatment, find out what kinds of games are popular at home. In general, choose activities that can be replicated in the client's environment. This will make treatment more meaningful and will assist with generalization and maintenance.

3. **Provide treatment in the client's natural environment.** Of course, this is not always possible or realistic. But, as much as possible duplicate your client's natural environment by using appropriate language, activities and materials.

4. **Do not schedule appointments on religious or cultural holidays.** Individuals who practice Christianity do not typically go to the dentist on December 25. Citizens of the United States do not usually attend speech therapy on July 4. Similarly, you may anticipate that clients of different religious and ethnic backgrounds may observe different holidays and events. You may not be aware of all the religious ceremonies or celebrations your clients participate in. In advance, ask your clients what days and dates are unacceptable for clinical appointments.

5. **Modify treatment procedures to suit the client.** As noted before, practical exigencies may force you to initially select a standard treatment method with your culturally different client. However, as you learn from the initial treatment sessions, you are likely to modify the treatment sessions to suit the individual client. Some of these modifications may be dictated by the cultural background of the client. In all cases, be alert to the possibility that the methods may need to be changed because of the cultural and linguistic background of the client.

6. **Collaborate with family members and other professionals.** Engage other people in your clients' treatment. In the educational setting, work closely with the classroom teacher and other educational specialists. In the medical setting, collaborate with other health care professionals. Involve family members in treatment and train them to work appropriately with your client in the home and community.

7. **Keep accurate and detailed records of treatment methods and their outcome.** You are required to keep detailed records of treatment sessions with all clients. However, with clients of culturally diverse backgrounds, this requirement is more pressing because even a method with demonstrated effectiveness may fail. You may have to make constant modifications in treatment methods. It is important that you document these modifications and their effects, so that future treatment of clients with similar cultural background may be facilitated.

8. **Learn to appreciate your clients' culture and language differences.** As you work with clients with multicultural backgrounds, it is hoped that you will learn new information about different cultures and languages. Although evaluation and treatment is individualized for each client, your knowledge of linguistic differences and varying cultural practices will be useful across clients. You will become more sensitive to clients' beliefs and more observant of behavioral variations and how they all affect assessment and treatment variables.

9. **Share your experiences with clients of differing cultural backgrounds with other clinicians.** The profession is still learning about assessing and treating clients with different cultural and linguistic backgrounds. Eventually, your professional experience in assessing and treating clients of varied backgrounds will be valuable to other clinicians as well. Therefore, when you gain experience in working with varied clients, share it with your colleagues.

There is a great need to conduct treatment efficacy research involving clients of varying linguistic and cultural backgrounds. Although some attention has been paid to assessment issues in multicultural speech-language pathology, very little attention has been paid to the potential need for unique treatment procedures for multicultural populations. Therefore, it is essential that clinicians employ empirically supported treatment procedures and make careful measurements to document their effectiveness. Dissemination of treatment outcomes with multicultural populations is equally important.

Working With an Interpreter

Earlier we noted situations that require the use of an interpreter. The interpreter helps obtain information, assists with evaluation, and helps report information to clients and family members. There are two basic types of interpreting: **consecutive interpreting** and **simultaneous interpreting**. In consecutive interpreting, an individual talks, pauses, and then the interpreter translates. In simultaneous interpreting, the interpreter translates as the individual talks. As with all aspects of assessment and treatment of communicative disorders, you will learn to use interpreters effectively as you gain more experience and knowledge. As a starting point for learning to work effectively with an interpreter, follow these suggestions:

1. **Use the same interpreter as much as possible.** If you are able to use the same interpreter on a number of occasions, both you and the

interpreter can benefit (ASHA, 1985). You will not need to spend as much time training the interpreter. Your interpreter will know your expectations and thus is likely to assist you most effectively.

2. **Use an interpreter from the same ethnic background as the client, if possible.** A qualified interpreter from the same cultural or ethnic background as your client may help you establish rapport more quickly, provide more accurate interpretation, and give valuable insights into your client's culture (Cheng, 1991).

3. **Meet with the interpreter in advance.** Even if you are working with an interpreter you have used before, arrange to meet with him or her a few minutes before the scheduled assessment time. Schedule sufficient time so you can review the planned assessment and discuss the unique aspects of the client to be evaluated. You also can clarify your expectations of the interpreter's performance. The interpreter may offer information on the client's cultural background that may be helpful in selecting assessment procedures. The extra time also may be used to provide any needed training to the interpreter.

4. **Train the interpreter to administer any new tests you will be using.** Review tests the interpreter will be administering or assisting with. After you have explained the test administration guidelines, role play test administration to help the interpreter gain experience with the test. This will give you an opportunity to correct any problems, such as improper prompting or cueing. Also, your interpreter will have a chance to ask questions and clarify any misunderstanding of your instructions.

5. **Discuss the testing format with the interpreter.** Give your interpreter an overview of the planned assessment schedule. Tell the interpreter that you may alter the assessment plan if necessary. Describe potential modifications.

6. **Describe what you want the interpreter to do in clear and simple language.** Allow time to discuss the expected skills. Include information regarding client confidentiality. Remind your interpreter that you will be the only one to make evaluative comments and diagnostic statements.

7. **Let the interpreter ask questions or make comments before meeting with the client.** You will want your interpreter to have enough time to clarify any needed information. Also, as noted before, your interpreter may have valuable information to provide about your client's culture or language.

8. **Arrange a comfortable environment.** All participants in a session (e.g., you, the client, and the interpreter) should be able to make eye

contact with each other. As you know, when talking to a client through an interpreter, you should maintain eye contact with the client. Consider that in some cultures, direct eye contact is a sign of rudeness or aggression, so adapt the intensity of eye contact as necessary.

9. **When you meet with the client, introduce yourself and the interpreter to the client.** When communicating with the client, you, not your interpreter, should take the lead. To introduce your interpreter correctly, find out in advance how the interpreter wants to be addressed.

10. **Describe your role and that of the interpreter to the client.** Do not assume that the client will automatically distinguish your role from that of your interpreter. In simple language, tell them what you will be doing and how the interpreter will help.

11. **Talk to and look at the client, not the interpreter.** Although you will not ignore the interpreter's presence, most of your comments and questions will be made while looking at the individual they are addressed to. To show your interest (and gain information through observation) maintain appropriate eye contact with the client and the accompanying persons when you talk. When the client or the accompanying persons talk, continue to maintain the eye contact, even when you must wait for interpretation to understand what has been said.

12. **Use brief sentences or paragraphs.** Remember, to accurately translate information, your interpreter must be able to recall everything you speak. Try to keep your utterances short, but do not omit any critical information. If you routinely work with the same interpreter, you may be able to increase the length of your comments. Your interpreter will become familiar with the structure of your clinical sessions and with the vocabulary used.

13. **Use a normal rate of speech and allow sufficient pauses.** Do not speak too rapidly. Again, the interpreter must be able to remember and understand what you have said (Cheng, 1991).

14. **Do not allow others to talk during the interpreting process.** You may be in a meeting with several other professionals. Even though they may not understand the client's language, during the interpreting process, everyone should be listening.

15. **After the session, discuss the session with the interpreter.** Get unclear or confusing information clarified. Also, give the interpreter an opportunity to make comments and ask questions. Learn as much as possible from the interpreter about the client's culture and communication. If you will use the interpreter again, add any sugges-

tions you have for enhancing the interpreter's skills in administering tests or translating questions and answers.

16. **Thank the interpreter for his or her assistance and pay for the service.** The interpreter is a professional. Treat your interpreter with respect. Acknowledge his or her help. If appropriate, pay your interpreter.

As our discussion so far suggests, working with clients of differing cultural backgrounds requires more than the usually required technical competence in the traditional assessment and treatment procedures. The core competence in working with diverse populations is a **broader cultural understanding**. This core competence serves as a foundation for you to learn other skills. For instance, when you have the basic multicultural competence, you can modify your professional behavior and techniques to suit individual clients with differing linguistic and cultural backgrounds.

A broader cultural understanding requires more than studying linguistic differences. True, it is necessary to understand how Black English or Spanish-influenced English differs from the standard English on phonologic, syntactic, morphologic, and pragmatic variables. However, such a knowledge in itself is not sufficient to develop cultural sensitivity and understanding. Literature on multiculturalism in speech-language pathology tends to be overly concerned with linguistic differences. As a student clinician, you should go beyond the linguistic differences. An understanding of people requires a basic study of history, geography, religion, and literature. Minimally, you should read a few books from the culture you are trying to understand. An excellent means of cultural education is to read a few literary classics from the culture.

A more personal means of learning about other cultures is to foster friendship with persons of other cultures. Students have an excellent opportunity to do this as many programs in communicative disorders now have both students and faculty who are from diverse cultural backgrounds. If you see diversity around you as an opportunity to broaden your cultural understanding and educational base, you will be enhancing your skills in working with people of diverse cultures.

PART II

Clinical Methods in Speech-Language Pathology

In Part I you learned how clinical practicum in speech-language pathology is organized. You also learned some of the rules and guidelines a student clinician must follow.

In Part II you will find an overview of how to treat adults and children who have various communicative disorders. Selection of target behaviors, treatment procedures to increase desirable communicative behaviors, procedures to decrease undesirable behaviors, and methods to promote maintenance of communicative skills are described.

7

Target Behaviors Across Disorders

Typically, you start treatment only after you have selected target behaviors for your client. Occasionally, you may experiment with a few different targets before you finalize them. In either case, formal treatment begins only after the skills you want to teach your client have been carefully selected.

Your starting point for selecting target behaviors depends on what you find out about your clients. You must first determine if the clients assigned to you have been assessed or treated at your clinic or have received any kind of clinical services at another clinic.

If the clients have received services at your clinic, you should carefully read the reports in the files. The files may contain an initial assessment (diagnostic) report, treatment reports, progress notes, and reports from other professionals. These reports help you make a rough evaluation of each client's status.

If the clients were newly referred to the clinic, you should assess them before starting treatment. Assessment procedures were described briefly in Chapter 5. Therefore in this chapter, you learn about selecting target behaviors for clients of all ages who have many types of communicative disorders.

Selection of Target Behaviors

A **target behavior** is a generic term that means any skill or action you teach a client or a student. The term is applicable to educational and medical settings. Anything a clinician teaches regardless of the professional setting is a target behavior. Therefore, it includes the whole range of skills from the normal pattern of swallow for patients with dysphagia to the appropriate use of morphological skills by a child with language delay.

You need to select target behaviors for several reasons: **First, you need to teach multiple targets to most clients.** If clients need to learn only one or a few targets, there probably is no reason to choose. However, most persons with communicative disorders are unable to produce many target behaviors. A child with an articulation disorder, for example, may not produce several phonemes. Another child with a language disorder may not produce many classes of verbal behaviors, including grammatic, semantic, or pragmatic features. Similarly, adults with aphasia, people who have had a laryngectomy, persons who are dysarthric, and children with cerebral palsy or hearing loss are unable to produce many target behaviors that are essential for everyday communication.

Second, most clients cannot learn multiple targets at once. You need to select a few behaviors for the initial treatment and continue to teach only a few behaviors at a time. You teach more complex behaviors to clients as they master simpler behaviors. Therefore, to teach most of the missing communicative behaviors, the clinician must make some initial choices. Making such choices is the selection of target behaviors.

Third, multiple targets should be sequenced. Again, this requires careful selection of behaviors. You must design a logical sequence of treatment. A sequence is necessary, because some behaviors best serve an immediate purpose of improving communication, with others capable of being deferred to a later stage in treatment. For example, it is better to teach children who are nonverbal such words as *Mommy, Daddy, juice,* or *car* than it is to teach *red, sofa,* or *triangle.* For an adult man with aphasia, it may be better to teach the forgotten name of his wife than it is to teach the name of the local football team in which he never had interest.

Fourth, some behaviors *need* to be taught before others. This, too, means selection of target behaviors. For persons who are nonverbal, it is necessary to teach a basic set of words before teaching word order or other syntactic features. Many morphologic or syntactic features are useless when a child has no basic vocabulary. Nouns and verbs need to be taught before many grammatic morphemes can be taught. For example, you cannot teach prepositions (in, on, under) to a child who does not name anything. You cannot teach the auxiliary verb *ing* to a child who does not produce any main verbs (*walk, eat*). Similarly, for children who do not produce certain speech sounds, it may be necessary to teach them at the word level before teaching them at the phrase or sentence level. Therefore, the clinician must choose target behaviors at all stages of treatment.

Approaches to Target Behavior Selection

The two main approaches to selecting target behaviors are the normative and the client-specific. In the well-established **normative approach**, you select target behaviors that are appropriate for the client in view of his or her age and the age-based norms. For example, if a 4-year-old child does not produce language behaviors appropriate for 4-year-olds, then those behaviors are the targets.

In the more recently developed **client-specific approach**, the targets that make an immediate and significant difference in the client's communication are selected regardless of the norms. In this approach, you do not necessarily follow the table of norms to select target behaviors. You teach behaviors that best serve a client's communicative, educational, and social needs. A study of the client's environment and the educational and social demands made on that client is likely to suggest relevant and useful target behaviors.

The client-specific approach is suitable for choosing targets that are **culturally and linguistically appropriate** for the individual client. Because this approach requires a careful study of each individual client, the cultural and linguistic background of the client can be assessed for the relevance of target behaviors. As we noted in Chapter 6, choosing a culturally and linguistically appropriate service model is important in the practice of speech-language pathology.

In some cases, the normative and the client-specific approaches may suggest the same target behaviors for a given client. However, in many other cases, the targets may be different. The client-specific approach is more demanding than the normative, because it requires a greater study of the individual client and his or her family and cultural background.

The two approaches contrast more for children than for adults and more in the case of speech and language targets than for other targets. More research is needed to find out the best approach to selecting target behaviors. This means that clinicians cannot automatically assume that norms are the best targets for children. Some evidence suggests that target behaviors that are especially relevant for a client may be better generalized and maintained than those that are selected with no particular regard to the needs of the client (Hegde, 1993). The client-specific approach makes clinical sense, because it takes into consideration the uniqueness of each client. Therefore, for the most part, the following guidelines on selecting target behaviors are based on the client-specific strategy.

Guidelines on Selecting Target Behaviors

Use the following guidelines to select target behaviors. The guidelines apply to various disorders of communication.

1. **Select behaviors that will make an immediate and socially significant difference in the communicative skills of the client.** Select target behaviors that will improve the client's social communication, academic achievement, and occupational performance. In treating a child with misarticulations, select those sounds that are most frequently used in conversation and misarticulated by the child and whose correct production will most improve intelligibility. In treating clients with language disorders, select words that will immediately help the client achieve basic communication. In treating clients with vocal abuse, select the most frequently exhibited abusive behaviors for reduction.

2. **Select the most useful behaviors that may be produced and reinforced at home and in other natural settings.** Such behaviors are likely to be sustained over time. Behaviors that fulfill the needs of a client tend to be produced and reinforced in home and other natural settings. Behaviors that help a client meet the demands made on him or her also tend to be produced and maintained in natural settings.

3. **Select behaviors that help expand communicative skills.** Teach words that can easily be expanded into phrases and sentences. Although all words can be expanded, some expansions may be more significant for a client than other expansions. For instance, persons with language impairment who learn such adjectives as *big* and *little* and such nouns as *cup* and *car* can expand them into *big car*, *little cup*, and so forth. Such expandable words provide more meaningful communication than what is possible with *triangle* or *refrigerator*.

4. **Select behaviors that are linguistically and culturally appropriate for the individual client.** Find out what kinds of vocabulary, language structures, and pragmatic communication patterns are valued in the culture and the family. For instance, in teaching a set of basic words to a child who lives in an extended family, kinship terms may be more important than a set of words that name objects. Talk to the parents, spouses, and other family members before you finalize the target behaviors for a client from a diverse cultural background.

Potential Target Behaviors Across Disorders

In this section, you will find a range of potential target behaviors that may be appropriate for clients of all ages and disorders of communication. You must remember that the suggested behaviors generally are appropriate, but the final selection depends on an individual client's (a) environment, (b) communicative level before starting treatment, and (c) communicative needs.

Frequent shifts are common in the theory and clinical practice in all areas of speech-language pathology. Therefore, you must read articles in various journals to find out current trends and recent advances in both what to train and how to train. Also, note that student clinicians select target behaviors for their clients only after consulting with their clinical supervisors.

A practical consideration is that each supervisor has his or her views on what to train and how. Since you want to learn various approaches, find out your supervisor's approach. Read the books or articles your supervisor recommends. A more advanced student clinician always can discuss a different approach that she or he wishes to try. Mostly, the student clinician will get the supervisor's approval to try something different. But a good start is to first learn what the supervisor has to offer.

Sometimes, student clinicians wonder whether they should use an approach learned in an academic course that may not agree with what the clinical supervisor recommends. Generally, supervisors would like you to apply your academic knowledge to clinical practice. However, some supervisors may have strong opinions about certain approaches. Therefore, discuss the different approaches with the supervisor.

If your supervisor also has taught your academic course on a disorder, review the class notes and the text used in the class. When you discuss the potential target behaviors for your client with a disorder of articulation, for example, you should review your course information. If it is still current, review the textbook you used. If it is not, read a more recently published book on articulation and phonology. When you discuss your client with your supervisor, you should be knowledgeable about the disorder under discussion.

Articulation and Phonological Disorders

The first few clients assigned to most undergraduate student clinicians may have articulation or language disorders. This is because, in the typical undergraduate academic sequence, courses on articulation disorders and language disorders are likely to precede courses on other communicative disorders. Therefore, the very first client you treat may have a disorder of articulation or language. We, therefore, start with articulation and phonological disorders.

Obviously, a client with an articulation disorder does not produce or only inconsistently produces certain speech sounds. Equally obvious is that the treatment targets are those sounds that are not produced correctly.

However, as you have found out from your academic courses, the nature of articulation disorders makes the process of selecting treatment targets a bit more complicated.

Most of the complications are due to theoretical shifts in the study of articulation and its disorders. Because of changing theories, the treatment targets for clients with articulation disorders have changed dramatically over the past few years, although some fundamentals have remained the same. Some of the changes may not be as substantial as they initially appear, but shifts in theories have suggested apparently dissimilar treatment targets for clients with articulation disorders. Student clinicians need to learn different approaches that are supported by clinical data. Therefore, the major approaches to selecting articulatory target behaviors are summarized here.

An overview of assessment of articulation was described in Chapter 5. It was pointed out there that an analysis of your assessment or reassessment data will show the types and variety of speech sound errors made by a client. You summarize the number of sounds in error, the frequency of those errors, and the types of errors. Further analysis may be made of the patterns of errors. The pattern analysis may depend either on distinctive feature theory or phonological theory. This analysis sets the stage for selecting treatment targets.

Selection of Individual Sounds for Training. Most experts agree that a mild disorder of articulation does not require a pattern analysis. Patterns may be discovered when the child misarticulates many phonemes, thus forming classes of misarticulations that are handled more efficiently as error groups. When this is not the case, the traditional sound-by-sound approach will be adequate.

Select **individual sounds** for training when one or more of the following conditions are met:

- The child's speech is generally intelligible.
- Only a few sounds are in error.
- The errors of articulation are caused by such organic factors as cleft palate, velopharyngeal insufficiency (VPI), and neurological involvement.

The meaning of *only a few sounds in error* is not always precise. The critical point is that the phonemes in error do not form significant patterns based on distinctive features or phonological processes. A few errors, even if they share distinctive features, may be handled efficiently within the sound-by-sound approach. Patterns or relations are unlikely in case of just a few misarticulations. Also, the analysis of a negligible pattern that may underlie misarticulations of a few phonemes may not add much to treatment economy or efficiency.

> ### Take the following steps to determine target behaviors through the sound-by-sound analysis:
>
> **1.** Find out if each phoneme is produced correctly or not.
> **2.** Classify errors as either substitutions, distortions, or omissions.
> **3.** Find out the word positions in which the sounds are misarticulated.
> **4.** Select the initial target sounds for training and write your target behavior statements in objective and quantitative terms.
> **5.** In the case of a child who is bilingual, multicultural, select the phonemes based on a clear understanding of the phoneme use in the client's language.

The following is an example of a target behavior statement for a child who substitutes /w/ for /r/ in all word positions:

> The target is the correct production of /r/ at 90% accuracy in conversational speech produced at the clinic and the child's home. The correct productions should be observed in all word positions and in at least three consecutive speech samples each containing a minimum of 20 opportunities for producing the target phoneme.

Note that the example of target behavior description specifies:

1. Quantitative criterion of performance (*90% correct*);
2. Response mode (*conversational speech*);
3. Response setting (*clinic and the child's home*)
4. Number of speech samples in which the target behavior productions are documented (*three samples*); and
5. Number of opportunities for producing the target phoneme in each sample (*20*).

The quantitative criteria mentioned in the example of target behavior description are only suggestive. Each of those criteria may be modified. A different response setting may be specified. For example, depending on the client, classrooms or work places may be the settings in which the target phoneme productions are documented. Discuss these criteria with your clinical supervisor who may suggest alternatives.

In writing target behavior statements, avoid such phrases as: *the client will produce /s/ in conversational speech.* Whether the target behavior will be learned or not will depend on many variables. Also, state when the client will meet the goal in probabilistic terms, not by a certain date. It is acceptable to make such probabilistic statements as: *the phoneme or phonemes are expected to be learned in 3 months of therapy given twice weekly in 30-minute sessions.*

Selection of Sound Patterns for Treatment. Theories of normal and disordered sound production have described several patterns, clusters, or classes. When a theory describes patterns of misarticulations, the treatment goal is their elimination. When a theory describes patterns of normal sound production, then the treatment goal is to teach the missing patterns to a client. Three patterns are available for selection: (1) patterns based on place-manner-voice analysis, (2) patterns based on distinctive features, and (3) patterns based on phonological processes.

Patterns Based on Place-Manner-Voice Analysis. This older method of classifying speech sounds into patterns is based on how the sounds are normally produced. In the place-manner-voice analysis, errors of substitution are classified according to similarities in the place of articulation, manner of articulation, or in the presence or absence of voicing. In this method, you find patterns in multiple substitutions that are based on **the place, manner of articulation**, or the **feature of voicing**.

Take the following steps to find patterns based on the place-manner-voicing analysis:

1. Find out all substitution errors of the client.
2. Group those substitutions that are based on place of articulation. For instance, a child may substitute lingua-alveolars for linguadentals (e.g., d/ð); or linguavelars may be substituted for lingua-alveolars (e.g., k/t; g/d).
3. Group substitutions that are based on manner of production. Sounds produced in one manner may be substituted for sounds produced in another manner. For instance, a child may substitute stops for fricatives (e.g., b/v; t/s; p/f) and glides for liquids (e.g., w/r; w/l).

4. Group substitutions that are based on voicing features. A child, for instance, may substitute voiced sounds for voiceless sounds (e.g., b/d; g/k).

5. Teach one or more sounds from each group. Probe to find out if untrained sounds in the group are produced without training (generalization). For example, teach a few fricatives to a child who substitutes stops for fricatives; teach a few voiceless sounds to a child who uses voiced sounds instead. Find out if the untrained fricatives or untrained voiceless sounds are produced. If not, teach them as well. Generalization may or may not occur; if it does, you will save clinical training time. Still, you should extend treatment to nonclinical settings for maintenance.

6. In the case of clients who are bilingual-bicultural, make this analysis with a firm knowledge of the phonology of the clients' language.

See Chapter 8 for training procedures. How to probe for generalization also is described in that chapter.

The following is an example of a target behavior description for a client who substitutes voiced sounds for voiceless sounds:

> The target is the correct production of voiceless sounds [specify them] in all word positions at 90% accuracy in conversational speech evoked at the clinic and at the child's home. The correct productions should be observed in at least three consecutive speech samples. Each speech sample should have at least 20 opportunities for producing the target phoneme.

When you write a target behavior statement for a pattern of misarticulation, you must **list the individual sounds** as well. Just saying that you will teach voiced sounds or fricatives will not be specific enough. It is likely that not all sounds in a category are in error. Even if they are, you do not teach a category or a pattern directly. You teach concrete individual sounds that belong to a conceptual category or pattern.

Patterns Based on Distinctive Features. In the 1970s, the distinctive feature approach to articulation training was researched frequently. Although researched less frequently in recent years, you may wish to learn this approach by using it with a client or two. **Distinctive features** are unique characteristics that distinguish one speech sound from the other. A feature system proposed by Chomsky and Halle (1968) has been used widely. Using a binary system of pluses and minuses, Chomsky and Halle have described 11 distinctive features of English consonants.

The distinctive feature analysis is not much different from the traditional place-manner-voice analysis (Elbert & Gierut, 1986). What is new about it—the binary system—is only a superficial application of a quantitative method with very little mathematical meaning. However, clinical training is the only way to test the validity of distinctive features. If they are valid, untrained sounds with the same features as the trained sounds should be produced on the basis of generalization. Therefore, you can do some informal clinical experimentation while using this approach. A client who is trained on a few sounds that share a set of features should begin to produce other missing sounds that have the same features without training. Reliable baselines and continuous treatment data will help you determine if this happens in treatment.

Take the following steps in using distinctive features to find patterns of misarticulations:

1. Find out all the errors of your client.
2. Determine the distinctive features shared by the phonemes in error.
3. Group misarticulated sounds on the basis of shared (common) distinctive features.
4. Teach a few sounds from each group. Probe to see if untrained sounds within the group are produced without training. If they are, reinforce them and implement a maintenance procedure.
5. Make a distinctive feature analysis of a bilingual client's misarticulations with a firm knowledge of the linguistic and phonological features of the relevant language.

The following is an example of a target behavior description for a client who substitutes nonnasal sounds for nasal sounds (d/n; b/m; g/ŋ). The assumption is that the client has not mastered the distinctive feature nasal or has not mastered the contrast between nasal and nonnasal sounds:

The target is the correct production of nasal sounds (/n,/m/, and /ŋ/) in all word positions at 90% accuracy in conversational speech evoked at the clinic and at the child's home. The correct productions should be observed in at least three consecutive speech samples. Each speech sample should have at least 20 opportunities for producing the target phoneme.

Note, again, that you should specify the sounds that you plan to teach. Do not write: *I will teach stridency*. Instead, list the sounds that share the feature stridency. You cannot teach a distinctive feature directly. You only can teach some sounds that have certain features. The value of the method, as pointed out, is in monitoring potential production of untrained sounds. The system simply makes it easier to track the effects of treating some sounds on other, untrained sounds.

Patterns Based on Phonological Processes. Most experts now recommend a phonological approach to organize target behaviors for persons with multiple misarticulations resulting in limited speech intelligibility (Bernthal & Bankson, 1993; Hodson, 1980; Stoel-Gammon & Dunn, 1985). There are several phonological process analyses that are not totally compatible. Ultimately, your systematic clinical work will help you select the one that has worked the best. Eventually, you may modify an approach in light of your experience and use it consistently. Meanwhile, clinical research may show that a particular approach is better than others. During your clinical practicum, you may experiment with different approaches or use the one suggested by your supervisor.

You should know the basic phonological processes to select the appropriate processes for a given client. Though there is no full agreement among experts on the total number of processes, the following are most frequently described in the literature and are categorized as shown (Bernthal & Bankson, 1993; Stoel-Gammon & Dunn, 1985).

Frequently used phonological processes include the following:

I. Syllable Structure Processes. In these processes, the structure of syllables is changed.

Final consonant deletion. Certain final consonants are omitted.

[ba] for *ball*; [da] *Daddy*.

Unstressed syllable deletion. An unstressed initial or medial syllable is omitted.

[medo] for *tomato*; [təfon] for *telephone*.

Reduplication. A syllable, part of a syllable, or a monosyllabic word is repeated.

[wawa] for *water*; [gogo] for *go*.

Epenthesis. Addition of an unstressed sound, often the vowel [ʌ].

[bʌ lak] for *black*; [bʌɪg] for *big*.

Cluster reduction. Most frequently, omission of a sound in a cluster of sounds; sometimes, one of the sounds of a cluster may be deleted and another may be substituted.

[bu] for *blue*; [cod] for *cold*; [no] for *snow*; [fi] for *tree*.

II. **Substitution Processes.** In these processes, target sounds are replaced by other sounds. These processes often involve changes based on place of articulation or manner of articulation.

The following two processes are based on **a shift in place of articulation**:

Fronting. A sound typically produced in the back is replaced by the one produced in the front of the oral cavity.

[ti] for *key*; [su] for *shoe*.

Backing. A sound typically produced in the front is replaced by the one produced in the back of the oral cavity.

[gu] for *do*; [kæn] for *tan*.

The following processes are based on **a shift in the manner of articulation**:

Gliding of liquids. A glide is produced instead of a liquid; observed also in consonant clusters.

[wʌn] for *run*; [bwo] for *blow*.

Stopping. A stop is produced instead of a fricative or an affricate.

[tʌn] for *sun*; [du] for *zoo*.

Affrication. An affricate is produced instead of a fricative.

[tʃu] for *shoe*; [tʃʌn] for *sun*.

Deaffrication. Affricates are replaced by sounds of other kind.

[sap] for *chop*; [dʌmp] for *jump*.

Vocalization. A vowel, typically [o] or [u] is produced instead of a syllabic liquid.

[nudu] for *noodle*; [zipu] for *zipper*.

Denasalization. A nonnasal sound is produced instead of a nasal sound (the manner of production may be similar for the target and the substituted sound).

[bud] for *moon*; [deis] for *nice*.

Glottal replacements. The glottal stop is produced instead of a sound in the final or intervocalic position.

[baʔl] for *bottle*; [tuʔ] for *tooth*.

III. **Assimilation Processes.** In these processes, one sound becomes more like another sound. In progressive assimilation, a sound is assimilated to a previous sound as in [bup] for *boot*; in regressive assimilation, a sound is assimilated to a subsequent sound, as in [bʌmp] for *jump*. Several kinds of assimilation processes are described:

Velar assimilation. A nonvelar sound changes into a velar sound.

[kok] for *coat* (progressive); [kek] for *take* (regressive).

Nasal assimilation. A nonnasal sound changes into a nasal sound.

[mani] for *bunny*; [nʌn] for *done*.

Labial assimilation. A nonlabial sound changes into a labial sound.

[pɪp] for *pit*; [bup] for *boot*.

Prevocalic voicing. A voiceless consonant in prevocalic positions is voiced.

[dam] for *Tom*; [bepɚ] for *paper*.

Devoicing of final consonants. A voiced consonant in final word positions is devoiced.

[bæk] for *bag*; [nos] for *nose*.

Metathesis is an additional phonological process in which sounds are transposed.

[ɛfəlʌnt] for elephant.
[æmənəl] for animal.
[bæksɪt] for basket.

Take the following steps to analyze and select phonological processes for intervention:

1. Select one phonological analysis procedure, as there are several somewhat incompatible approaches.
2. Following the procedure prescribed by the selected approach, record continuous speech samples, transcribe the samples, and make a process analysis.
3. Select processes and the involved target sounds for intervention. Remember, you teach specific sounds to eliminate a process.
4. In the case of a client who is bilingual, make phonological process analyses only with a firm knowledge of the clients' language and phonological features.

Most experts recommend that your initial targets should be those processes that:

- Most reduce intelligibility;
- Include sounds from different classes;
- Are outgrown soonest by normally developing children; and
- Tend to persist in children with multiple misarticulations.

When you have selected a process for remediation, write target behavior descriptions that specify what sounds will be taught. Do not simply state that the "goal of treatment is to eliminate final consonant deletion." It is both abstract and negative. Also, the reader would not know what you do to eliminate a process. Instead, specify the process to be eliminated and the sounds to be taught. For example:

The treatment goal is to eliminate the final consonant deletion process by teaching the correct production of the following consonants in word final positions: [*list the phonemes*]. The final criterion is at least 90% accuracy in the production of the target phonemes in three conversational speech samples recorded in nonclinical settings.

Note that no phonological process is eliminated without training certain individual phonemes. Also, phonological processes are theoretical ways of grouping errors; they should not be confused with treatment methods. Therefore, you should not write that: *I will be using the phonological method of treatment.*

Language Disorders

What to teach children with language problems was controversial during the times when theories of language were changing rapidly. When speech-language pathologists began to study Chomsky's transformational generative grammar in the 1960s and 1970s, other language targets seemed inappropriate. Some years later, when the semantic theory of language became popular, teaching vocabulary or grammar was considered a dated practice. Finally, when the pragmatic theory was hailed as the latest revolution in the study of language, teaching anything other than pragmatic rules was considered passé.

Though theoretical diversity persists, the magnitude of theoretical shifts has diminished. Although we are always looking over our shoulders for that next revolution, we have learned in recent years that new theories did not eliminate the need to teach what the old theory said we should. New theories only listed additional behaviors to teach. Obviously, it would be foolish to claim that we do not have to teach vocabulary or grammatical morphemes or syntactical features just because of an emphasis on pragmatic aspects of language. Because **pragmatics** is the study of social use of language, a client who does not produce words, phrases, and sentences at all has no use for pragmatics. You cannot use what you do not have. Clinically, pragmatic concerns are especially important at an advanced stage in therapy. Having established certain language behaviors, you promote their naturalistic production (McCormick & Schiefelbusch, 1990; Nelson, 1993; Owens, 1992; Reed, 1994; Schiefelbusch & Lloyd, 1988; Warren & Rogers-Warren, 1985).

In treating most if not all disorders of communication, you shape the final target behaviors from simpler behaviors. Clinicians continuously build more complex behaviors by integrating simpler ones. This is especially true of language because it is the most integrative of all communicative behaviors. Clinicians build this abstract, integrative structure by teaching simpler, concrete responses.

Student clinicians need not wonder about the final target behavior for people who are language impaired. It is always the same: **personally significant and socially useful verbal skills**. This final target often is theoretical and sometimes not achieved. Each client reaches a certain level of proficiency in learning those skills. But there is no question that we would like to take clients who are language impaired to the highest level of performance in naturalistic settings that can be achieved with the best possible techniques.

Student clinicians often wonder about the starting point. A general rule that applies to all clients is that it depends on the client. The initial selection of targets depends mostly on the existing language repertoire of a client. This is true of children and adults with language problems that may have varied etiology or associated conditions. In many children, the diagnosis may be language delay or disorder. In other children and most adult clients, it may be a language disorder associated with neurological disease or damage. In clients of any age, language disorder may be associated with mental retardation, autism, hearing impairment, physical disabilities, or other conditions. In each case, you should find out the client's communicative repertoire and build on it. A careful analysis of your assessment data will help you select the initial target behaviors.

Language Targets I. Basic Vocabulary.   For many infants and children with language delay, the initial verbal targets are a set of words. Although you should not select some standard set of canned target words for all clients, you can use a few general guidelines to select words that give a good starting point for language treatment.

Take the following steps in selecting a set of basic vocabulary for teaching:

1. **Concrete words that name specific things or actions.** For the initial targets, do not select generic or abstract words. For instance, do not try to teach such words as *toys*, *food*, or *clothes*. Instead teach specific words like *car*, *milk*, and *sock*.
2. **Names (nouns) of manipulable objects.** Teach names of toys (*car, truck, ball, balloon, train, choo choo*) the child plays with. Also, teach words that name food items (*milk, juice, cookie*), clothing and personal belongings (*shirt, sock, shoe, hat*), and names of family members (*brother, sister, mommy, daddy, grandma, grandpa*).
3. **Names of animals and pets.** Teach these names and later integrate them into short stories to expand the vocabulary and to teach sentence structures.
4. **Verbs.** Select commonly used verbs (*run, jump, hop, walk, push, laugh, smile, eat, drink*). Represent them by action that might help keep the child's interest in therapy. Once taught, use the verbs to teach basic sentence structures.

5. **Adjectives to describe objects and people.** Teach simple adjectives (*big, small, tall, short, red, green*) that can be used later to expand the client's utterances.
6. **Culturally and linguistically relevant words.** For all clients, select words that are appropriate for the cultural and linguistic background of the client.

Language Targets II. Phrases. Teach phrases when the child can produce several single words. Initially, teach two-word phrases. As the child learns more phrases, increase the number of words in utterances until the child is ready to learn morphological and syntactic elements of language.

Take the following steps to select phrases as targets to teach:

1. **Simple phrases.** Combine already learned words to form the initial target phrases to teach. For example, teach two-word utterances that are a combination of adjectives and nouns the child reliably produces (*big bull, little car, red sock*).
2. **Two-word utterances.** Combine nouns and action verbs you already have taught the client. You may teach such phrases as *boy run, kitty jump, baby eat.*
3. **Two- or three-word utterances.** Form these by combining already learned and yet to be learned words. Requests or mands are excellent for this kind of target responses. For example, teach such combinations as *want milk, more juice, cookie please,* and so forth. Other targets may include nouns and verbs: *ball hit, boy hit ball,* and *push car.*

Language Targets III. Morphological and Syntactic Elements. Start morphological training when a child can produce phrases. While teaching morphological elements, you may continue to teach new words and multi-word phrases to expand the child's verbal repertoire. Before you can teach syntactic structures, you need to teach several grammatical morphemes.

Select the following morphological features for training:

1. Morphological features that help build a language repertoire. See what features may be integrated into the existing lan-
(continued)

guage responses. You know the selected responses should be useful to the individual client so they are likely to be produced and reinforced at home.

2. **The present progressive *ing*.** This is one of the early morphological features to teach. Use the already taught noun and verb combinations to teach the use of the present progressive. For example, you could teach *boy running, Daddy coming, frog jumping, kitty eating*, and so forth.

3. **Prepositions** (*car* in *box, book* on *table*), regular plurals (*two cups, my cookies, give me marbles*), possessives (*Daddy's hat, Mommy's coat, Kitty's tail*), articles (*I want a cookie, give me the ball*), regular past tense inflections (*I missed it, he jumped, she smiled*), and irregular past tense words (*he went, I ate, she broke*).

4. **Morphological features that help expand the multi-word utterances into syntactically more correct utterances or complete sentences.** Expand the previously taught phrases into longer utterances by adding additional grammatical features. For example, by adding the auxiliary verb *is*, you can expand the multiword utterances into such sentences as *the boy* is *running, the man* is *working, the girl* is *smiling* and so forth. Copula also will help expand phrases into sentences (*The man* is *nice, the lady* is *beautiful, the dog* is *big, the cat* is *small*). Expand phrases used to teach prepositions into sentences (*car is* in *the box, book is* on *the table*).

5. **Pronouns.** Teach them by using other, already taught sentence structures (she *is walking*, he *is eating*, it *is coming*; this *is my coat*, that *is your hat*).

6. **Other grammatical morphemes and syntactic structures.** Select those that help form complex forms of sentences. For example, teach questions involving *who, what, where, why, how*, and *when*. Also, teach negative sentences involving *no, not, nothing*, and so forth.

7. **Grammatical morphemes and syntactic structures that are culturally and linguistically appropriate.** For clients who are bilingual and bicultural, select grammatical morphemes and syntactic structures with a clear knowledge of the clients' primary language and cultural background.

Language Targets IV. Functional Units and their Social Use. So far, we have described various structural elements of language that are appropriate for early and intermediate training. In the more advanced stages of language treatment, broader functional or pragmatic units should be taught. Always remember that the final goal of language intervention is to promote appropriate conversational speech in natural settings.

In speech-language pathology, **functional units** have two different meanings. In **pragmatics, functional units** mean language structures that have different speaker intentions and listener effects. Sometimes also called speech acts, functional units may express needs or feelings, control other persons, establish communication, and so forth. Other functional units include utterances that call for attention, request information, give information, request action, and respond to requests. Pragmatic structures especially relevant to conversational speech include topic initiation, topic maintenance, turn taking, and conversational repair (James, 1990; Owens, 1991, 1992). As you can see, pragmatic (functional) units are not based on the structure of language as morphologic or syntactic units are. Instead, they are based on what they do for both the speaker and the listener.

Functional units that have another meaning are described in the behavioral analysis of language. Like pragmatics, behavioral analysis also describes language in functional units. These units are not based on the structure of language. However, the **functional units in behavioral analysis** are based on a cause-effect analysis. That is, verbal behaviors are divided into different groups because the responses belonging to those groups have different causes. In a general sense, this is what pragmatic units are supposed to be, but may or may not be. From the very beginning, behavioral analysis has emphasized functional units as against structural units of language. Although initially rejected by both linguists and speech-language pathologists, alike, the basic logic of the behavioral analysis is now being appreciated, especially in language intervention (Warren & Rogers-Warren, 1985).

The basic logic of the behavioral analysis is that meaningful units of language are not structures, but cause-effect (functional) units that describe what a speaker said, why it was said, and what effects it had on the listener (Skinner, 1957; Winokur, 1976). Therefore, a functional unit specifies not just an utterance, but the circumstance under which it is produced and the effects that follow. A functional unit of verbal behavior is defined as a causal relation between an utterance, its antecedent, and its consequence. The utterance may be described structurally: It may be a word, a phrase, a sentence, and so on. The antecedent may be either an event in the environment or an internal, typically motivating state of the speaker (hunger or pain, for instance). The consequence is the effect the utterance has on a listener or listeners.

Although there are important differences between them, both pragmatics and behavioral analysis have drawn attention to **meaningful**

units of speech as they are produced in specified conditions to produce specified effects. If speech is useful, it is precisely because it affects the behavior of other persons. Language is a tool only in this sense: You can accomplish something with it. Children with language disorders lack that powerful social tool. Therefore, in language intervention, you eventually must teach conversational skills that give such children a means to express themselves and to influence others.

Research continues to be done on teaching behavioral and pragmatic functional units. These units will be refined as clinical data emerge. Also, you will find new targets as researchers describe and evaluate them.

Select the following pragmatic language categories for target behaviors:

1. **Requests or mands.** In pragmatics, requests are subdivided into requests for action, information, objects, and so on. In the behavioral analysis, all requests, commands, demands, and similar utterances are classified into single functional response units called mands. It is possible that when a client learns to make certain kinds of requests, other kinds of requests will be made without further training. Obviously, this can happen only when the client produces the basic words to make any kind of request. If not, you must first teach selected words. As you do with any other response category, teach one or two types of requests or mands and probe to see if the client begins to produce other kinds of requests or mands.

2. **Tacts or descriptive statements.** Children and adults with limited language do not readily describe or talk about events in their environment. They may not comment on things and objects that evoke speech from most people. Statements that describe and comment on things, events, and persons are called tacts in the behavioral analysis. Such statements are excellent pragmatic targets to teach. In teaching them, you should often include the conversational skills described next.

3. **Topic initiation.** This skill is emphasized in pragmatic research. Persons with language impairment do not readily start talking about a topic. Topic initiation requires that the speaker be the first one to introduce a new topic for conversation. However, with most clients with language impairment, you will have to say something to have the child begin con-

versation on a topic. For example, you may have to ask questions on a topic to prompt the client to begin talking.

4. **Topic maintenance.** Once the client begins to initiate conversation, topic maintenance becomes an appropriate target to teach. Again, persons with language impairment tend not to stay on a topic of conversation. They may shift from one topic to another without saying much about any of them. To overcome this problem, you can target progressively longer durations of speech on targeted topics of conversation.

5. **Turn taking in conversation.** Conversational speech requires that two or more individuals take turn in speaking and listening. Each person engaged in conversation is both a speaker and a listener. A person who plays only one of these roles is not a good conversational partner. Therefore, it is necessary to teach persons with language impairment to talk and to listen in an alternating manner.

6. **Conversational repair.** This is another conversational skill described in pragmatics. Many persons with language impairment fail to do something when they do not understand what is said to them. This may be why they do not continue a conversational topic. Normally, the listener who does not understand a speaker suggests this in some way to the speaker. The listener may say "tell me more about it," "I don't understand," "please speak louder," and so forth. Such statements prompt the speaker to simplify, change words, expand, and repeat to modify the utterance in these and many other ways. Both the listener actions and the speaker modifications are involved in conversational repair. Teach clients to request more information, to ask for clarification, or to say "I don't understand."

7. **Narrative skill.** A more complex language skill is to narrate events, stories, and experiences in a cohesive and chronologically correct manner. Obviously, before you target narrative skills, you must have taught many other skills, including vocabulary, morphologic features, and syntactic aspects of language.

8. **Culturally appropriate pragmatic communicative behaviors.** Pragmatic communicative behaviors are heavily culturally determined. Therefore, select pragmatic features for training only after you have made a clear analysis of the cultural communication patterns of a multicultural client.

Voice Disorders

Voice disorders include many kinds of problems. Some are related to abnormal vocal fold actions, others to oral and nasal resonance, several to physical diseases, and many to general behaviors of the client that have an impact on the health of the vocal folds. After a medical examination and a careful voice assessment, you determine the nature of the disorder and the target behaviors to be trained to eliminate that disorder (Boone & McFarlane, 1998; Case, 1996; Wilson, 1987).

Target Behaviors in Disorders of Phonation. Some disorders of phonation are caused by physical problems or diseases. Among these are paralysis and ankylosis, carcinoma, varieties of laryngeal tumors and lesions, infections, and papilloma. Other disorders of phonation are caused by abuse or misuse of the vocal mechanism.

In treating disorders of phonation that have physical causes, the necessary medical or surgical treatment is first carried out. Then the voice therapy techniques are used to improve the functioning of the vocal mechanism. When surgery removes the laryngeal structures, as in laryngectomy, you should integrate new ways of phonation or new sources of phonation into the voice therapy. In treating disorders of phonation attributable to vocal abuse or misuse, you must change the vocal and general behavior of the client. Because a majority of voice disorders are related to vocal abuse or misuse, a major task of the voice clinician is to change vocally abusive behaviors and to modify patterns of misuse.

> ### Select the following targets to treat disorders of phonation:
>
> 1. **Respiration training.** Use this target when there is evidence of faulty use of the airstream during phonation and continuous speech. A specific target is a deep enough inhalation to sustain utterances of typical length. Sustained exhalation while prolonging certain vowels is a common target.
> 2. **Muscular effort.** Some patients have difficulty in approximating their vocal folds because of unilateral cord paralysis, general fatigue, and myasthenia. Such patients need to exert muscular effort in achieving vocal fold approximations. A specific target is to teach the client to push on the arm of the chair on which he or she is sitting and phonate simultaneously. Hard glottal attacks also have been targeted for such cases.

3. **Esophageal speech.** This is a target for patients who have undergone laryngectomy. In teaching esophageal speech, target either the injection or inhalation of air; in some cases, the two may be combined. In injecting air into the esophagus, the patient is asked to first impound some air in the oral cavity and then push it back. The production of plosive consonants are especially helpful in this process. In inhaling air into the esophagus, the patient rapidly takes in air while keeping the esophagus relaxed and open. The air passing through the esophagus produces vibrating sound that is articulated into speech sounds.

4. **Phonation with artificial larynx.** An alternative target for the laryngectomee, phonation with artificial larynx, involves the use of mechanical devices to produce sound that is articulated into speech sounds.

5. **Relaxation.** When there is evidence of excessive muscular tension affecting the voice of the patient, muscular relaxation might be a useful target. Systematic relaxation of specific muscle groups is targeted.

6. **Vocal rest.** This is a target for patients with infectious or traumatic laryngitis. The patient is asked to refrain from speaking and whispering.

7. **Altered head positions.** Changing the head position while speaking often results in better voice. You must try different head positions to find a position that promotes best voice quality. Extended, flexed, or tilted head positions have all been noted to change the voice.

8. **Elimination of vocally abusive behaviors.** Target for reduction:
   a. Yelling and screaming
   b. Smoking
   c. Coughing and frequent throat clearing
   d. Excessive talking, singing, crying, or laughing
   e. Talking too much with allergic reactions and upper respiratory infection
   f. Talking in noisy situations

9. **Elimination of vocal misuse.** Reduce:
   a. Frequent use of hard glottal attack
   b. Excessively loud speaking
   c. Habitual speaking with inappropriate pitch levels
   d. Continuous speaking or singing for extended durations

(continued)

10. **Culturally appropriate vocal behaviors.** In selecting specific vocal behaviors for your multicultural voice client, consider cultural patterns of communication. For instance, an artificial larynx may or may not be culturally acceptable to certain clients. Discuss your treatment strategy with the client, the family, or both to place it within the cultural context.

Target Behaviors in Disorders of Loudness and Pitch. The term disorders of loudness and pitch is self-explanatory. Disorders of loudness include both excessive loudness or insufficient loudness of voice. Disorders of pitch include too high or too low a pitch for a given person.

Select the following target behaviors in treating disorders of pitch:

1. **Increased loudness.** This is a target for clients who speak excessively softly. Select a client-specific level of loudness.
2. **Decreased loudness.** This is a target for those who speak with excessive loudness. Again, select loudness level that is appropriate for the client.
3. **Higher pitch.** In the typical case of high-pitched male voice, target a client-specific lower pitch.
4. **Lower pitch.** In the low-pitched female voice, target a higher pitch. The target pitch is relative to the client's typical pretreatment pitch.

Target Behaviors in Disorders of Resonance. Disorders of resonance include hypernasality, hyponasality, and reduced oral resonance.

Select the following targets in treating disorders of resonance:

1. **Reduced nasal resonance on non-nasal speech sounds.** This is a target for many clients including those with hearing impairment, velopharyngeal incompetence, cleft palate, and paralysis of the velum associated with cerebral palsy, stroke, and other neurological problems. A predominant voice problem in these clients is hypernasality.

> 2. **Increased nasal resonance on nasal speech sounds.**
> This is a target for clients with hyponasality (denasality). People with hearing impairment, among others, may need this target.
> 3. **Increased oral resonance.** In some cases of resonance disorders, lack of oral resonance is a dominant problem. In them, you increase oral resonance.

Disorders of Fluency

Apparently, disorders of fluency are treated in many different ways. Historically, the targets in stuttering treatment programs have varied because of the numerous definitions of stuttering. Among other targets, increased self-confidence, reduced anxiety, resolution of social role conflict, reduction of parental concern for normal nonfluencies, improved self-image, fluent stuttering, acceptance of stuttering, modification of negative attitudes, and resolution of repressed psychological conflicts have all been targeted. That these targets may not be appropriate is suggested by lack of documented evidence for their effectiveness in reducing stuttering (Bloodstein, 1987; Hegde, 1985; Ingham, 1984).

As with all disorders, consider the client's **cultural background** to assess the clients' or the family members' dispositions toward fluency and its disorders before planning a treatment program. Discuss the clients' and their family members' views of stuttering, its origin, and remediation. Your treatment strategy may partly be dependent on what you learn from them. For instance, if the parents believe that stuttering is not modifiable, you may have to counsel them and offer scientific and professional information.

In recent years, many effective treatment programs have been researched. Although different treatment packages differ somewhat from each other, almost all of them use some or all of the targets suggested here.

> **Select the following targets in treating stuttering:**
>
> 1. **Management of airflow.** This target behavior has two components. The first is a slightly exaggerated inhalation of air. The second is a slight exhalation of air through the mouth before starting phonation. Make sure the client does not impound the air in the lungs. A small amount of air must be exhaled as soon as the peak of inhalation is reached. You may use this target for most persons who stutter, but especially with those whose stutterings are associated with mismanaged airflow.
>
> *(continued)*

2. **Gentle onset of phonation.** Teach the client to initiate phonation gently after the slight exhalation of air through the mouth. The phonatory onset should be relaxed, soft, and easy.

3. **Reduced rate of speech through syllable prolongation.** Reduce the rate of speech to a level where speech is free from stuttering. Note that the initial target speech rate is client-specific. Some have to slow down more than others to maintain a stutter-free speech. Do not reduce the rate by pauses between words or phrases; reduce it by syllable (mostly vowel) prolongation. Teach the production of phrases and sentences without gaps between words. The client should produce words as though they were a string of prolonged syllables without word boundaries.

4. **Normal prosody.** The rate reduction and explicit management of airflow and phonatory onset result in an unnatural fluency. Therefore, in the final stages of treatment, shape normal prosody including a near-normal rate, intonation, and rhythm.

5. **Maintenance of fluent conversational speech in natural settings.** This is the final target. Make sure that at the time of dismissal, the client is close to 98% fluent in the clinic. This high rate of fluency is not expected to be maintained in the natural settings. A minimum of 95% fluency must be maintained over time.

In the treatment of cluttering, another disorder of fluency, reduced rate and more deliberate articulation of speech sounds have been targeted. Teaching maintenance of intelligible and fluent speech in clutterers still is a major clinical challenge.

Neurogenic Communicative Disorders in Adults

Several types of communicative disorders are associated with neurological disease or damage. The dominant such disorders are aphasia, apraxia, dysarthria, and dementia.

Although some abnormal neurological condition is associated with these disorders of communication, the patients in this general group are highly varied. There are subgroups within each diagnostic category. Individual differences in subgroups are also significant as they are in all groups of persons with (or without) communicative problems. Therefore, a comprehensive description of target behaviors for adults and children with neurogenic communicative disorders is beyond the scope of this book. There are several books that you may read to understand the full range of target behaviors that may be selected for clients with neurogenic communicative disorders (Brookshire, 1997; Collins, 1991; Davis, 1993; Duffy, 1995; Hall, Jordan, & Robin, 1993; Helm-Estabrooks & Albert, 1991; Johns, 1985; LaPointe, 1997; Lubinski, 1991; Rosenbek, LaPointe, & Wertz, 1989; Yorkston, Beukelman, & Bell, 1988).

For neurologically affected persons who are bilingual or bicultural, it is important to have a general understanding of the first language and the cultural patterns of communication before a treatment plan can be developed. As with all disorders of communication, target behaviors selected for neurologically involved patients should be **culturally appropriate**. To do this, it is necessary to analyze the premorbid levels of education, cultural experience, and family interaction. In the case of bilingual persons, you will have to determine the language in which the treatment should be offered.

Target Behaviors for Patients With Aphasia. **Aphasia** is an impairment in understanding, formulating, and expressing language caused by brain damage. Before selecting target behaviors, the complex pattern of neurological and verbal deficits must be evaluated carefully. The individual patient's pattern of deficits will determine the selection of target behaviors. Select them only after a careful assessment of the type of aphasia, the patient's predominant problems, his or her communicative needs, and chances of some immediate success at communication. Select behaviors that are meaningful and pragmatic for the patient.

Select the following commonly suggested target behaviors for many patients with aphasia:

1. **Auditory comprehension of spoken language.** Initially, ask patients to point to named pictures, objects, or body parts. Ask yes/no questions. Later, ask for correct responses to phrases and sentences. Ask them to follow instructions. Gradually increase the complexity of speech presented to the patients.

2. **Naming responses.** Select names of objects, persons, and actions that are of immediate use to a client. Besides synonyms and antonyms, rhyming words, spelling selected words, and completing sentences with target words may all be useful targets.

(continued)

3. **Phrases and sentences.** Initial targets may be useful phrases and simple sentences. Subsequently expand the repertoire by adding a variety of sentence forms or functional units including mands (requests, commands, demands), tacts or declarative statements, wh-questions, yes-no questions, passives, and other forms. Include specific morphologic features necessary for these verbal expressions.

4. **Pragmatic aspects of language.** Teach such conversational behaviors as turn taking, topic maintenance, and narration as found appropriate.

5. **Gestures paired with verbal expressions.** If it improves communication, pair ordinary gestures or a formal system of gestures (e.g., AMERIND) with words and sentences.

6. **Writing.** Copying letters, words, and sentences; writing from dictation and spontaneous writing are the typical targets, often taught in that order.

7. **Reading skills.** First, teach reading isolated words that are useful to the patient. Next, teach silent reading (and comprehension) of materials of high interest and pragmatic value. Select reading passages from graded materials. Target more complex and longer reading passages as the patient's comprehension of read information improves.

Target Behaviors for Patients With Verbal Apraxia. **Verbal apraxia** is a motor speech disorder involving difficulty in initiating and executing movement patterns necessary to produce speech, even though there is no paralysis, weakness, or discoordination of speech muscles. It is a disorder of both articulation and prosody (Rosenbek, 1985). The difficulty is thought to be due to impaired motor planning of speech.

Damage to the motor programmer in the brain may cause apraxia of speech. Apraxia also may result from edema or damage to tissue surrounding the motor programmer. Apraxia may be associated with aphasia and dysarthrias as well. In such cases, treatment targets include those that are appropriate for aphasic and dysarthric patients.

Select the following commonly suggested target behaviors for patients with verbal apraxia:

1. **Nonspeech movements.** Target these for patients who cannot imitate speech sounds and syllables. Select those movements that are related to speech: tongue protrusion, blowing, biting the lower lip, pressing the two lips together, tongue tip movements, and so forth. These often are appropriate initial targets for patients with severe apraxia. However, generally, do not start with nonspeech movements unless attempts at starting treatment with speech movements have failed.
2. **Misarticulated but correctly imitated speech sounds.** The initial speech sounds to be treated may be those that are imitated or correctly produced with fewer trials.
3. **Sounds that are produced with visible movements of the articulators.** These also are good initial targets.
4. **Singletons and clusters.** Generally, treat them in that order, but consider the pattern of errors of individual patients.
5. **Most frequently occurring sounds.** Treat them first. Target sounds that are used less frequently or rarely for later treatment.
6. **Stressed syllables.** Select these for treatment, if your patient's performance on them is better than that on unstressed syllables. This is true of some patients.
7. **Gesturing and writing.** These are targets especially in the case of severely apraxic patients.
8. **Rhythm.** Use it as in the Melodic Intonation Therapy.
9. **Normal prosody.** Teach normal sounding intonation by systematically varying it during sentence production and continuous speech.

Target Behaviors for Patients With Dysarthrias. **Dysarthrias** are a group of speech disorders that are caused by impaired muscular control of the speech mechanism. This impairment, in turn, is caused by brain injury or various neurological diseases. Besides muscular control problems, the symptoms include respiratory, phonatory, resonance, articulatory, and prosodic problems. There are different types of dysarthrias, although, they share many common characteristics. Targets selected for a client depend on the predominant type of dysarthria and the pattern of difficulties.

Select the following commonly targeted behaviors for most dysarthric patients:

1. **Appropriate posture and tone and improved strength of muscles.** Relaxation is targeted when there is hypertonia. Induce postural adjustments that facilitate improved speech. Improved strength of the general musculature may be targeted by the physical therapist, but the speech-language pathologist's target is improved tone of muscles involved in speech production.

2. **Improved respiratory management for speech.** Improved muscle strength and appropriate postural adjustments are interrelated with this target. Teach controlled and sustained exhalation that helps produce sustained and louder speech.

3. **Improved phonatory behaviors.** Treat hyperadduction through relaxation training and hypoadduction through increased muscular effort by such means as pushing exercises.

4. **Improved articulatory skills.** Achieve improved intelligibility of speech through articulation training. Targets are syllables and words produced at slower rate rather than the production of specific sounds.

5. **Improved resonance characteristics.** To achieve this target, reduce hypernasality and increase oral resonance.

6. **Improved prosody.** Teach improved rhythm, stress, and intonation of speech. You may have to teach speech rate control as well.

7. **Nonverbal or augmentative means of communication.** For the severely impaired persons who do not benefit from verbal communication training, teach nonverbal means of communication. For others, teach augmentative means to supplement oral speech.

Target Behaviors for Patients With Dementia. **Dementia** is an acquired neurological syndrome associated with persistent or progressive deterioration in intellectual functions and behavior. Dementia is frequently associated with such neurological diseases as Alzheimer disease, Pick disease, and Parkinson disease. Dementia is diagnosed when at least three of the following five functions show evidence of impairment: (1) memory, (2) visuospatial skills, (3) emotion or personality, (4) language, and (5) cognition. Symptoms across individuals may vary; variations are especially marked at different stages of dementia. Therefore, the target behaviors selected also will depend on the kinds of impairment a patient exhibits. In the advanced stages of dementia, treatment often is limited to clinical management.

Select the following target behaviors for patients with dementia:

1. Maintenance of memory skills to the extent possible.
2. Simple daily routines.
3. Writing down instructions and information.
4. Maintaining a written list of activities.
5. Keeping records, documents, phone numbers, and so forth in an invariable place.
6. Maintaining personal care habits.
7. Management of interpersonal relations to the extent possible.

In all cases and especially in the advanced cases of dementia, the treatment target often may be the family members.

Select the following targets for treating the family members of patients with dementia:

1. Better understanding of the strengths and limitations of the patient in communicative situations (through counseling).
2. Use of gestures, facial expressions, posture, and other cues to supplement verbal expressions.
3. Clear and direct speech.
4. Asking *yes* or *no* questions (not open-ended).
5. Simple, redundant speech with short sentences.
6. Structured living environment.
7. Conversations on familiar and simple topics.
8. Specifying the referents of speech.
9. Nonprovoking behavior to reduce emotional outbursts.
10. Reduced demand on the patient.

Neurogenic Communicative Disorders in Children

A major group of children with neurogenic communicative disorders are classified as having cerebral palsy. These children will have suffered brain injury in the prenatal and perinatal period. However, brain injury suffered later in childhood may not be classified as cerebral palsy.

Brain injury in children is different from that in adults mainly because of their still developing neuromuscular system and communicative behaviors. Even so, many common effects are seen in adults and children with neuropathologies. Children with neuropathologies are a diverse group, with varied etiological factors, symptoms, and subgroup classifications. Target behaviors selected for a child depend on these factors. Therefore, you should select target behaviors after a careful assessment of both the neurophysiological status and communicative behaviors. Neurologically affected children typically need physiotherapy to improve muscle functioning. Some speech-language pathologists with special training in techniques that promote neuromotor development may combine some of those techniques with communication training methods. Because neuropathologies affect all aspects of speech, treatment targets include the fundamental processes of speech.

Select the following target behaviors for children with neuropathologies:

1. **Respiratory management for speech.** Teach the client to inhale a sufficient amount of air for speech, then exhale in a controlled manner to sustain phonation and speech, and to maintain a rhythmic pattern of inhalation and exhalation.
2. **Appropriate phonatory behaviors.** Target appropriate loudness, pitch, and voice quality.
3. **Improved resonance with or without surgical or prosthetic treatment.** Reduce hypernasality and nasal emission, and increase oral resonance.
4. **Improved articulation and intelligibility.** Teach specific speech sounds that are difficult for the individual client. Teach visible sounds, correctly imitated sounds, and sounds that are correctly produced in some contexts before other sounds. You also may consider speech muscle training to improve your client's strength, tone, and range of motion.
5. **Improved prosody.** Target appropriate stress and intonation to reduce monotonous speech.

Target Behaviors for Children with Developmental Apraxia. In some children, a form of articulation disorder is diagnosed as **developmental apraxia of speech** (Hall et al., 1993). Although adults with apraxia of speech show evidence of brain injury, children with a diagnosis of developmental apraxia of speech do not. Therefore, this diagnostic category is controversial (Thompson, 1988).

Select the following target behaviors for children diagnosed with developmental apraxia:

1. **Nonspeech movements of oral structures.** These targets should be related to speech movements.
2. **Imitation of speech sounds.** Initial targets should be visible sounds and the trials should be massed. But do not linger on these targets, because isolated sound productions are not a problem for the person with developmental apraxia.
3. **Syllables and words in which the articulatory breakdowns occur.** If the breakdowns occur only in phrases and sentences, start treatment at this level. Use words that require back-to-front and front-to-back articulatory placement (e.g., *back/cab*).
4. **Reduced rate of speech.** The target sounds in words and sentences must be produced at a slower rate and with even stress to achieve improved intelligibility.

Target Behaviors for Persons With Hearing Impairment

Hearing impairment varies from a minimal loss to profound deafness. The degree of effect on communication depends on various factors, including the age of onset, the type and degree of loss, the quality and the time of initial intervention, and many others. Even mild hearing impairment in infancy is a potential cause of speech and language problems. Severe to profound loss almost always creates significant problems of speech, language, resonance, prosody, and intelligibility.

Complete audiological and otological examinations and a thorough assessment of all aspects of communication are essential before you select target behaviors for your client who is hearing impaired. Compared to those who are hard of hearing, the deaf require a more intensive as well as extensive treatment program. The deaf need training on all aspects of speech and language production. Also, these speech and language targets are part of a carefully developed program of aural rehabilitation whose major components are the use of amplification, auditory training, and working with the family members

> ### Select the following speech and language behaviors for persons with communicative problems associated with hearing impairment:
>
> 1. **Oral language.** For the infant with hearing impairment, an early, home-based, language stimulation is started first and formal language training is initiated as soon as practical. Basic vocabulary and morphologic, syntactic, and pragmatic aspects of language are all targets.
> 2. **Speech production and improved articulation.** For the infant, the period of language stimulation is also the period of speech stimulation. The child constantly hears the speech sounds in syllables and words. Later, formal speech training is started. Teach all misarticulated target sounds; among these, fricatives, affricates, and those that are produced at the back of the mouth are especially important to teach. Also, teach correct productions of distorted vowels.
> 3. **Improved voice quality.** Children and adults who are deaf need extensive training in improving their voice quality. You may target reduced hypernasality, improved oral resonance, improved nasal resonance on nasal sounds, reduced nasal emission, and overall improved voice quality.
> 4. **Improved prosody.** With or without the help of biofeedback devices, teach improved rhythm and intonation of speech. Also, teach modified speech rate, smooth flow of words, and appropriate pitch and loudness.
> 5. **Nonoral means of communication.** For clients who cannot benefit from oral speech-language training, target nonoral means of communication. Some nonoral systems of communication are described in the next section.

Target Behaviors for Nonverbal Persons

Many children and adults with multiple physical and sensory disabilities may not master the skills of oral language needed for social communication. These people are the candidates for nonverbal means of communication.

Nonverbal persons may be candidates for several modes of communication, but most learn some oral speech. Therefore, in many children and adults, the selected nonverbal modes supplement oral speech and language. For this reason, these modes of communication are called **augmentative**. They augment (enhance, expand) oral speech. In persons with severe disabilities, the nonverbal means may be the primary mode of communication.

There are many modes of nonverbal communication. Each has its advantages and limitations. Select the one that suits a client after a careful assessment of his or her physical potential and limitations, communicative needs, cost of the system, and practicality (Musselwhite & St. Louis, 1988; Silverman, 1989).

The two major means of nonverbal communication are unaided and aided. **Unaided** means of communication do not require the use of equipment and include gestures, signs, mime, and facial expression. Incidentally, speech is also unaided communication, but our focus here is nonverbal means. **Aided** means of communication use graphic or physical symbols and equipment of various sorts, including mechanical and electronic devices. There are several unaided and aided systems of communication.

Select among the following frequently used unaided systems of communication:

1. **American Sign Language (ASL).** Considered a separate language with its own rule system, ASL is the most sophisticated and widely used system of nonverbal communication. You may teach this system to deaf persons, because most prefer it.
2. **Signed English.** In this system, signs stand for words and morphologic features. The signs parallel the word order of spoken English.
3. **Signed Exact English.** Another set of signs that closely follows the spoken and written forms of English.
4. **Amer-Ind Gestural Code.** This is not a linguistic or sign system; it is also known as American Indian Hand Talk. It has been used by peoples of various North American tribal bands to communicate with each other. It has been an excellent means of intercultural communication.
5. **Fingerspelling.** In this system, words are spelled by fingers; letters are represented by various handshapes.

Because some of the aided systems are based on computer technology, new systems are likely to emerge in the near future. You should keep in touch with recent developments and select the one that is most useful and practical for a particular client. Among the aided systems, some use symbols, pictures, and graphic devices whereas others involve electronic devices.

Select among the following aided systems of communication:

1. **Object display.** Teach the client to communicate by pointing to various objects displayed in front. Use real or miniaturized objects.
2. **Pictures, photographs, and line drawings.** Select commercially available packages or prepare them for individual clients.
3. **Traditional orthography.** English (or any other language) may be represented on a communication board. You may design boards with the letters of the language and some commonly used words and phrases. The display may be electronic.
4. **Blissymbolics.** These are a collection of semi-iconic and abstract symbols printed and pasted on a communication board. Teach individual symbols for single words and combination of symbols to form phrases and sentences. Because the symbols are not language specific, they may be read by speakers of any language.
5. **Rebuses.** In this system, words or parts of words are represented by pictographic drawings. Some of the drawings are combined with letters of the alphabet; others are more like pictures of the objects or persons.
6. **Abstract symbol systems.** There are several symbol systems that use abstract, geometric shapes whose meaning is established only by training; examples are Carrier symbols (Premack-type) or Yerkish Lexigrams. The Premack-type symbols are plastic shapes that may be arranged into phrases and sentences. The Yerkish Lexigrams contain nine geometric figures that may be combined to form messages.
7. **Braille and International Morse Code.** These use traditional orthography. Braille contains a set of tactile symbols (raised dots) traditionally used by persons who are blind. Morse code is a system of dots and dashes. Messages expressed in Morse code may be printed in English. You may use computerized electronic devices to translate and print Morse code messages.

8. **Speech generators or synthesizers.** These are electronic devices that store messages. The speaker can retrieve these messages and display them on small screens or deliver them through built-in speakers. A computer monitor may be used to display messages.

9. **Neuro-assisted devices.** Use these with the most severely disabled individuals who cannot use their hands or feet to point or type messages or activate switches by movement to deliver messages electronically. These devices do not require the speaker to move or act on the switching mechanism to generate messages. The body's electrical signals activate the device and generate messages. Both muscle action potentials and brain waves have been used to activate specially designed electric typewriters, teletypewriters, and computers. Currently, this technology is expensive and of limited use, but improvements may be expected.

Target behaviors described in this chapter should help you get started with most clients. In all cases, remember that the final treatment target is effective communication in natural settings. Throughout the treatment phase, periodically assess your client's status to find out what additional target behaviors must be taught to enhance communication. Follow the logic of moving from simple behaviors to more complex behaviors, from clinically controlled speech to speech controlled by natural events in the client's environment.

8

Treatment in Speech-Language Pathology: Concepts and Methods

In speech-language pathology, the term *treatment* includes medical and educational connotations of treating and teaching persons with communicative disorders. Most importantly, the term is used in its basic scientific sense. Treatment is an agent of change. To effect change is the main job of clinicians and educators. Any time you teach a new communicative behavior to someone or alter an existing one, you will have changed that person. Therefore, you will have treated that person.

All treatment or teaching methods are means of creating something that did not exist or changing something that did. We create or alter communicative behaviors. In speech-language pathology, **treatment** is rearranging communicative relations between speakers and their listeners. Success in treating communicative disorders depends on how effectively the clinician changes the way certain speakers and their listeners react to each other.

The rearrangement of the listener-speaker relation begins with the new ways in which the speech-language pathologist organizes his or her interaction with the client (Hegde, 1988, 1998b). The clinician manipulates stimuli and creates new stimuli that might increase the probability of appropriate communicative behaviors. For example, in a case of a child with a language delay, the clinician may bring and manipulate various objects, toys, pictures, and other stimuli that might set the stage for speech and language. The clinician may model the correct responses, ask the child to imitate those responses, prompt the child to say something, and perform other acts that might lead to a desirable response.

The rearrangement continues when the clinician responds to the child's attempts at communication in ways that are different from what the child has been accustomed to. Although the family members may have responded favorably to a nonverbal child's gestures, the clinician may not. Instead, the clinician may proceed quickly to teach words to replace gestures. When a child begins to reliably produce those target words, the clinician will expect the child to use words in communication, instead of gestures. The clinician may reinforce only the word productions. In this manner, the clinician may change the results of a child's communicative attempts. Words produce more favorable results than gestures. Consequently, the child's communicative attempts change for the better.

The final and probably the most important part of rearranging a communicative relation is to change the way family, friends, and others in the life of a client react to the client. In the case of a child with a language delay, the clinician teaches family members new ways of interacting with the child. These are the ways the clinician will have used to change the communicative behaviors by the child. Family members, teachers, and friends are taught to react the way the clinician reacted. These persons now should react differently to the child's gestures and words. These differential (discriminated) reactions help support and sustain the newly learned communicative behaviors and help eliminate old, undesirable behaviors.

Basic Methods of Treatment

To treat disorders of communication, you should perform the tasks:

1. **Evoke communicative behaviors.** Normally, no special procedures are required to evoke speech from speakers. Speech itself is a powerful stimulus. Also, events surrounding us and our internal body states provide additional stimuli to speak. However, these typical stimuli may be ineffective with persons who have a communicative disorder. Therefore, we need special stimuli to evoke speech.

2. **Create nonexistent communicative behaviors.** Many clients who seek treatment do not produce certain desirable communicative

behaviors. The task of the clinician is to create those behaviors. For example, a clinician who treats a child who has not acquired language must create verbal behaviors the child did not previously produce.

3. **Increase existing communicative behaviors.** Many other clients who seek treatment do have certain communicative behaviors in their repertoire, but the behaviors are not produced frequently enough. In such cases, the clinician's task is to increase the frequency of those behaviors. For instance, a person who stutters does speak fluently, but not often enough.

4. **Strengthen and sustain communicative behaviors.** Communicative behaviors created in the clinic or increased to a higher frequency may not be produced in the natural environment. Also, newly learned behaviors may not last. Therefore, before dismissing clients from treatment, the clinician must use procedures that help strengthen and sustain newly taught behaviors.

5. **Control undesirable behaviors.** Treatment also includes procedures that help decrease certain behaviors. These include undesirable communicative behaviors and such inappropriate behaviors as uncooperative behaviors, nonattending behaviors, crying, and other behaviors that interfere with treatment.

In this chapter, we describe procedures to create, evoke, increase, strengthen, and sustain communicative behaviors. In Chapter 9 we describe procedures to decrease undesirable and uncooperative behaviors.

How To Evoke Communicative Behaviors

Evoking procedures are special stimulus events needed to have clients in treatment produce speech. The frequently used evoking procedures include instructions, modeling, prompts, and physical stimuli.

Instructions

Instructions describe the skill to be learned. Technically, instructions set up the target behaviors. Therefore, instructions are the starting point of treatment. We often have to tell the young and the old what we want them to learn. Various instructions are used in treating disorders of articulation, language, voice, and fluency.

Instructions in Treating Articulation Disorders. In teaching the correct production of speech sounds, give instructions on how to produce them. Describe tongue positions, lip configurations, direction of airflow, mouth opening or closing, and other actions necessary to produce the target sounds. Also, describe the articulatory movements and contacts needed to produce the target sounds. While giving these instructions, model what you describe.

What follows is a sample of instructions given in treatment sessions designed to correct certain kinds of articulation disorders. You might find other examples in textbooks on articulation disorders.

Instructions to correct an interdental lisp

1. I want you to say /ʃ/(sh). While you are saying it, smile so your lips go like this (*demonstrate lip retraction*). Then, push your tongue toward your front teeth, like this (*demonstrate*). Let us see if your /ʃ/ (sh) changes for an /s/.
2. Let me hear you say /i/. OK, now make a long /i/ and as you make it, raise the tip of your tongue to blow the air through the teeth.

Instructions to teach the correct production of /l/

1. Put the tip of your tongue here (*demonstrate the correct tongue position for /l/*). Now say /ɑ/ as you lower the tip of your tongue. Did you hear [lɑ]? Good. Repeat that for me.
2. Look at the mirror. Open your mouth like this (*demonstrate a slight mouth opening to show the tongue placement*). Now say /l/.

Instruction to teach the correct production of /f/

1. Bite gently on your lower lip like this (*demonstrate*). Now as you do it, blow air like this (*demonstrate*).

Many other kinds of instructions are used in teaching the correct production of various speech sounds. When you select target sounds for a client, give some thought to how you might give instructions to produce them. Write the instructions down and practice their delivery along with demonstrations.

Instructions in Treating Language Disorders. Various aspects of language may be treatment targets for children with language delay or disorder, adults with aphasia, and children and adults with inappropriate language. In treating language disorders, instructions may be given about when to use the selected target language feature or element.

Children who have not learned language in the typical developmental process do not begin to produce elements of language when instructed about the rules of usage. For example, a child who does not produce the plural morpheme correctly will not produce it solely because the clinician has described the rules of plural usage. However, simplified descriptions of certain rules may be helpful when combined with other treatment procedures.

Different kinds of instructions may be equally effective in teaching various elements of language. Therefore, the following examples are only suggestive. You may experiment with other kinds of instructions for the same target behaviors:

Instructions to train the irregular plural morpheme

When you see one of these (*show a picture*), you say: Woman. Now, say: woman. Good. But when you see two like these, (*show a different picture*), you say: Women. Now say: women. Good.

Instructions to train the regular plural morphemes /s/

When you see one of these (*show a picture*), you say: cup. Now you say: cup. Good. But when you see two of these (*show a different picture*), you say: cups. Now say cups. Good.

Instructions to teach appropriate greeting responses

Look at the picture here. They are eating breakfast. When it is breakfast time, you say: good morning. Now say: good morning. Good. And look at this picture here. They are going to bed. When it is time to sleep, you say: good night. Say: good night. Excellent.

> **Instructions to teach correct recall
> of names to an aphasic person**
>
> When I show this picture (*the client's daughter*) and ask you who
> is this, say: Nina. Now say: Nina. Very good. But when I show
> this picture (*the client's son*), and ask who is this, say: Tom. Now
> say: Tom. That was correct!

In preparing instructions for a client in language treatment, do not describe grammar rules in linguistic terms, although, you will be teaching
behaviors that may seem to follow such rules. It is not helpful for a client
to hear you say that "Gerunds are special forms of verbs that end in *ing*."
The clients (and all speakers of any language) do not have to know the
name or definition of a grammatic feature to use it correctly.

In some cases, you may describe the conditions under which a feature
is used. For example, instead of describing the rules of verb usage, you
may demonstrate actions and describe them to show when certain verbs
are used. Whenever possible, make the conditions of usage concrete and
use pictures and arranged situations; when you instruct in rules of conversations, engage in conversations to demonstrate them.

Instructions in Treating Voice Disorders. Treatment of voice disorders in adults and children requires many instructions. Mostly, treatment
targets in voice therapy include changes in vocal quality, pitch, loudness,
or resonance. In all cases, first you must instruct your clients about the particular target and how to achieve it. Once the target behavior is established
in the clinic, you need to implement additional procedures to document its
reliable occurrence in the natural environment and to sustain it over time.
These procedures, too, require the use of instructions.

> **In treating clients with vocal hyperfunction**, sometimes
> changing the head position while talking may be beneficial. In
> such cases, you might give instructions such as:
>
> The position of your head while talking affects your voice. A
> change in head position may improve your voice. Let us try.
> (*Experiment with different head positions while the client produces
> prolonged vowels to see if a desirable change occurs.*) Now it sounds
> like your voice improves when you flex your neck downward
> so that your chin almost touches your chest. Keep your head in
> that position and say /i/. Does your voice sound better? Good.

In treating clients with reduced oral resonance, talking with a greater mouth opening is often recommended. In this case, explanation and instruction may be used:

When you talk with closed mouth, your voice sounds muffled. It sounds better if you keep your mouth open while talking. Let us try. Say /ɑ/ while you open your mouth widely. Drop your jaw and make the sound. Now close your jaw and make the same sound. Do you hear a difference? Good. Let us now practice making sounds and saying words while keeping the mouth open.

To reduce a child's vocally abusive behaviors, first you have to establish the frequency of those behaviors. For example, a child may spend much time playing with toy guns. While playing, he or she may also produce tensed and loud phonation.

To establish the baseline frequency of vocally abusive behaviors, you may instruct the parent:

During the next week, I would like you to chart how often your son plays with the toy guns making the loud sounds you have described to me. Also, chart how long he played each time. Record the date and the beginning and ending time of each episode. Once we know how often he engages in this behavior, we can design a plan to reduce it.

An adult man who has been treated to **talk with a lower pitch** in the clinic may be asked to document its maintenance in the natural environment. In this case, you may instruct the client:

I would like you to keep a record of how often you used your new pitch. Anytime you talked in your old pitch, make a note on this card (*give the client a recording sheet or card*). Also, anytime you lower the pitch, make a note. Make this kind of record for a week and bring it to the next session.

In preparing instruction for clients with voice disorders, first select the target vocal behavior and find out how that behavior may be facilitated. Make sure the selected facilitating technique works; experiment informally. Find out more about this approach in the section on **shaping voice characteristics.**

Instructions in Treating Fluency Disorders. In treating disorders of fluency, including stuttering and cluttering, instructions and demonstrations play a major role. In most stuttering treatment programs, you need to teach skills of fluent speech production. As described in Chapter 7, the most frequently used target behaviors include management of airflow, gentle phonatory onset, and reduced rate of speech through syllable stretching.

In teaching appropriate airflow management, give the following instructions:

I would like you to breathe-in a bit more air than the usual. Like this. (*Demonstrate a deeper than the usual inhalation.*) Then, immediately let a little bit of air through your mouth. Like this. (*Demonstrate a slight exhalation through open mouth.*) You try it. Make sure you do not hold the air in your lungs. As soon as you breathe in, breathe out a little bit of air.

In teaching gentle phonatory onset, you may instruct the client as:

Sometimes you start your sound abruptly and harshly. Your vocal cords work too hard when you do this. You experience too much muscular tension and effort when you start sounds abruptly and harshly. Instead, you should start your sound softly, easily, and with less effort and tension. Let us practice that.

In teaching rate reduction through syllable stretching, use the instructions:

You may have noticed that when you speak slowly, your fluency improves. Practicing a slower rate of speech is part of our treatment program. You don't want to slow down your speech by pausing between words. (*Demonstrate this.*) Instead, I would like you to reduce your overall rate by stretching the syllables of words. I want you to stretch most syllables, but the first syllable of the first few words in a sentence must be stretched more than the other syllables. Like this. (*Demonstrate syllable stretching.*)

A reduced rate also improves the fluency and intelligibility of a speaker with cluttering. In general, stuttering treatment procedures may be modified in treating cluttering.

How To Prepare Effective Instructions

The client understands the target behaviors only through your instructions and demonstrations. Unless you give effective instructions, the rest of the treatment procedures may be difficult to implement. Therefore, use the following general guidelines in preparing and delivering your instructions:

1. Select the target behavior.
2. Make an analysis of the target behavior. What topographic features distinguish the behavior? In other words, what is the shape or the form of the target behavior? How does it look, feel, or sound?
3. Find out how the target behavior can be evoked. Generally, simplify it so it can be produced by the client.
4. Write out instructions that help evoke the target behavior. Write them in simple, clear, and unambiguous words; whenever possible, use ordinary language. Especially for children, write instructions in words they can understand.
5. Do not talk down to the client. Modify your presentation depending on the judged level of the client's sophistication.
6. Rehearse the instructions. Once you gain experience, you can give instructions spontaneously. In the beginning of your clinical practicum, you should practice giving instructions before you give them to your client.
7. Do not read instructions to your client; do not deliver instructions too formally. Deliver instructions in a natural, conversational manner.
8. Make sure the client understands your instructions. Ask the client to repeat your instructions. See if the client can do what you ask him or her to do. If not, repeat your instructions, change words, add gestures, and demonstrate.
9. Repeat all or portions of your instructions whenever the client makes mistakes that suggest that the instructions are not remembered.
10. Give new instructions whenever you change the target behavior or you shift training to a higher level.

Modeling

Modeling, like instructions and other stimulus events, is a necessary part of treatment in communicative disorders. When the client does not respond correctly with instructions and other stimuli, you have to model the target response. Thus, **modeling** is the clinician's production of a client's target response. Clinical research has shown that modeling is an effective procedure in establishing many kinds of target behaviors. Therefore, modeling is one of the widely used methods of teaching new behaviors.

In some language treatment programs, the clinician may model target responses, but may not necessarily expect the child to imitate it. In most other treatment sessions, the clinician expects the client to imitate the modeled response. Note that modeling is the special stimulus provided by the clinician and imitation is the response given to this stimulus. Because imitation is a client's response, it never should be described as a treatment procedure. Modeling is a treatment procedure because it is provided by the clinician to evoke the imitated response.

Normally, a stimulus and its response are topographically different. For example, the stimulus "How are you doing?" is topographically different from the response "Fine, thank you." To be called imitation, a response should meet two criteria. First, **imitated response should be topographically similar to the modeled stimulus.** Ideally, the stimulus and the response should be identical. But in clinical training, modeling and imitation may not be identical, especially in the beginning stage. Yet, an acceptable imitation and its stimulus (modeling) should have a similar form. In case of vocal and verbal behaviors, the two should sound similar. If not, there is no imitation.

Second, **imitated response should follow the modeled stimulus immediately.** Although delayed imitation sometimes is described in the literature, the most clinically useful imitation is immediate. This is because the clinician can reinforce the immediately imitated response. Obviously, the clinician cannot reinforce the client who repeats the modeled response at another time and place. Possibly, no individual may reinforce that response.

Modeling in the Treatment of Articulation Disorders.   Probably, modeling is most frequently used in the treatment of articulation disorders. When the sounds are taught in words or in isolation, modeling is most useful. Most models are "live" in the sense that the clinician produces them in front of the client. However, taped models may be just as fine. They provide standardized stimuli; a collection of such stimuli may be useful in treating articulation disorders.

In treating articulation disorders, use modeling by:

1. First, giving instructions as described.
2. While giving such instructions, model both the articulatory movements and the target sound.
3. Ask the client to imitate the sound you modeled. Prepare a collection of taped models and use whenever necessary.

Modeling in the Treatment of Language Disorders. Modeling is necessary also in the initial stages of language teaching. In teaching words, grammatical morphemes, and various pragmatic behaviors, the clinician should model the target behaviors. A special feature of modeling language targets is that you should first ask a relevant question and then model the target (Hegde, 1998b). For example, in teaching the regular plural morpheme with the help of pictures, you should not just show the picture of two books and model "books" for the client to imitate. You should ask a question and then model the correct response. In the same example, you should ask a question such as "What do you see?" or "What are these?" and immediately model the response by saying "Say books." Similarly, in teaching words to children who are language delayed, you should show a picture or an object, ask a question, and immediately model the response. For example: "What is this? Say cat."

In treating language disorders, use modeling by:

1. Instructing the client about the modeling and imitation sequence.
2. Showing a picture or object.
3. Asking a relevant question.
4. Modeling the target response.
5. Fading or withdrawing modeling (but not the relevant question) as the imitative response is reliably produced.

When a question reliably precedes modeling, the correct response may be maintained later when modeling is withdrawn and only the question is asked. For example, assume a child consistently imitates "books," when you say "What are these? Say books." Then, you stop modeling and ask "What are these?" The child may say "books." If you did not ask the question before modeling the response, the question, introduced later, may not evoke the correct response because it is a new stimulus to which the child previously has not responded.

When the client imitates the target response consistently, you should stop modeling. Yet, when the modeled stimulus suddenly is stopped, even after the client has been imitating the target response, the response may not be produced. This is likely to happen especially when the modeled target responses are long, as they often are when the targets are grammatic features. Therefore, in many cases, you should **fade the modeled stimulus.**

In fading a modeled stimulus, progressively withdraw parts of it. Withdraw additional parts as the correct response is maintained. For example, in teaching the preposition *on*, you may have asked the question "Where is the ball?" and modeled "Say the ball is on the table." Note that the modeled stimulus is a long sentence that included other syntactic elements. In fading this modeled stimulus, first you should drop the last word. After asking the question, you model "Say the ball is on the . . .," and wait for the correct response. Ask the child to start with "The ball" as the likely response is just "table." If the child gives the correct response (the entire sentence), then on the next trial, drop another word by modeling only "Say the ball is on . . . ." Make sure the child repeats the whole target sentence. On each of the subsequent trials, drop one additional word of the modeled phrase until you ask only the question "Where is the ball?"

Modeling in the Treatment of Voice Disorders.   Various voice qualities and characteristics also need to be modeled before the client can fully understand them. For example, the desired pitch, loudness, vocal quality, and resonance characteristics must be modeled for the client. In some cases, the clinician may be unable to model a desired voice characteristic. For example, an adult male may not be able to model a target vocal pitch for a child or a woman. In such cases, the model voice may be tape recorded from another child or woman and played for the client to imitate. Also, clients themselves may provide voice models. A patient with too high a pitch may be able to produce a lower pitch with some help from the clinician. This desired pitch may be tape recorded and used as a model for the client to imitate. With appropriate software and such instruments as Visi-Pitch, many voice characteristics may be displayed on computer monitors.

In treating voice disorders, use modeling by:

1. Instructing the client in the modeling-imitation sequence.
2. Modeling the vocal target behavior.
3. Using taped models when necessary.
4. Tape recording the client's correct imitations.
5. Using the client's productions as models.
6. Fading modeling by asking the client to produce the target behavior; do not model.

Modeling in the Treatment of Fluency Disorders. In teaching such fluency skills as management of airflow, reduced rate of speech, and gentle phonatory onset to persons who stutter, you should first model each skill separately and then in combination. For example, you may start with inhalation and a slight exhalation before saying a word or two. Therefore, model as you describe inhalation and exhalation. You then add rate reduction by describing and modeling it. Model each of the subsequent targets that were described in Chapter 7.

> ### In treating fluency disorders, use modeling by:
> **1.** Instructing the client in the modeling-imitation sequence.
> **2.** In the beginning stages, modeling each of the specific fluency skills separately.
> **3.** Modeling a new skill when the earlier skill is correctly imitated.
> **4.** Modeling the combined skills in the sequence they are taught (e.g., airflow management and gentle phonatory onset).
> **5.** Modeling the entire fluency skills in words, phrases, and sentences.
> **6.** Fading modeling by asking the client to produce the target behavior; do not model.

How To Model Effectively

A clear model, produced by the clinician or a mechanical device, is effective in treatment and often necessary with most clients. With some clients, repeated modeling is indispensable. Use the following guidelines in providing effective modeling and to determine when to model, how much to model, and when to stop modeling.

1. Decide whether you will model the target response or whether taped or otherwise mechanically represented model will be used. Possibly, as clinical instrumentation becomes more sophisticated and more commonly used, mechanical models will be used more frequently. If your clinic has such instruments, use mechanical models.

2. If a client's own correct response can serve as a model, use it.

3. Model often in the early stages of treatment, because it is needed to establish the target behavior.

4. Model consistently and continuously in the beginning until the imitated responses are produced reliably. Use such objective criterion as production of five consecutively correct imitated responses before terminating modeling. Do not terminate modeling prematurely; this will unnecessarily increase the error rate.

5. Do not overuse modeling. Do not continue modeling when the client meets an objective criterion (such as five correctly imitated responses). Remember that the final target is not imitated responses but responses given to more natural stimuli.

6. Reinstate modeling when the client fails to give the correct response without it. Do not continue to evoke wrong responses by not providing the needed modeling. Reinstate modeling when two to four wrong responses are given on trials without modeling.

7. Instead of stopping suddenly, fade a complex and lengthy model. If the wrong responses return the instant you stop modeling, then drop the final element first and work your way backwards until all elements of the modeled stimulus are faded and only the question is asked.

8. Model every new target response when first introduced.

9. Model the same target response when training is moved to a higher level. For example, model the /s/ in words when you shift training from syllable to word level. Model the phoneme in phrases, and again in sentences when the training is shifted to these higher levels.

10. Reduce the frequency of modeling in the final stages of treatment. Use it least frequently when the target response is stabilized in conversational speech.

11. Ask the client to imitate your model promptly.

12. Reinforce the imitated responses. In the beginning, reinforce approximations of the model, but reinforce only promptly produced responses. On subsequent trials, reinforce progressively better approximations until the response matches the model.

Prompting

Prompts and models are similar in one important respect. Both are special stimuli that precede the target response. In all other respects, models and prompts are different.

A prompt is often a partial stimulus; whereas a modeled stimulus is full-fledged. For example when you model, you might say "Jimmy, say *the cat is jumping*"; but when you prompt the same response, you might say "Jimmy, *the cat is* . . . ." and wait for the response. All models are direct stimuli; they display the full response. **Some prompts are indirect stimuli**; they only suggest the target response instead of displaying it. For instance, to model a slower rate of speech for a person who stutters, you have to speak slowly to fully display it. But to prompt it, you may give a hand signal to suggest a slower rate. Some prompts may contain parts of the target response while others may contain no part of it. For instance, your prompt "Jimmy, *the cat is* . . .," contains some parts of the target response. But a hand gesture to slow down the rate of speech contains no part of the target response.

Some prompts are a special feature of modeled responses. For example, you might place an extra vocal emphasis on the target preposition *on* when you model: Say *the ball is **on** the table*. This vocal emphasis is a prompt within a modeled stimulus. Such an emphasis makes the target response more distinct than without the emphasis. Other ways of making a target response embedded in a string of responses distinct include increased vocal intensity, varied pitch, slower delivery than the rest of the words in the string, and injecting a pause just before its production (Hegde, 1998b).

Several **other kinds of prompts are nonverbal.** Gestures and motor behaviors, while suggesting the target response, can prompt responses. When you teach verbs, you can demonstrate action to prompt the correct word response. For example, the word jump may be prompted by a hopping motion demonstrated by your hand. You may prompt the correct production of a phoneme by showing the correct articulatory posture without saying the sound or the word. For example, you can prompt the correct production of /m/ in "Mommy" by pressing a client's lips together.

Prompts should be strong enough to evoke the desired response, but not unnecessarily strong, loud, or long. A prompt is a gentle hint. It is a minimal clue sufficient to evoke a response. Most clients find subtle prompts more acceptable than boisterous prompts. If a brief and quiet hand gesture can prompt a slower rate of speech in a person who stutters, do that and avoid lengthy verbal prompts or exaggerated nonverbal prompts.

Clients can maintain their target responses better, if their family members learn to prompt. The clinician teaches the family members to provide such prompts. These prompts used in natural settings are especially subtle. Clients are likely to find loud and lengthy prompts in these natural settings unpleasant or embarrassing, because such clues are obvious to other persons.

Like modeling, prompts also should be faded. When you observe a few consecutively correct responses to prompts, stop prompting to see if the responses will be maintained. If not, reinstate prompts. Fade prompts by reducing their topography. For example, make a particular hand gesture progressively smaller until it is completely faded out. A lengthy verbal prompt (e.g., *What do you say for this?*) may be reduced by using only some of the words or by word substitutions (e.g., *You say . . .* or *This is . . .*).

In treating articulation disorders, use prompts in the following manner:

1. Initially, prompt by naming the sound (*this word starts with an es*).
2. Use emphasis on the target sound to prompt it.
3. Later, prompt by showing only the silent articulatory positions.
4. Fade the prompts as the client becomes proficient in producing the target sounds.

In treating language disorders, use prompts as:

1. Partial modeling to prompt language structures.
2. *What do you say for this?*
3. Nonverbal prompts as movements and gestures that suggest verbs and other language targets.
4. Fade the prompts.

In treating voice disorders, use prompts as:

1. A brief model to prompt a vocal quality or characteristic.
2. Various hand gestures to prompt higher or lower pitch.
3. Other hand gestures to prompt increased or decreased vocal intensity.
4. Such nonverbal prompts as touching nose to suggest nasal resonance.
5. Fade the prompts.

In treating fluency disorders, use prompts as:

1. Prompts for each of the specific skills separately.
2. Such nonverbal prompts as hand gestures to suggest reduced rate of speech.

3. Suggesting airflow management by such nonverbal prompts as touching your nose or the chest.
4. Prompting gentle phonatory onset by touching your laryngeal area.
5. Fade the prompts.

How To Prompt Effectively

Prompting at the right time with the right clue will reduce the frequency of wrong responses. Use the following guidelines in using this technique effectively:

1. Whenever appropriate, use partial modeling to prompt the target responses. This will help fade modeling and will keep the correct response rate high.
2. Give your prompts promptly. Delayed prompts may promote delayed responses. The earliest sign of a hesitation or a wrong response is your clue to prompt.
3. Prompt more frequently in the beginning stages of treatment. Gradually reduce frequency as the correct responses become more stable and the responding becomes faster.
4. Prefer a subtle or short prompt over a loud or lengthy prompt. Prefer a silent, gestural prompt over a verbal prompt.
5. Fade prompts by making them progressively subtler or shorter.
6. Teach family members to prompt the target behaviors in a subtle manner.

Physical Stimuli

Instructions, modeling, and prompts can help evoke target behaviors in most clients. But some clients need additional stimuli. Children and adults in language therapy often need physical stimuli. In teaching words and various elements of grammar, pictures or objects may be necessary to evoke target responses. Physical stimuli may be helpful in articulation treatment as well.

Such physical stimuli as pictures and objects may be used to evoke speech in the beginning stages of treatment. In the final stages, you should evoke continuous conversational speech from all clients. Target behaviors must be stabilized in conversational speech to promote maintenance. Children who are reluctant to talk may begin to talk when you show them pictures in storybooks.

How To Effectively Use Physical Stimuli

Most adult clients with conversational skills do not need physical stimuli to evoke target responses or to maintain continuous speech. There should be no need for physical stimuli in the advanced stages of treatment when conversational speech should be the target. However, when concrete representation of target responses is needed, physical stimuli are unavoidable. Therefore, use the following guidelines in the selection and use of physical stimuli:

1. Prefer objects over pictures. If at all practical, ask the child to bring the relevant stimulus objects from home.

2. Select pictures that are three-dimensional, colorful, and realistic. Find them in popular magazines.

3. Use pictures and objects in the early stages of treatment. In later stages, especially when continuous speech is evoked, do not use pictures or use them sparingly. When the child is capable of continuous speech, do not use pictures. Find other ways of making the child talk. Talk about what interests the child.

4. If you need to use pictures in storybooks, read the story to the child and ask him or her to retell the story while looking at the pictures.

5. Discontinue the use of pictures as soon as possible. Do not overuse pictures in the later stages of treatment when conversational or more naturalistic speech should be evoked.

Creating New Responses

Many clients with severe physical disabilities resulting in communicative impairments cannot imitate modeled responses. Because of neurological problems, clients may be unable to move their articulators. Children who are nonverbal also are unable to imitate verbal responses. In treating such clients, you cannot just model the target response and expect them to imitate it. A response that is not even imitated is nonexistent in the client's repertoire. You need procedures to create new responses that do not exist.

Shaping or **successive approximation** is a highly researched method of creating new responses. The method allows you to shape a nonexistent complex response from simple responses that do exist in the client's repertoire. In each of several successive stages of treatment, you teach a simple response that takes the client one step closer to the final target response.

Breaking a target response into its simpler components is the key to shaping it (Hegde, 1998b). Even the most severely involved client may be able to make some movement that is remotely related to the target response. You then start with this movement and shape something more complex out of it by adding other components. The basic idea in shaping is that you teach what the client can learn in each step. But, you do not just evoke random responses that the client happens to learn. You teach responses that are systematically related to the final target behavior. Each new response mastered by the client should be a move in the right direction.

Manual guidance is physical assistance in shaping a response. When the client cannot make a physical movement at all, you may have to manually assist that movement and reinforce the client for any success. In manual guidance, you gently but firmly make a movement happen. For example, a boy with a severe articulation disorder may not move his tongue tip for an articulatory position. But the movement is possible, it is only not probable. Therefore, you may take a tongue depressor and move the tongue tip in the desired direction. A woman with aphasia may have great difficulty in moving her hand to point to a message on an electronic display, but the movement can be assisted by taking her hand and pointing to the message. When a boy who is profoundly retarded does not open his mouth to produce a vowel, you apply a downward pressure on the chin to make the jaw drop so the mouth is opened. A man with a high pitched voice does not produce or imitate voice of lower pitch, but as you apply a slight finger pressure on the thyroid cartilage when he produces a prolonged vowel, his pitch may drop. These are all techniques of manual guidance that help shape a target response.

Shaping Correct Articulation

To shape target phonemes, analyze them to identify their simpler components. Then, find out if the client can perform any of the components that may be used to shape the target phoneme. For example, if your client, a boy with a severe articulation problem, cannot produce a phoneme in words, can he produce it in syllables? If not in syllables, can he produce it in isolation? If not in isolation, can he move the tongue tip in the right direction? Can he make an appropriate lip movement? Can he make any kind of movement of the articulators? Can he open his mouth? If not, can you make him open his mouth with manual guidance? Can you make his tongue or lips move with manual guidance?

In treating articulation disorders, use shaping by:

1. Defining the final or the terminal target sound or syllable production.
2. Finding a simple response that the client can perform and that is related to the final target sound or syllable production.
3. Specifying intermediate responses that should be shaped.
4. Shaping the simplest response first by modeling and imitation.
5. Adding intermediate responses.
6. Continuing to shape until the final target sound or syllable production is achieved.

Shaping Language Behaviors. Children who are nonverbal and those with severe movement problems are excellent candidates for shaping. Simple, single-word utterances are the most likely initial targets for these clients. The most difficult part of treatment will be this initial stage of establishing a set of basic words. The need for shaping is greatest in this stage.

In teaching word productions to children who are nonverbal and thus do not imitate words or syllables, first you should find an articulatory movement that can be made. For example, a girl who is nonverbal may be able to open her mouth with manual guidance. With some gentle, downward pressure exerted on her chin, you may get her to open her mouth. Next, as the mouth opens, you may ask her to expel some air through the mouth. Model this and give some manual assistance; a slight push on the abdomen as the mouth opens will result in some audible expulsion of air. This audible airflow may be a basis to shape an /h/. In the successive stages, you can shape the articulatory movement for /l/ and /o/. You gradually can shape these responses into a *hello*.

In treating language disorders, use shaping by:

1. Defining the final or the terminal language response (such as the production of a word).
2. Finding a simple response that the client can perform and that is related to the final target sound or syllable production.
3. Specifying intermediate responses that should be shaped.
4. Shaping the simplest response first by modeling and imitation.
5. Adding intermediate responses.
6. Adding additional language elements to shape phrases and sentences.

Shaping Voice Characteristics. Many clients with voice disorders may be unable to imitate target voice characteristics. Therefore, shaping is a primary technique of voice therapy. In effecting changes in fundamental frequency (pitch), vocal intensity (loudness), oral or nasal resonance, hard glottal attacks, hoarseness, and harshness you may have to use shaping in the initial stages of treatment.

Clinicians also use manual guidance in voice therapy, which is often described as digital manipulation in textbooks on voice disorders (Boone & McFarlane, 1998; Case, 1996). In this procedure, your application of a slight finger pressure on the thyroid cartilage as the client produces a prolonged vowel tends to lower the pitch. The lower pitch is a result of increased mass of vocal folds due to their shortening as the digital pressure pushes the thyroid in the backward direction. Once the client achieves a lower pitch on a vowel, you must shape the pitch in producing words and phrases. The new pitch must be practiced in successively longer utterances until it is sustained in conversational speech.

In experimenting with different head positions that might facilitate a more normal sounding voice, manual guidance may be necessary. You might manually help the client change the head position to change a certain characteristic of voice. Keeping the head straight, tilting it toward the left or right side, or flexing the neck in a downward direction are all useful in changing vocal characteristics. In some cases, along with instructions and modeling, manual guidance also may be necessary.

A male speaker's high pitch is reduced in small steps. Any reduction in pitch is reinforced initially. In subsequent steps, speaking with progressively lower pitch is reinforced. The process is continued until the most desirable pitch is established. In most cases, the first step might be to produce a slightly lower pitch on single words. In the next step, the new or even lower pitch is practiced while speaking short phrases. Finally, the lower pitch is used in sentences and conversational speech. A sequence similar to this may be effective in shaping other voice targets.

In shaping target voice characteristics, you might use mechanical devices that give automatic feedback to the client. For example, Visi-Pitch, PM 100 Pitch Analyzer, and Phonatory Function Analyzer may be used in modifying the pitch of a client. An instrument called Tonar II may be used to modify nasal resonance (Boone & McFarlane, 1998). These devices work on the principle of shaping. In each successive step of treatment, the client achieves a progressively higher or lower pitch, decreased or increased nasal resonance, and so forth.

In treating voice disorders, use shaping by:

1. Defining the final or the terminal voice quality or characteristic (such as a specified vocal pitch or loudness).

(continued)

2. Selecting a simple response level at which the desired vocal target may be imitated (such as in producing a sound, syllable, or word).
3. Specifying intermediate responses that should be shaped (words, phrases, sentences).
4. Shaping the simplest response first.
5. Adding intermediate responses.
6. Shaping the desired vocal target in conversational speech.

Shaping Fluency. In treating stuttering and cluttering, skills of fluent speech are shaped in sequenced steps. Whether it is management of airflow, gentle phonatory onset, or reduced rate of speech, you must take one skill at a time and shape it. Then you put them together and have the client practice the skills starting at the one- or two-word level. As the client maintains fluency, you introduce more complex responses until the client practices fluent speech in conversational speech outside the clinic. This sequence of treatment also is based on shaping.

To reduce stuttering, you must teach interrelated skills, each carefully shaped and then integrated. In the beginning, you may start with inhalation and slight exhalation before phonatory onset. This skill may be practiced without phonation. Then, you add gentle phonatory onset. Ask the client to produce a syllable or a word. When the airflow management and gentle onset are established, add rate reduction by syllable stretching. Target single words at this stage. Before saying the word, the client should inhale, exhale slightly, achieve smooth onset, and speaks by stretching the syllables. The client should stretch especially the initial syllables and vowels.

When single word utterances are free from stuttering, ask the client to produce two-word phrases. Monitor all the skills taught so far. If the client maintains speech free from stuttering, have the client practice skills of fluent speech while producing sentences and conversational speech.

An important part of most stuttering treatment programs is to shape normal sounding prosody when stutter-free speech is established. Rate reduction through syllable stretching induces a monotonous speech that is unacceptable in the natural environment. The client is unlikely to speak at that slow rate outside the clinic. This means that fluency may not be maintained. To strengthen fluency at near-normal rate of speech, you should fade the excessively slow rate and shape normal prosody.

By allowing the client to slightly increase the rate, you can make sure that fluency is maintained while shaping normal prosody. In carefully planned steps, allow the rate to increase. Typically, increased rate brings back normal patterns of intonation. In some cases, you may have to shape intonation as well. Shaping pitch variations in conversational speech will usually be effective. Excessively slow speech tends to be too soft. Therefore, shaping louder speech will also help in reducing monotone.

In treating fluency disorders, use shaping by:

1. Defining the final or the terminal target level of fluency behavior (such as less than 5% dysfluency in conversational speech).
2. Selecting a simple response level at which the client can practice the skills of fluency (words or phrases).
3. Selecting the first fluency skill to be shaped (airflow management).
4. Shaping the skill at the simplest response level.
5. Specifying intermediate skills that should be shaped (rate reduction, gentle phonatory onset, maintaining the airflow throughout an utterance).
6. Shaping the intermediate skills.
7. Shaping the skills of fluency in conversational speech.

How To Effectively Use Shaping

As you have seen, carefully planned steps in which progressively more complex communicative behaviors are shaped are essential in the treatment of speech, language, voice, and fluency problems. Therefore, use the following general guidelines in shaping target communicative behaviors:

1. Select the final target behavior for the client. Make an analysis of this behavior so you know how to simplify it. Remember that the simplification of a target behavior is client-specific. That is, the same target phoneme, language feature, voice characteristic, or skill of fluency will have to be simplified more or less and in different ways to suit each individual client. But you should know the several ways of simplifying target communicative behaviors.

2. Experiment with each client to find out what relevant response the client can imitate. This will be the initial response to be taught. If a more complex response related to the final target can be imitated, do not select a simpler response. Simplify a response only to the extent needed, not to the extent possible. This is because you have to move the client through the simpler to the more complex final response. Generally, the more complex the initial level, the faster the treatment progress.

3. Teach progressively more complex responses; but always make sure the client is moving in the direction of the final target response.

4. Use instructions, modeling, and manual guidance at each step of training.

5. Reinforce imitated responses. To begin with, accept approximations of modeled responses. Subsequently, reinforce more accurate productions. Do not reinforce the initial and intermediate responses excessively. If you do, you will have difficulty moving the client to higher levels of training. Stabilize only the final target response.

6. Fade modeling and instructions. Also, fade any undesirable aspects of the shaped response. For example, fade the slow rate and the monotone of the treated stutterer. Fade any unusual postures you may have taught to sustain a certain voice quality.

Increasing the Frequency of Responses

Instructions, modeling, and shaping are useful in creating nonexistent communicative behaviors. But these procedures will not be effective if the client's responses do not meet certain consequences. A client's response may be a crude approximation of the modeled response, a perfectly imitated response, or a correct, unimitated response. In each case, the response may not last if certain environmental consequences do not follow it.

How to make certain consequences follow a response is the topic of this section. These consequences help increase the frequency of newly established responses. The consequences also help strengthen and sustain responses taught in treatment sessions. In this section, you will learn about procedures to increase the frequency of new responses. In the next section, you will learn about procedures to strengthen and sustain responses.

Positive Reinforcement

Normally, what the listener does when a speaker says something is the consequence for the speaker's speech. One person (a speaker) may say "Hi!" and the other (listener) may either say "Hi!" or ignore the speaker. The child might say "Mommy!" and the mother may pick up the child. Therefore, in everyday conversations, one person's speech is followed by another person's speech or nonspeech behavior. These behaviors are the consequences of speech. And, these consequences will determine if the speaker will say the same thing next time.

In treatment, especially in the initial stages, the communicative behaviors and what follow them are not as naturalistic as they typically are. For one thing, the communicative behaviors may be either absent or not effective—that is why the client is seeking help from the clinician. A child who is nonverbal, a woman with aphasia, a man with a laryngectomy, and a person who stutters each need to do something different in their attempts at communication. Therefore, clinicians set up target behaviors for them. Normally, you only respond to a speaker's communicative behavior. But clinically, you also teach your clients what or how to say and then you react to their communicative attempts in ways that are *clinical*. These clinical ways of reacting to client's speech or attempts at speech are the consequences that either increase or decrease the client's speaking behavior.

There are two kinds of consequences. One kind, when it follows a response, makes the response more likely under similar circumstances. The other kind makes the response less likely in the future. These consequences help decrease undesirable behaviors and are described in Chapter 9.

Those consequences that follow a response and increase its frequency are called **positive reinforcers.** The procedure of increasing responses by making positive reinforcers follow them is called **positive reinforcement.** To increase the frequency of new target responses, you must reinforce them positively.

Because no event will reinforce a response all the time, you should constantly evaluate their effects to see if they continue to reinforce. Initially, you should select a potential reinforcer, arrange it as an immediate consequence for a response, and watch what happens. Count the number of responses produced by the client when the consequence is being used. If the response rate increases, then you call that consequence a reinforcer. If the response rate did not increase, your potential reinforcer was not a reinforcer for that client on that occasion. Note that reinforcers always are defined after they are demonstrated to increase a response rate.

There are many types of potential positive reinforcers (Hegde, 1998b). All are known to be effective some of the time with some clients under certain conditions. Most of them will work with clients on certain occasions. However, what worked with a client during one treatment session may not work in another session. What worked with one client may not work with another client. Some of the consequences are more powerful than others. No consequence will work with every client every time.

Primary Reinforcers. Events that increase a response rate because of their biological (survival) value are called primary reinforcers. Potential primary reinforcers include food and drink.

In some cases, a response followed by food may be learned faster. It is often pointed out that food is an unnatural reinforcer for communicative behaviors. When a little girl correctly names the family dog the first time, no one puts some applesauce in her mouth. However, some communicative behaviors are reinforced primarily. For these behaviors, only the primary reinforcers will do. For example, your requests for food and drink are reinforced primarily. Therefore, it is not correct to say that speech and language behaviors are never primarily reinforced. It is correct to say that some speech and language behaviors are reinforced primarily and most are reinforced socially.

During treatment, clinicians use primary reinforcers for clinical reasons, not because they are natural. Food and drink may be used when other, more natural events do not have an effect.

In using primary reinforcers:

1. Use food and drink only when other reinforcers do not work. Expect to use them with infants and with persons who are nonverbal and profoundly retarded.
2. Before selecting primary reinforcers, discuss it with the client or, more likely, with the family members. Consider their objections or recommendations about the kinds of food to use. Select healthy food items. Avoid foods that are not recommended for medical reasons.
3. Ask parents to withhold the reinforcers before the session. Better yet, arrange treatment sessions around snack time or lunch time so that the infant or the child is motivated for your primary reinforcer.
4. Always use social reinforcers with primary reinforcers. For instance, praise a child for the correct response as you offer a sip of juice.
5. Eventually, fade the primary reinforcer and keep only the social reinforcers.

Social Reinforcers. Reinforcing effects of some events depend on past experiences. These events reinforce because of their association with other kinds of reinforcers. Events that reinforce because of past experiences are called **social**, or **conditioned, reinforcers.**

Social reinforcers are natural reinforcers for many kinds of verbal responses. In everyday communication, social reinforcers are used frequently. In communication, attention to a speaker, a smile, a nod, a touch, a pat on the shoulder, verbal approval, verbal praise, and other kinds of verbal and nonverbal responses from the listener can be potential reinforcers.

Therefore, they are preferable in treatment sessions. Even when you use primary reinforcers, you also should use social reinforcers. This means that social reinforcers are used in all stages of treatment.

In using social reinforcers:

1. With infants and clients who are profoundly retarded, use smile and touch along with primary reinforcers. Add praise and other verbal stimuli as they seem to gain reinforcing value for the client.
2. Use social reinforcers naturally. When you say "Good boy!" or "Excellent job!" or "I like that!," smile and show proper emotional expressions that go with such statements. You should sound and look happy when a correct response is produced. Use appropriate patterns of intonation so you do not sound like a robot when praising the client.
3. As you fade primary reinforcers, keep the social reinforcers.

Conditioned Generalized Reinforcers. Certain events that have a more pervasive effect on behavior are called **conditioned generalized reinforcers.** These events become reinforcing because of their association with other reinforcers. In that respect, conditioned generalized reinforcers are similar to social reinforcers.

The two are different only in one respect. An ordinary social reinforcer has to effect a change by its own power. However, a conditioned generalized reinforcer can affect a response through several other events or objects that may be gained by it. For example, a token, which is a conditioned generalized reinforcer may be effective because it can be exchanged for a variety of other reinforcers. A token is not just a token. It can mean anything you say because it can be exchanged for many other reinforcers. But verbal praise is only verbal praise. Either it is effective or it is not.

You can use plastic chips for tokens that may be exchanged for other reinforcers the child chooses in a session. Similarly, check marks entered in a booklet or stars and stickers pasted on a sheet of paper, points accumulated, marbles given, and coins earned may be exchanged for chosen reinforcers. You can use anything as a token, provided it is dispensed easily for correct responses and exchanged later for a reinforcer. This points out one important requirement of such conditioned generalized reinforcers as tokens: You should always have backup reinforcers. If you cannot afford to do that, do not use tokens. A clinician who is simply giving tokens or stickers is not to using conditioned generalized reinforcers.

Tokens are the most flexible of the reinforcers. For the child who does not respond to juice, you can offer an opportunity to play if a certain number of tokens are earned. If this does not work, you can offer to read a story for the same tokens. You may offer still other choices for the child: a small toy, a piece of gum, a walk through the clinic with you.

In using conditioned generalized reinforcers:

1. Consider the cost of a backup reinforcement system before you design a token system. Your clinic may not have any funds to purchase backup reinforcers. Do not promise a child that the parents will back up your tokens unless the parents previously have agreed to it.
2. Always have some backup reinforcers.
3. Ask the child to choose the reinforcer at the beginning of the session.
4. Tell the child how many tokens are needed to receive the backup reinforcer.
5. Do not set the number of tokens too high. The child must be able to exchange tokens for the chosen backup. If not, all the correct responses given in the session may be technically unreinforced. Therefore, set a number the child is likely to achieve.
6. Do not limit your backups to toys, food, and other tangibles. Such activities as reading a story to the child, working on a puzzle, listening to music, or taking a walk on the campus may be just as effective.

Feedback. Both adults and children wish to know how well they are doing in therapy. When that information is systematically given to them, their performance or movement toward a target may be reinforced. The information given back to a person or a mechanical system about how the person or the system has been performing is called **feedback.** Feedback is a reinforcer when it increases the rate of response or some quality of it.

Feedback became a powerful tool in changing behavior with the invention of mechanical feedback devices. These devices are especially helpful in giving information about neurophysiological activities that can not be readily observed. For example, without the help of a mechanical device, you cannot give feedback to a person about the electrical activity of muscles. Such information given back to a person about his or her neurophysiological activities through a mechanical device is called **biofeedback.**

Biofeedback is used in treating stuttering and voice disorders. Several mechanical devices are available to monitor phonatory onset, continuous phonation, and muscle tension. Several kinds of electronic units help reduce the rate of speech in those who stutterer by giving delayed auditory feedback (DAF) of their speech. Newer instruments give feedback on phonatory onset and airflow management. Electromyographic instruments help reduce a speaker's muscle tension.

Biofeedback has been successful especially in treating voice disorders. As mentioned earlier, such instruments as PM 100 Pitch Analyzer, the Phonatory Function Analyzer, and the Visi-Pitch give feedback to clients on their vocal pitch and their attempts at changing it. Nasal resonance problems may be altered by the Nasometer, which displays a ratio of oral and nasal resonance. In gradual steps, the client can increase the ratio in favor of the target resonance.

Increased use of computers in treatment will make mechanical feedback more common in therapy. Yet, feedback given to clients in treatment need not be mechanical. You may tell a man who stutters that his rate of dysfluency in the previous 5 minutes of conversation was 15% compared to 17% in the previous session. You may inform a woman that her hoarseness has been reduced some 50% over the past three sessions. A boy in articulation treatment may learn that his correct production of /s/ has increased from 30% to 90%. Such information about performance levels is feedback and when used systematically, it can increase the rate of responses.

In using feedback, follow these guidelines:

1. Always give informational feedback in a comparative manner. Say where the client was and how close the performance is to reaching the final target or some intermediate criterion of performance.
2. In working with children, show progress graphically. Use colors whenever practical. If available, use computers that provide colorful displays on the progress and movement toward the target.
3. Give feedback throughout the session so you can make it contingent on responses.
4. Combine mechanical feedback with verbal praise.
5. Do not continue to give negative feedback when the client makes little or no progress. Something is not working right. Perhaps you should change the treatment procedure or further simplify the target response.

High Probability Behaviors. An interesting fact about behavior is that **one action of a person can reinforce (increase) another action of the same person.** The behavior that reinforces is of high probability. That is, it is exhibited frequently. The behavior that is reinforced (increased), is of low probability. It is exhibited infrequently. The unique aspect of high probability behaviors as reinforcers is that both the reinforcer and the reinforced are the behaviors of the same person.

In using high probability behaviors to reinforce low probability behaviors, the clinician does not give anything except an opportunity to perform that highly desired behavior. But that opportunity is given only when the client performs what he or she is not likely to perform. Thus, the clinician increases the frequency of an unlikely behavior.

Target communicative behaviors are of low probability. The goal of treatment is to increase their frequency. To do this, first you must find a behavior that the client exhibits frequently. Does the client frequently paint, sing, read, listen to music, ski, go to movies, or talk to friends on the phone? Can any of these actions be used to reinforce target communicative behaviors under treatment?

Some high probability activities can be allowed in the treatment session itself. You may give a child 2 or 3 minutes to read a brief story or a part of a story after a certain number of correct responses are given. Opportunities to draw or paint, put puzzles together, listen to a song played on a tape recorder are among other activities that can be used to reinforce target responses in the clinic.

Opportunities for other behaviors cannot be provided in the clinic. The child cannot ski or see a movie in the treatment room. Often, these are the behaviors of highest probability with the greatest reinforcement potential. These behaviors may occur days or weeks after treatment sessions in which the target responses are produced. High probability behaviors in such cases are at best delayed reinforcers.

To bridge the gap between the eventual high probability behavior and the target responses, use a token system. Reinforce each correct response with a token. Require a certain number of tokens to engage in that cherished behavior. Obviously, in case of children, you should have the approval of parents who will make such opportunities available. In case of adults, you should have some system to verify the client's compliance with the arrangement.

> ### In using high probability behaviors as reinforcers:
>
> **1.** In talking with parents and clients, always try to find potential high probability behaviors.

2. When you use one, find a way to control unauthorized opportunities for it. You do not have a reinforcer if the client gets to ski every weekend regardless of the number of tokens earned.

3. In the beginning, require a number of tokens that will assure the opportunity for the high probability behavior. Increase the required number of tokens in gradual steps.

4. With young children, give brief but frequent breaks for the high probability behaviors.

5. Do not avoid using a behavior that takes extra time to complete. A longer story may be read in chunks. A complex puzzle may be completed in stages. Require a small number of tokens to read a few paragraphs or to fit a few pieces of the puzzle.

Instructions, modeling, shaping, and reinforcing consequences discussed so far help you create new responses and increase the frequency of new and existing responses. But to strengthen and sustain those responses, you need to use reinforcers in certain ways. Next we discuss those procedures.

Strengthening and Sustaining Target Behaviors

To strengthen and sustain responses you shape or increase, you must use reinforcers differently in different stages of treatment. A pattern of reinforcement arranged for a pattern of responses is called a **schedule of reinforcement.** One kind of schedule must be used to create and increase responses and another kind to sustain and strengthen them.

In a **continuous schedule**, every response is reinforced. This schedule is necessary in the early stage of treatment when the response needs to be shaped or increased to a higher frequency. A continuous schedule is helpful in establishing a behavior, but not in sustaining it. A continuously reinforced response is susceptible to extinction when reinforcement is stopped. After dismissal, the client may not maintain the target responses because of infrequent reinforcement or lack of it in the natural environment.

A paradoxical effect of reinforcement schedule is that responses are strengthened more when they are *not* reinforced continuously. On an **intermittent schedule**, some responses are reinforced and others are not. There are many patterns of reinforcement and nonreinforcement resulting in many intermittent schedules.

In a fixed-ratio schedule, a response is reinforced after a fixed number of unreinforced responses have been made. For example, a fixed ratio of 10, abbreviated FR10, means that you reinforce every 10th response. This schedule creates a pattern of 9 unreinforced responses and a 10th reinforced response.

A fixed-ratio schedule is easy to use and is used frequently in clinical and educational work. After a period of continuous reinforcement to establish a target response, you should switch to a fixed-ratio schedule. For example, you may initially reinforce a child continuously for naming a set of pictured stimuli. When the child's correct response rate increases substantially, say from 10% to more than 50%, you may shift to an intermittent schedule. Your first intermittent schedule may be an FR2 (every second response is reinforced). When the response rate shows a further, significant increase, you may switch the schedule again, perhaps to an FR5. A fixed ratio allows you to make a progressive reduction in the amount of reinforcement delivered for correct responses.

In a variable-ratio schedule, the number of responses required before giving a reinforcer varies around an average. Compared to a fixed ratio of 5, in which every fifth response is reinforced, in a variable ratio of 5 (VR5), an average of 5 responses are required before a reinforcer is given. Because the schedule is based on an average, the actual number of responses required on any given occasion will vary. You may reinforce the 7th response on one occasion and the 3rd on the next. The variable ratio is not a random method of reinforcement. The variable ratio is determined beforehand and reinforcers are given so as to conform to an average number of unreinforced responses.

Variable ratio produces a strong response rate. Whenever possible, use this schedule in the latter stages of treatment. Use a variable ratio schedule especially when you monitor the target behaviors in conversational speech.

Typically, a schedule specifies which behavior will be reinforced and how frequently. But there is an unusual schedule that specifies which behavior will *not* be reinforced. This schedule is called the **differential reinforcement of other behavior (DRO).** Sometimes, what matters most is that a client not exhibit a certain behavior. In such cases, there can be one or a few unacceptable behaviors, with many other acceptable behaviors that could be produced instead. So your schedule specifies what behavior or behaviors will not be reinforced. This means that many other alternative behaviors can be reinforced.

Suppose you are working with a small group of children and a boy in the group refuses to sit in his chair. He moves around and disturbs other children working on their assignments. In this case, not sitting in the chair is the troublesome behavior; instead the child could be reading, sitting quietly, working on his arithmetic, coloring, and so forth. Therefore, you tell the child that he will be reinforced provided that he does not leave the chair. You reinforce any of the desirable behaviors, including just sitting in the chair.

Two other frequently discussed schedules are the fixed interval and the variable interval. Although the ratio schedules are based on the number of responses that go unreinforced between reinforcers, the interval schedules are based on the time that lapses between reinforced responses. In a **fixed interval schedule (FI)**, an invariable period of time lapses between any two opportunities for presenting a reinforcer. In a **variable interval schedule (VI)**, the amount of time that lapses between two such opportunities is varied around an average.

An important thing to remember about the interval schedules is that the reinforcer is not automatically given after the specified fixed or variable time interval passes. The lapse of the interval creates an opportunity for reinforcement. The first response made after the interval is over is reinforced. That first response may or may not be made precisely at the end of the interval. Always remember that a reinforcer must be given immediately after a response is made.

Interval schedules have not been used frequently in treating communicative disorders, although they have some potential. In treating voice and fluency disorders, you can use interval schedules. For example, a stuttering speaker's fluent speech may be reinforced on a VI10 s (variable interval of 10 seconds). In this schedule, you reinforce if the speaker maintains fluency during 10-second intervals on the average. Similarly, a speaker with hoarseness may be reinforced for clear voice on a fixed or variable time schedule.

How To Effectively Use Reinforcement Schedules. Generally, variable ratio and variable interval schedules produce stronger responses than fixed ratio or fixed interval schedules. But all intermittent schedules produce stronger response rates than the continuous schedule. There are several other reinforcement schedules that may be helpful in treating various disorders of communication. See Hegde (1998b) for details.

In using different reinforcement schedules:

1. Begin with continuous reinforcement. During response shaping and modeling, reinforce every correct response.
2. When nonimitated response rates show a substantial increase over baselines, switch to a fixed-ratio schedule.
3. Start with a small ratio, perhaps an FR2.

(continued)

4. Increase the ratio in small steps as the correct response rates continue to increase.

5. Use a large ratio during conversational speech. An FR10 or larger should work. If possible, use a variable interval ratio.

6. If a switch to a thinner schedule of reinforcement causes a decline in the correct response rate, lower the schedule.

7. Use DRO when many desirable behaviors are incompatible with one or a few undesirable behaviors.

Sequence of Treatment

Treatment is started after you have assessed the client's communicative behaviors and selected the target behaviors. However, before you begin treatment, you must establish baselines of target behaviors.

Baselines of Target Behaviors

Baselines show a client's pretreatment response rates. Baselines are necessary to assess the client's improvement with treatment. The client's progress may be judged continuously against the baselines.

The assessment data are not enough to evaluate the client improvement in treatment because the data may be dated by the time you start treatment. More importantly, measures of communicative behaviors taken during assessment are limited, not repeated and, hence, are of questionable reliability. Therefore, you need to establish baselines just before starting treatment to get current, reliable, and comprehensive data on a client's status before treatment.

In baserating behaviors, **measures are repeated** to establish reliability. For example, instead of taking one conversational speech sample to assess articulation, language features, or stuttering, you take two or more samples to find a somewhat stable rate of those behaviors. Because you can focus only on the immediate target responses, you can afford to take more extensive measures than it is possible during assessment. For example, during assessment, you wish to find all phonemes in error; having already determined this during baserating, you only use in-depth measurement for only a few of the misarticulated phonemes that are targeted for immediate treatment. You baserate new phonemes when you are ready to teach them. This method always gives you both reliable and current pretreatment response rates.

To obtain comprehensive baselines, **responses are sampled adequately.** For example, it is not sufficient to give one or two opportunities to produce a phoneme or a grammatical morpheme. Typically, this is all a standardized test can do. Therefore, you must prepare an adequate number of stimulus materials to evoke the target responses on repeated trials. For baserating speech and language targets, roughly 20 stimulus items are needed to measure the production of target responses. When combined with repeated speech and language samples, such measures reflect pretreatment response rates more accurately than test results.

How to Baserate Target Behaviors. Use the following guidelines to baserate target behaviors:

1. Baserate only those behaviors that you plan to teach immediately. Repeat a baseline before teaching any behavior, even if it was baserated a few weeks earlier. Because behaviors tend to change, only a baseline taken just prior to treatment is valid.

2. Write instructions to the client. Also, write questions to evoke the target responses. You need questions to evoke responses to pictured stimuli. Select physical stimuli (pictures or objects).

3. Plan how you might take conversational speech samples. To sample language structures adequately, you should direct conversation so that opportunities for producing infrequently used language structures are presented. **See Appendix H for guidelines on taking and analyzing speech samples.**

4. For an articulation or language client, write at least 20 response exemplars for each target behavior. An exemplar may be a word, phrase, or sentence that contains a target response. For instance, the word *soup* or the phrase *hot soup* or the sentence *I like soup* contains the /s/, a potential target response for a child who misarticulates it. Each of those three is an exemplar. Similarly, in teaching the present progressive *ing*, you might have such exemplars as *walking*, *boy walking*, and *boy is walking*, and so forth. Your exemplars may be of one kind only. You may have 20 words, phrases, or sentences depending on the initial level of training. They are likely to be words or phrases.

5. Present the 20 stimulus items on discrete trials. A discrete trial gives the client one opportunity to produce the target response. Typically, you show the picture or object, ask a question, and wait for the response. Also, baserate imitative responses on a set of trials in which you model the responses after asking the question.

6. Take an adequate conversational speech sample. Ask the client or parents to supply taped conversational speech samples from home to assess the target behavior rate in extraclinical situations.

7. Record each response on a recording sheet. See **Appendix R for a sample discrete trial baseline recording sheet.**

8. In case of articulation and language clients, calculate the percentage correct response rate separately for discrete trials and for the conversational speech samples. Also, calculate the response rates separately for clinical speech samples and home samples. For fluency clients, calculate the percentage dysfluency rates based on the number of words spoken. For voice clients, you may calculate durations of conversational speech that are free of problems and those durations that are characterized by such problems as hoarseness or nasality.

9. If any two measures for the same response mode and situation are not comparable, repeat the measures. For instance, if two clinic speech samples show different baselines, then you need to repeat them. Similarly, if two home samples disagree widely, you need additional home samples. Home and clinic samples may vary in case of stuttering and voice characteristics. But the response rates should not vary much in case of articulation and language.

10. Write objective statements to summarize the baseline data. Such objective statements help evaluate the effects of subsequent treatment by giving a quantitative specification of a client's status before treatment:

> The child's correct articulation of /s/ in conversational speech, measured across three samples, was 20%. Each sample contained at least 10 opportunities to produce the phoneme.

> The client's rate of dysfluency on two home samples of at least 2,000 words each was 13% and 15%.

> The client's longest fluent utterances, measured over two conversational speech samples of 800 words each, typically lasted 10 seconds. (*Note:* this is a durational baserate of fluency. The measure is a statistical mode—which is the most frequently occurring event—not an average.)

The client's voice was judged hypernasal on 90% of utterances that did not contain nasal speech.

The client was hoarse 90% of the time she spoke during two baserate sessions. She spoke at least 500 words or more in each session. (*Note:* another durational baserate measure).

The patient did not recall the names of 5 of his close relatives, including his wife. The patient was asked to name them on three occasions—each separated by 24 hours.

Ten percent of the words spoken by the patient were jargon.

Table 1 shows the correct production of seven grammatic morphemes recorded across three samples. (You can present data in tabular form. In this case, you list the grammatic morphemes and the percentage correct production rate for each of them. A similar table may be prepared for a client's multiple misarticulations.)

Initial Treatment Sequence

Number of Target Behaviors. After establishing baselines, begin teaching the target behaviors. The first question you face is: How many behaviors can I teach in individual sessions? There is no single rule that you can follow in all cases. Much depends on the disorder of the client, severity of the disorder, the general learning ability of the person, age, education, and other subject characteristics. But equally important are the clinician's expertise, the duration of sessions, and whether the client is treated individually or in a group.

To start with, try the following recommendations; if they do not work, you should analyze the data to find out what went wrong:

1. Be ready to initiate training on 3 to 5 phonemes in syllables or words.
2. Plan on initiating training on 2 to 4 grammatical morphemes, syntactic structures, and other language features.
3. Be prepared to instruct and model all the basic skills of fluency in the first full session of treatment. If the session lasts at least 30 minutes, you should be able to go over the skills and initiate practice on all of them. In the case of persons who learn fast, you may be able to move from the single-word level to two-word phrases or even to short sentences in one or two sessions.
4. Expect to instruct and model the target behaviors and initiate training on voice targets in the first treatment session. If you use a feedback instrument, be ready to fully demonstrate it and start training the client on it. Depending on the client's learning rate, you may be able to move from word to phrases and sentences in the first session or two.

Structure of Treatment Sessions.   Treatment sessions may be highly structured or loosely structured. The argument you often hear about tight versus loose structure of treatment sessions is not that important. Two factors dictate the structure of treatment sessions: the client and the stage of treatment. First, a client who is minimally verbal or nonverbal or has multiple misarticulations often responds better under a structured format. Many neurologically involved patients also perform better with a structured format. Children with attention deficits need structured formats.

Second, during the early stages of treatment, most clients benefit from structured format. They can better focus on target behaviors and get used to the clinical process sooner if it is structured and somewhat simplified. However, during the latter stages of treatment, all clients need the loose format. During these stages, the target behavior is more likely to be conversational speech, which cannot be implemented within a structured, discrete-trial format.

In essence, use the tight structure if the client needs it, but use the loose structure if the client can handle it. In the latter stages of treatment, always use the loose structure, so the treatment resembles communication in natural settings.

Discrete Trial Procedure.   The initial training is better started with some structure, especially when the targets are narrowly defined articulation and language targets. Therefore, in most cases, use the structured discrete trial procedure to establish the target speech and language responses. The discrete trials are less useful or not at all needed in treating fluency and voice problems.

See Appendix M for steps in administering discrete treatment trials. In the treatment of articulation and language disorders, a discrete trial consists of (1) stimulus presentation, (2) asking a question that normally evokes the target response, (3) modeling, (4) giving a few seconds for the client to respond, (5) consequating the response, (6) recording the response, (7) marking the end of the trial by pulling the stimulus away, and (8) starting the next trial after a few seconds.

Practice the stimulus presentation so that you can administer each trial quickly and efficiently. Instruct, ask questions, and model responses as described earlier. In evaluating consequences, make a quick judgment about the accuracy of the client responses. If the response is correct, immediately reinforce it. If it is wrong, use one of the response reduction procedures described in Chapter 9. Record every response of the client on a recording sheet (See Appendix M for a sample).

Movement Through the Treatment Sequence

When the treatment is working, you will see systematic increase in a client's target behaviors. As this happens, you begin to make important clinical decisions. To take a client from the initial imitation of a narrowly defined target response to the final stage of conversational speech in natural settings, you must move from one stage of treatment to the next.

Each movement is progress. But each movement requires a clinical decision. A wrong decision made at a juncture might retard the client's progress. For example, if you spent too much time reinforcing the isolated production of a phoneme, it may be difficult for you to move the client on to the word level of training. The following general guidelines should help you make decisions to move to a different level of training. The guidelines are also clinical criteria of movement through stages of treatment.

Criteria for Clinical Decisions

When Do I Stop or Reinstate Modeling?

1. Stop modeling when the client imitates the initial target response on at least five consecutive trials.
2. Reinstate modeling when you observe incorrect responses on three to four trials with no modeling. Again, stop modeling after five correctly imitated responses. If you have to stop and reinstate modeling repeatedly, continue modeling until the client gives 10 or more imitated responses. Alternatively, see if the client can give correct responses if you continued a little longer without modeling.

Training Criteria for Target Response Versus Behaviors. To understand some of the subsequent criteria, you should make a distinction between a target response and a target behavior. As you know, you use some 20 words in teaching a phoneme. The production of each word that contains the target phoneme is a target response; the correct production of the phoneme in varied contexts and in conversational speech is the target behavior. Likewise, in teaching a grammatical morpheme, you may have some 20 or so sentences that contain that target morpheme. The production of each sentence is a target response; the production of the morpheme in varied contexts and in conversational speech is the target behavior.

Each specific response is an exemplar of the target behavior. The word soup is an exemplar of /s/ (or another phoneme in it). The word *walking* is an exemplar of the present progressive. Production of the phoneme /s/ and the present progressive in varied contexts and in natural settings are target behaviors.

When we say that a client has multiple articulation targets to learn, we do not mean the 20 or so sentences for each phoneme; we mean the number of phonemes to be taught. Similarly, when we say the child has multiple grammatic morphemes to learn, we do not mean any particular word or sentence that contains a morpheme; we mean such classes of responses as the regular plural, present progressive, an article, a preposition, and so forth (Hegde, 1998b).

You also can think of a target behavior as a group of similar responses and a target response as any one of those responses. We teach the more concrete individual responses to have the client master the more abstract target behavior.

When Is a Target Response Tentatively Trained?

A target response is tentatively trained when the client gives at least 10 consecutively correct, nonimitated responses. Suppose you were teaching a child the present progressive *ing* in words. Perhaps you were teaching four words with the target feature in it. When the child correctly produces the word *walking* 10 times in a row, you could consider that response (not the behavior) to have been tentatively learned.

Extend this logic to (1) a child under articulation training and (2) a man under voice therapy who is being trained to say individual words without nasal resonance.

> *Explanation of the Criterion.* This is a highly tentative criterion. Much work needs to be done to complete the teaching of the target behavior, but the client has met a tentative training criterion on one exemplar (response). You should stop training an exemplar at some point, and this is a suggested point. You can redefine this criterion just as appropriately as 15 or 20 consecutively correct responses.

When Is a Target Behavior Tentatively Trained?

A target behavior is tentatively trained when the client meets a tentative **probe criterion** of at least 90% correct response rate on probe trials.

The tentative training criterion for a target behavior is based on an external procedure. That is, you cannot decide that a behavior (the /s/, the present progressive, oral resonance, normal voice quality) is tentatively trained because the responses on selected training words or phrases have been correct. Instead, you conduct a probe.

Probe Procedure. To find out if the behavior meets the probe criterion, conduct probes. A **probe is a procedure** to find out if a trained response is produced on the basis of generalization. For example, a phoneme trained in a few words may be correctly produced in other, untrained words. A grammatical morpheme trained in a few sentences may be produced in other, untrained sentences. To say that a behavior is tentatively trained, you must document this generalized production.

Hold a probe when you have trained four to six target responses (e.g., four words or phrases). You may probe through discrete trials or speech samples. On **discrete trial probes**, you alternate the trained and the untrained stimuli. For example, of the 20 words you had baserated for teaching /s/ in words, assume that you have used 4 words in training. The client has met the tentative training criterion on each of those words. Now you probe to see if /s/ is tentatively trained. First, prepare a probe list on which the first word is the one already trained. The second should be one of the words not used in training. The third is again a trained word, followed by an untrained word. Reuse the trained words until all the untrained words have been alternated with them.

Do not model any words on probe trials. Show pictures to have the child name them or ask the child to read the printed words on the probe list. Reinforce the correct production of the trained words as you will have done on training trials; do not evaluate consequences to right or wrong productions of the probe words.

Count the number of correct productions of untrained words only; ignore productions of trained words. Calculate the percentage of correct untrained word productions. This is your probe response rate. If this is at least 90%, you may assume that the target behavior has been tentatively trained.

Tape-record a brief conversational speech sample, making sure that at least 20 opportunities were available for producing the target behavior. Count how many were correctly produced. Calculate the percentage correct probe rate for the conversational speech to see if it meets the criterion.

Use the same probe criterion at the level of words, phrases, or sentences. When you have completed training in sentences, use only the conversational speech probe to calculate the percent correct probe response rate.

Note that a behavior is trained only when some untrained exemplars of that behavior are produced correctly. You can use the same procedure to probe various language targets. For clients who stutter or for those who have voice problems, probes should be conducted at the relevant level of response topography (phrases, sentences, conversational speech). Record the responses without evaluating consequences to any of the behaviors. Measure the target behaviors of interest in the same way you did during baserate sessions. Calculate the percentage of probe response rates (e.g., percentage dysfluency rate or the percentage of utterances without hoarseness) and compare them against the percentages recorded during baserate sessions. **Appendix I shows a sample probe recording sheet.**

When Do I Make Topographical Shifts in Training?

Topographical shifts are made when you move to words from syllables, to phrases from words, and to sentences from words. These topographical shifts are necessary in the treatment of most disorders of communication.

It is likely that in most cases, you will have started training on three or four behaviors. The initial topographical level of training on most if not all of these behaviors may be syllables or words. The level is rarely conversational speech. But the final topographical level is always conversational speech.

The progress on multiple target behaviors under training is likely to vary. Each behavior is shaped through its own topographic sequence. One behavior may move through fewer sequences than the other. Some behaviors will meet the tentative training criterion sooner than others.

Make the first topographic shift when a behavior meets the tentative probe criterion at the initial response level. For example, when the initial probe shows 90% correct production of /s/ in untrained words, shift training to phrase level. When the phoneme production is 90% on probe phrases, shift to sentences. When the probe for sentences shows 90% correct, move to more natural conversational speech. Move again to more natural settings when within the clinic, the target phoneme is produced at 90% accuracy on conversational probes.

When one of the target behaviors meets the final criterion or any time you have extra treatment time, select another behavior for training. Start with a simple topography and move through a sequence.

Design a similar or modified sequence to training language features, fluency, and voice characteristics. Note that the probe criterion may be higher for fluency. Generally, 90% fluency is too low. A probe criterion of 97 or 98% is desirable.

What Do I Do When Probe Criteria Are Not Met?

A client may fail the probe criterion at any level of training. When this happens, give additional training at the same level. For example, the child who fails the tentative probe criterion at the word level of a phoneme training, should be trained on new exemplars. Teach two to four new exemplars before you probe again. In some cases, especially when you already have trained 8 to 10 exemplars, a few additional training trials on all of the trained exemplars may be sufficient to have the client meet the probe criterion.

When Is a Target Behavior Finally Trained?

A target behavior finally is trained when its production in conversational speech in natural settings is acceptable. Different criteria may apply to different communicative behaviors. Phonemes and language structures may be considered finally trained when they are produced in conversational speech at 90% accuracy. Fluency may be considered trained when the client's rate of dysfluencies in conversational speech in extraclinical situations does not exceed 3% or 4%. Normal voice characteristics may be considered trained when they are sustained at least 90% or 95% of utterances or of speaking time.

The target behavior is finally trained when the client is ready for dismissal. You dismiss the client from services only when the communicative behaviors are produced under natural conditions.

The various criteria described so far are suggested guidelines for making clinical decisions. They have worked in clinical research. But always remember that no criterion is a rule you cannot violate and that all criteria depend on client performance. Design your criteria that are supported by clinical data. Each client's response rates you record are your clinical data. These data are your ultimate guiding principles.

9

Controlling Undesirable Behaviors

I n Chapter 8, one of the treatment tasks described was to reduce the frequency of undesirable behaviors. While implementing procedures to increase desirable communicative behaviors, you may use procedures that reduce undesirable communicative responses. In many cases, you also must reduce undesirable general behaviors that interfere with treatment.

Often, undesirable communicative behaviors are the ones the client or the parents complain about. They are the behaviors that need to be replaced by appropriate communicative behaviors (Hegde, 1998b).

Behaviors To Be Reduced

Reduce the following **undesirable or inappropriate** communicative behaviors while working with your clients:

1. **Disorders of language.** Undesirable communicative behaviors to be reduced in clients with language disorders include among others: gesturing; crying or fussing when something is wanted; using inappropriate words or semantic, syntactic, and/or morphologic features; and inappropriate use of language in social situations.

2. **Articulation and phonological disorders.** Misarticulation of isolated speech sounds or patterns of misarticulations are the behaviors to be reduced.

3. **Voice disorders.** The behaviors to be reduced include breathiness, hoarseness, harshness, inappropriate pitch or loudness, hyper- or hyponasality, hard glottal attacks, and vocally abusive behaviors.

4. **Disorders of fluency.** In the initial stages of stuttering treatment, behaviors to be reduced include dysfluencies, speech rate, abrupt initiation of sound, inappropriate management of airflow, muscular tension associated with speech production, and avoidance of words and speaking situations. In the latter stages of treatment, you need to reduce monotonous and excessively slow speech that was targeted in the initial stages. In treating persons with cluttering, you need to reduce dysfluencies, imprecise articulation, excessively fast rate of speech, and poor organization or formulation of sentences.

You will encounter a wide array of undesirable general behaviors that **interfere** with treatment progress. Among others, you should reduce such behaviors as:

1. **Inattention.** Especially a problem with children, inattention and distractibility interfere with treatment. Unless you reduce these behaviors, you cannot concentrate on fostering the desirable target behaviors.

2. **Crying, fussing, and other emotionally laden conduct.** These are among the strong disrupters of the treatment process. They can be emotionally upsetting to the clinician who does not know how to handle them.

3. **Out-of-seat and other uncooperative behaviors.** Children who begin to move around in the therapy room, crawl under the table, or simply wiggle around in their seats cannot focus on treatment targets.

4. **Absenteeism.** A larger problem is a no-show or frequent cancellation of treatment sessions. Obviously, clients who do not attend treatment sessions cannot be helped.

5. **General unresponsivity.** Many clients show a generalized unresponsivity to treatment. Stimuli and treatment processes do not interest them. In such cases, lack of motivation for responding and working with the clinician seem to be the main problems that interfere with the treatment process.

Many clients interweave undesirable behaviors with appropriate responses. The undesirable communicative behaviors, such as the undifferentiated gestures of the nonverbal and the speech sound errors of a child with misarticulations may be more frequent in the beginning, but decline as treatment proceeds. Probably the best way of reducing undesirable communicative behaviors is to increase the desirable counterparts. For instance, the most effective way to reduce misarticulations is to increase correct productions of speech sounds.

Undesirable general behaviors that interfere with treatment often need some special procedures. An occasional interfering behavior is not a serious problem. At times, children wiggle in their chairs and fail to pay attention to the stimuli presented. These may be controlled easily by instructions and reinforcement. But when the client consistently exhibits interfering behaviors, you must take special steps.

Assessment of the Maintaining Causes of Undesirable Behaviors

If you can assess the potential maintaining causes of an undesirable behavior, you can reduce or eliminate them more efficiently. It may not always be possible to find out what maintains undesirable (or desirable) behaviors. It is difficult to say how stuttering, misarticulations, inappropriate or inadequate language, and voice quality deviations are maintained. Similarly, it is often not clear why a child is crying, wiggling in the chair, or exhibiting other interfering behaviors.

You can take some steps prior to starting treatment to find out potential maintaining variables. While establishing baselines, you may introduce the variable you suspect is maintaining an undesirable behavior to see what happens. Baselines that also are used to find out the maintaining causes of behaviors being measured are called **functional analysis baselines** (Mason & Iwata, 1990). A functional analysis helps you determine causes of behaviors.

In hindsight, successful treatment sometimes tells you what maintained an undesirable behavior. For example, you may find out that a nonverbal child's undifferentiated gestural or vocal attempts at communication have decreased after learning useful and effective verbal communication. A child who can request something in words is less likely to cry, fuss, or point to things wanted. In such a case, you might think that parental reinforcement maintained the undifferentiated attempts at communication.

In applied behavioral analysis, scientists have made systematic attempts at finding maintaining causes of some interfering behaviors. For example, studies of experimental analysis of self-injurious or self-stimulatory behaviors have suggested that these and possibly other undesirable behaviors may be maintained by either positive reinforcement, negative reinforcement, or automatic reinforcement (Durand & Carr, 1987; Iwata, Pace, Kalsher, Cowdery, & Cataldo, 1990; Repp, Felce, & Barton, 1988).

Most often, **attention is the positive reinforcer** that maintains undesirable behaviors. A teacher who otherwise ignored a child may promptly attend to a child's misbehavior, thus inadvertently reinforcing the troublesome behavior. These behaviors are most effectively reduced by **extinction** (withholding attention).

To find out if an undesirable behavior is maintained by positive reinforcement first measure the frequency of the behavior prior to treatment. Then, you pay attention to it to see if the frequency of the behavior increases. You then withdraw attention to see if the frequency of the behavior decreases. If the behavior increases as you pay attention and decreases as you ignore it, then the behavior is most likely maintained by positive reinforcement.

Negative reinforcement maintains an undesirable behavior when that behavior terminates an aversive event. For example, a child, faced with a difficult task the clinician demands (an aversive event), may exhibit an undesirable behavior (Weeks & Gaylord-Ross, 1981). Observing this behavior, the clinician may stop making those demands. In this case, the child escaped from the difficult task by exhibiting undesirable behavior. This is negative reinforcement. One way of reducing such negatively reinforced undesirable behaviors is to prevent escape by not terminating the task demand. The clinician should continue to make the demands and reinforce compliance.

To find out if an undesirable behavior is maintained by negative reinforcement, you can present some difficult tasks and see if the behavior increases in frequency. If it does, the behavior most likely is maintained by negative reinforcement. For example, you might present a series of trials on which a nonverbal child who frequently exhibits undesirable behaviors is asked to imitate relatively long and unusual words, a difficult task for the child. Having failed to give correct responses on repeated trials, the child may begin to exhibit the undesirable behavior (e. g., leaving the chair, crawling under the table). These behaviors are the child's way of escaping from a difficult (hence aversive) task demand. The escape negatively reinforces the undesirable behaviors.

Automatic reinforcement is presumed when behaviors do not seem to have environmentally generated maintaining causes. Neither externally delivered positive reinforcement nor negative reinforcement seems to account for the frequency of the behavior under observation. Therefore, undesirable behaviors are presumed to generate neural consequences that reinforce those behaviors. Lack of stimulation and activity frequently are cited reasons for undesirable behaviors that are maintained by automatic reinforcement. In these children, providing opportunities for play and other kinds of activities and for manipulation and exploration of toys and other materials tend to reduce their undesirable behaviors.

To find out if undesirable behaviors are maintained by automatic reinforcement, you need to leave the child alone in a room and see if the behaviors occur. Automatic reinforcement is most often presumed in case of stereotypic or self-stimulatory behaviors. An autistic boy may rock himself endlessly when left alone. It is difficult to point out positive or negative reinforcement for such behaviors. A reasonable assumption is that such self-stimulatory behaviors generate their own neural consequences that are reinforcing.

General Strategies for Decreasing Undesirable Behaviors

Procedures that reduce behaviors make no distinction between desirable and undesirable or good and bad behaviors. Behaviors are so described from a personal and social viewpoint. Procedures that decrease behaviors may decrease any behavior: desirable, undesirable, good, or bad. Therefore, the prudent clinician's job is to apply response reduction procedures to only the undesirable behaviors.

Most textbooks on behavioral treatment procedures classify response reduction procedures as extinction and punishment. Several procedures typically described under extinction and various forms of punishment are included here and are considered appropriate for therapeutic use. Behavior therapists have repeatedly emphasized that the scientific and therapeutic meaning of punishment does not share the negative connotations of punishment in everyday language. Nonetheless, we wish to minimize the use of the term punishment because its scientific meaning constantly is confused with its everyday meaning of a collection of many painful, exploitative, and vain procedures that most societies and governmental agencies employ. Also, the response reduction procedures recommended here do not include all of the punishment procedures researched in behavioral analysis. Therefore, we have taken a more descriptive approach in classifying response reduction procedures that you may use in clinical treatment.

We classify the response reduction strategies as either direct or indirect. This classification depends on whether a treatment contingency is placed on the behavior to be reduced or on another behavior. In the **direct response reduction strategy**, you place a contingency on the behavior to be reduced. Obviously, you use a contingency that reduces the rate of responses. In the **indirect strategy**, you place a contingency on a desirable behavior whose increase will have an indirect effect of decreasing an undesirable behavior. Note that the behavior to be reduced is not directly manipulated. Also, you use a contingency that increases a behavior. An important point to remember is that an undesirable behavior may be reduced by increasing a desirable behavior.

Another important point to remember is that only direct response reduction procedures may be defined as those that reduce behaviors. Although indirect procedures also help us reduce behaviors, they are not response reduction procedures. The indirect procedures increase responses; they are reinforcement procedures. You should not say that we use reinforcement procedures to decrease behaviors. By definition, reinforcement procedures increase behaviors. When used in a program of response reduction, the reinforcement procedures increase desirable behaviors. Presumably, this makes the undesirable behavior unnecessary. This is an important reason for classifying some response reduction strategies as indirect.

In the following sections, we return to this distinction to make it clearer to you. Specific procedures and examples show how a contingency is placed either on the behavior to be reduced or on a different behavior to be increased. Always, the behavior to be increased is productive and desirable.

Direct Strategy for Decreasing Behaviors

In the direct strategy, you concentrate on an undesirable behavior and place a contingency on it. The effect of this contingency is to directly reduce that behavior (Hegde, 1998b).

There are several procedures in which the behavior is directly reduced. These procedures fall into two major categories: stimulus presentation and stimulus withdrawal. We describe specific procedures under these categories.

Stimulus Presentation

Responses may be reduced by **presenting a stimulus immediately after a response is made.** Research has shown that several response-contingent stimuli can reduce behaviors. When they do, the stimuli typically are considered punishing. **Punishing stimuli** are those that reduce the future probability of a behavior.

Verbal stimuli most frequently are used in reducing behaviors. Such verbal stimuli as "no," "wrong," and "not correct," can reduce behaviors if presented immediately after the production of an incorrect response. Most clinicians indicate to the client in some way that a given attempt to produce the target response was not acceptable. The indication may be more or less subtle. The clinician may shake his or her head in a disapproving manner, show other facial or hand gestures of disapproval, or use explicit verbal stimuli. In all cases, the clinician will have used stimulus presentation as the method of reducing the undesirable response.

By themselves, verbal stimuli may not be effective. However, when combined with strong reinforcers for desirable behaviors that are shaped in carefully designed incremental steps, verbal stimuli may be sufficient to reduce undesirable behaviors. If you did not use verbal or gestural means of saying that the response was not correct or fully acceptable, the client's incorrect responses may persist.

How To Use Stimulus Presentation.   Take the following steps in using stimulus presentation as the method of response reduction:

1. **Present the verbal stimulus soon after the response is made.** To do this, you must make quick evaluations of the correctness of client responses.
2. **Present the verbal stimulus in a firm and objective manner.** Say "no" in such a manner to reinforce that you mean it. You should not sound unsure. The message, not necessarily the voice, must be clear and loud.
3. **Do not use an angry tone.** You should not give an emotional response to the incorrect response. Your tone should be objective and devoid of emotionality.
4. **Vary the words you use.** Do not use the same "no" or "wrong" throughout an entire session.

Stimulus Withdrawal

Immediately after a response is made, you may **withdraw a stimulus that presumably maintains or increases that response.** While you present stimuli that weaken a response, you withdraw stimuli that reinforce it. In reducing responses, stimulus withdrawal may be more effective than stimulus presentation.

There are three specific procedures of stimulus withdrawal: time-out, response cost, and extinction. In all three, reinforcing events or consequences are withdrawn or made unavailable.

Time-Out.   A frequently used method of behavior reduction is time-out from reinforcement. **Time-out** is a period of time during which all reinforcing events are suspended contingent on response and, as a result, there typically is a decrease in the rate of that response.

The clinically useful forms of time-out include exclusion and nonexclusion time-out. In **exclusion time-out**, the child is excluded from the current setting and the stream of activities. For example, you might ask a child to sit in the corner the instant he or she exhibits an undesirable behavior. All activities are terminated; the child is told to sit quietly. In this case, the setting is changed from the regular seating place to the corner. This is exclusion time-out.

In **nonexclusion time-out**, an undesirable behavior is followed immediately by cessation of all activity, but there is no physical movement and there is no change in the setting. For example, in stuttering treatment, you signal the client to stop talking for 5 seconds as soon as you observe a dysfluency or stutter. You avoid eye contact for the duration. At the end of the duration, you signal the person to resume talking. In this case, it is presumed that talking is reinforcing and interruption and silence are aversive. This aversive consequence is the presumed punisher that reduces the behavior on which it is made contingent. As you can see, nonexclusion time-out is time-out from the ongoing activity only; the person is not removed from the immediate setting and the activity is the presumed reinforcer.

Many research studies have shown that time-out can reduce several forms of undesirable behavior. Unfortunately, time-out is also most often misused. Careless use of time-out may have a paradoxical effect on behavior: the behavior might increase in frequency. This is likely to happen when the time-in period and setting are not reinforcing and the time-out duration and setting are. Avoid the following conditions under which **time-out may increase the undesirable behavior:**

1. **Time-out provides unintended negative reinforcement.** An uncooperative behavior may bring relief from aversive treatment trials. For instance, as soon as fussing begins, you send the child to the corner. But this action terminated treatment difficult trials, which were the cause of fussing (just what the child ordered, one might say). Consequently, the child's fussing behavior is negatively reinforced. When you resume treatment, the child may exhibit the undesirable behavior with added strength, because this is how he or she can terminate treatment trials.

   Treatment may be aversive because (a) target behaviors are too difficult for the child or (b) selected positive reinforcers given for the desirable behaviors are not working as such. The desirable behaviors do not increase and you say "no" to the child all too frequently because of wrong responses.

2. **Time-out provides unintended positive reinforcement.** During time-out, the child may pull a small toy from his or her pocket and begin to play. A picture on the wall may provide positive reinforcement, when you send the child to a corner. When asked to sit outside a classroom or treatment room, the child may enjoy watching people walking by or some activity going on outside. These events may positively reinforce the child's undesirable behavior because it is only through those behaviors that the child gets to watch reinforcing stimuli or outside activities. As soon as treatment is resumed, you may see an especially strong display of the undesirable behavior. Obviously, this troublesome behavior is the ticket to outside fun.

Advantages of Time-out. Prudently and sparingly used, time-out has many advantages. Compared to several other response reduction procedures, time-out is only mildly aversive. It is not a difficult procedure to learn and use. Brief time-out periods do not waste much teaching time. Therefore, consider using time-out to reduce undesirable behaviors in your client.

How To Use Time-out

Take the following steps in developing an effective and safe time-out procedure:

1. **Avoid too brief or too long durations of time-out.** Durations that are too long may be ineffective, because they may allow opportunities for other behaviors and take valuable time away from treatment. An appropriate duration depends on the nature of the behavior to be reduced. In reducing stuttering, for example, 5- to 10-second durations may be effective; longer durations are unnecessary. In controlling more global uncooperative, destructive, or inattentive behaviors, longer durations may be necessary. In most speech and language treatment sessions, the duration would not exceed 5 minutes.
2. **Try to avoid exclusion time-out, as it is the least desirable procedure.** Do not use it unless you have tried nonexclusion time-out, extinction, response cost, and other procedures first and have found them ineffective.
3. **Signal the beginning of the nonexclusion time-out with a stimulus.** For example, you may raise your index finger to signal to a stuttering person that a 10-second time-

(continued)

out has begun and that speech must be terminated. In exclusion time-out, a young child may be guided physically to a time-out area without any signal. But in all cases, either a verbal statement or a nonhuman sound such as a buzzer should announce the end of the time-out period.

4. **Try to avoid physical contact in administering exclusion time-out.** If the child complies with your instruction to go to the time-out area, do not use physical contact. Ask the child to go to the designated area and stay there until the end of the time-out period. Physically guide the child to the area only when the child does not comply.

5. **Use time-out on a continuous schedule.** Impose time-out on every instance of an undesirable behavior. Do not use an intermittent schedule, especially in the beginning of the response-reduction program. Intermittent scheduling may be useful in later stages of training when the undesirable behavior is of low frequency and you wish to keep it that way.

6. **Remove all reinforcers from the time-out area.** When you use exclusion time-out, the area to which you send the child to spend the time-out should not contain reinforcing objects, people, or events. For instance, do not ask the child to sit in a hallway full of people and events. Failure to follow this rule is the main reason why sending a child to his or her own room for misbehaving usually is ineffective. Typically, a child's room is full of reinforcers.

7. **Release the client from time-out only when the undesirable behavior has been stopped.** If the child continues to fuss in the corner, extend the time-out until the child becomes calm.

8. **Enrich the treatment situation with powerful and varied reinforcers.** Time-out is more effective when the return to the teaching situation is highly reinforcing and the time-out situation is dreary and unreinforcing. You will be in serious trouble if the situations are reversed.

Note that time-out will not reduce all behaviors in all clients. Besides, you should constantly watch for paradoxical effects. When you observe even a slight increase in the undesirable behavior being subjected to time-out, you should find an alternative procedure to reduce that behavior.

Response Cost. **Response cost** is a procedure of reducing behaviors through response-contingent withdrawal of reinforcers. The client must give up a reinforcer every time an undesirable response is made.

Time-out and response cost are similar in that both deprive the client of some reinforcers. But their procedures are different. In time-out, you arrange a brief duration of no reinforcement of any kind; during this time, there is no responding; the person may even be moved to another scene that lacks reinforcers. In response cost, you take away a specific, tangible, reinforcer the client has earned or has been given; there is no particular interruption of responses; the client does not move physically.

Response cost is implemented most effectively and efficiently in a token system. Tokens are presented and withdrawn depending on the behavior. At the end of a treatment session, the remaining tokens are exchanged for a back-up reinforcer.

Response cost may be either the lose-only type or earn-and-lose type. In the **lose-only** type, you give the client a certain number of tokens at the beginning of a session. These tokens are not contingent on desirable behaviors; therefore, the client does not earn them. During the treatment sessions, you withdraw a token for every undesirable response. You may reinforce the desirable responses with verbal praise and other such social reinforcers that you cannot take back.

In the **earn-and-lose** type of response cost, all tokens are contingent on desirable behaviors. That is, the client must earn them by exhibiting desirable behaviors. While earning them, the client also loses a token for every instance of an undesirable behavior. In this case, both the desirable and the undesirable behaviors evoke the token contingency.

Either the lose-only or the earn-and-lose method may be used individually or in small groups. When used with groups, any individual's undesirable behavior will cost the group a token. The group earns tokens only when all members exhibit the desirable behavior.

Like all other response-reduction procedures, response cost may be ineffective or may increase the rate of undesirable response under certain conditions. **You must carefully avoid the following problems in designing a response-cost system for your clients:**

1. **Low token loss preceded by high loss may be ineffective.** Typically, you withdraw one token per undesirable response. But in some cases, to make it work, you may have to withdraw multiple tokens per response. If you do this, you should not start with a high number and then go down. For instance, you should not first take away 5 tokens per undesirable response and then only 2. The reduced token loss condition may be ineffective.

2. **The client may run out of tokens.** Then there is nothing to lose and you do not have response cost to reduce the behavior.

3. **Loss of tokens may cause emotional responses.** If such responses do not subside quickly, use another method of response reduction. You should not carry the method to a point where you struggle with the client to take tokens away or that the child is in tears.

4. **The undesirable behavior may increase because of attention.** When you take a token away, you also pay immediate, contingent attention to the undesirable response. If the response increases, use another procedure.

Advantages of Response Cost.   Along with time-out, response cost is a widely researched method of reducing undesirable behaviors. It is known to be very effective, socially acceptable, and less aversive than some of the other methods of behavior reduction.

How To Use Response Cost

Take the following steps in designing a response-cost procedure for your client:

1. **Prefer the earn-and-lose method to lose-only method.** This method allows you to systematically reinforce correct and cooperative behaviors through tokens earned, while reducing undesirable behaviors through tokens lost.
2. **Give more tokens than you take back.** To this end, simplify the target response and shape it, if necessary. The child should experience more success (reinforcers) than failures (token loss). At the end of the session, the child should be left with some tokens to be exchanged for back-up reinforcers.
3. **Withdraw tokens promptly.** There should be no delay between the undesirable response and token withdrawal.
4. **If necessary, increase the number of tokens withdrawn per response.** Do this when a single or fewer token withdrawals are not effective. But do not decrease the number of tokens withdrawn.
5. **Avoid client indebtedness.** If you find yourself withdrawing enough tokens to result in client debt, switch to another response reduction method.

As with any response-reduction procedure, watch for excessive emotional responses and paradoxical increase in undesirable behaviors. Always be prepared to use another response-reduction procedure.

Extinction. In **extinction**, consequences that reinforce a behavior are withheld. Note that extinction is not a punishment procedure, yet response cost and time-out are. But all three procedures have the same effect on the behavior: reduced frequency. We have grouped extinction along with response cost and time-out to point out that in all three, the locus of contingency management is the undesirable behavior. Though the three procedures are direct compared to procedures that reduce undesirable behaviors by increasing desirable ones, extinction of positively reinforced behaviors is less direct than response cost and time-out. But the extinction of negatively reinforced behavior, as you will find out shortly, is a direct procedure.

In extinction, you do nothing to help sustain the behavior so the behavior is reduced. It is a response-weakening procedure that removes reinforcing consequences. Therefore, you can use this procedure only when the behavior to be reduced is either positively or negatively reinforced. Your functional analysis baselines might suggest that the behavior is indeed maintained by these kinds of reinforcement.

Children's **uncooperative behaviors** are prime targets for extinction. Such interfering behaviors as crying, fussing, frequent verbal requests to go to the bathroom or see the parent waiting outside, irrelevant talking (the "you know what?" type of interruptions), and many other similar behaviors are maintained by clinician's unintended reinforcement. The reinforcement may be positive or negative. The clinician may positively reinforce repeated verbal requests to go to the bathroom by paying attention. But leaving the treatment room for the bathroom is a negatively reinforced behavior. The child who leaves the treatment room terminates unwanted treatment. This is negative reinforcement. Note that if the child begins to leave the treatment room, you cannot just ignore the behavior. You need to prevent escape, thus depriving the child of negative reinforcement. **Prevention of escape** is sometimes described as escape extinction (Iwata et al., 1990). This procedure implies that extinction is not always a passive or indirect procedure.

Advantages of Extinction. Used correctly, extinction is an effective method of reducing undesirable behaviors. Consider it for reducing many crying, undesirable interruptions, and similar problem behaviors.

How To Use Extinction

Take the following steps in using extinction:

1. **Discuss the problem and the extinction procedure with the parents.** Some parents may be alarmed to see you sitting still when their 3-year-old child is loudly and tearfully crying "Mommy!." If they understand what you are doing and why, they may tolerate the procedure. Extinction is slow and unpleasant for both the child and for those who administer it or watch it.

2. **Find out what reinforces the undesirable behavior.** Try to find out if the behavior is reinforced positively, negatively, or with a combination of the two. Also, find out if the behavior is reinforced independent of what you do. For example, a child who leaves the chair and goes to the chalkboard to scribble may be reinforced independently of your actions. Also, the child is reinforced negatively (escaping from your teaching) and positively (scribbling on the chalkboard). In this case, even if you avoid all interactions with the child to eliminate reinforcement, the behavior still may persist because of negative and positive reinforcement.

3. **Remove positive reinforcers inherent to your actions as promptly and fully as possible.** Withdraw all attention from undesirable behavior. Avoid eye contact; sit motionless. Be firm, wait it out; do not change anything. For example, once you initiate extinction for crying behavior, do not lecture, do not admonish, do not cajole, do not try to charm the child, do not try to talk the child out of crying.

4. **Remove positive reinforcers that are unrelated to your actions.** If the child on the floor begins to play with a toy, look at pictures, examine your bag, and so forth, remove the objects promptly and then sit motionless.

5. **Remove negative reinforcers as promptly and fully as possible.** Prevent the child from leaving the seat, walking around or out of the treatment room. Do not stop treatment because the child asks interrupting questions. Do not answer such questions as "Do you know what?" If you answer such questions, you will have positively reinforced such interruptive questioning and negatively reinforced the escape behavior that terminates your teaching.

6. **Do not terminate the extinction procedure when you see an extinction burst.** There usually is a temporary increase in the rate of a response when extinction is initiated. This is called the extinction burst. It often scares the clinician, who quickly turns attention to the client. Do not do this. Continue to withhold reinforcers by sitting motionless and the behavior will eventually subside.
7. **Reinforce desirable behavior promptly and lavishly.** For example, the instant the child stops crying or fussing, you should smile, hug the child, wipe the tears, praise, give a token, and reinforce the child in other ways. Make the desirable behavior pay off better for the child than the undesirable behavior.

A Word of Caution. *Behaviors that are reinforced automatically and those that are destructive or aggressive are **not** candidates for extinction.* You cannot ignore a self-stimulatory behavior and expect it to diminish. Such behaviors are automatically reinforced by their sensory consequences. Aggressive behavior, though facing extinction, might still hurt others. Besides, the behavior itself is not likely to be reduced because of the reinforcement it receives (the effect on others). Do not use extinction to reduce these behaviors.

Indirect Strategy for Decreasing Behaviors

In the direct strategies of stimulus presentation and stimulus withdrawal (extinction, time-out, and response cost), one places the treatment contingency directly on the undesirable behavior to reduce its frequency. To the contrary, **in the indirect strategy**, one replaces the undesirable behaviors by desirable behaviors. You do not place a treatment contingency on the undesirable behavior at all. This approach is so indirect that you do nothing specific to the behavior to be reduced.

The main feature of the indirect strategy is that you reinforce desirable behaviors, increase them, and, as a consequence, decrease the undesirable behaviors. In a sense, you use reinforcement to control undesirable behaviors; by reinforcing desirable behaviors, you weaken undesirable behaviors. But you should never make the mistake of saying that, "I use reinforcement to decrease undesirable behaviors." Reinforcement only can increase behaviors. When you use reinforcing procedures, the behavioral reduction is a by-product. Undesirable behaviors decrease only because other behaviors increase. Therefore, you might say that, "I use reinforcement to increase some behaviors so that other behaviors are decreased."

The use of reinforcement to increase some behaviors while other behaviors decrease as a result is known as **differential reinforcement.** The term *differential* suggests that it is not the straightforward reinforcement of some behavior. There is a differential effect of the reinforcement procedure. Although some behaviors increase because of the reinforcement, others decrease as a by-product. This is the meaning of differential reinforcement.

There are several differential reinforcement procedures to help you increase some behaviors that can have a concurrent effect of reducing other behaviors. The difference between some of them is subtle and probably not crucial. But if you understand the difference, you will be a sophisticated user of response reduction procedures. The following four differential reinforcement procedures are important: differential reinforcement of other behavior (DRO), differential reinforcement of incompatible behavior (DRI), differential reinforcement of alternative behavior (DRA), and differential reinforcement of low rates of responding (DRL). All of these increase certain behaviors and thereby decrease certain other behaviors.

Differential Reinforcement of Other Behavior (DRO). In this procedure, you **reinforce a child for not exhibiting a specified undesirable behavior** for a particular duration. For example, you may reinforce a child for not wiggling in the chair for 2 minutes. If the child desists in the behavior for that entire duration, you may give the child a token. Gradually, you can increase the duration for which the child should refrain from the undesirable behavior. A child who frequently interrupts you during treatment may be asked not to do it for a period of several minutes. The child is then reinforced for compliance. An aggressive child may be told that he or she will receive a token, if physically or verbally aggressive behavior stops for a certain duration.

The examples of DRO show that what is reinforced is left open. The procedure does not require a particular desirable behavior to earn reinforcers. The child need not do anything in particular to get reinforcement; he or she must simply refrain from doing something (the specified undesirable behavior). An aggressive or hyperactive child, for example, may need to sit quietly for the specified duration to earn reinforcers. But the child may also read, color, work on mathematical problems, or put puzzles together to earn the reinforcer. You look for these and many other forms of acceptable behaviors, none specified ahead of time, to reinforce. Any one of several desirable behaviors and the omission of the specified undesirable behavior results in reinforcement.

Differential Reinforcement of Incompatible Behavior (DRI). In this procedure, you **reinforce behaviors that are incompatible with the undesirable behavior.** Unlike the DRO, in which no specific desirable behavior is required, a behavior that is topographically incompatible with the undesirable behavior is required in DRI and reinforced when it occurs. A child who is verbally abusive may be reinforced for nonabusive, socially acceptable verbal expressions. A child who snatches toys from other children may be reinforced for giving his or her toy to playmates.

Note that abusive expressions are incompatible with socially acceptable expressions in that both cannot be produced at the same time. Similarly, snatching and sharing do not occur simultaneously. Therefore, when the desirable behavior is increased with reinforcement, the incompatible undesirable behavior should decrease. To use DRI, you must find a response that cannot coexist with the undesirable behavior and target that for reinforcement.

Differential Reinforcement of Alternative Behavior (DRA). In this procedure, you **specify and reinforce a behavior that is an alternative to the undesirable behavior.** Note that an alternative desirable behavior is not necessarily incompatible with the undesirable behavior to be reduced. In DRA, the desirable behavior is just an alternative to, but not incompatible with, the undesirable behavior. For example, you may find out that a child often is disruptive because of lack of academic or social skills. In this case, you may target specific reading or writing skills and adaptive social skills that the child will enjoy more than the disruptive behaviors.

One drawback with the DRA procedure is that because the desirable behavior is not incompatible with the undesirable behavior, both may be exhibited. While learning better academic and social skills, the child may continue to disrupt. In such cases, it is necessary to teach behaviors that are incompatible with the undesirable behavior. For instance, reinforcing the child to sit quietly for periods of time would be incompatible with disruptive behavior.

Differential Reinforcement of Low Rates of Responding (DRL). In this procedure, you **reinforce the child when the frequency of undesirable behavior is below the baseline level.** In DRL, you shape the undesirable response down until it is eliminated or reduced to a manageable level. The procedure gradually reduces the behavior. For example, you find out that during treatment sessions, a child asks, "Are we done yet?" once every 2 to 3 minutes. You can then set a criterion of no more than 2 interruptions in a 10-minute interval. Normally, the child would have interrupted some 3 to 5 times during this interval. You can reinforce the child, if during the previous 10 minutes, the child had interrupted you only 2 times or less. In using this procedure, you must make sure that you do not reinforce the child soon after an interruption.

Differential reinforcement, especially the DRO, DRI, and the DRA, are procedures that help you replace undesirable behavior with desirable behaviors. In these procedures, while reinforcing desirable behaviors, you make sure that you do not reinforce undesirable behaviors. Therefore, a common theme of these procedures is that (a) the client gains access to reinforcing affairs through desirable behaviors; (b) the undesirable behaviors do not get reinforced anymore; (c) consequently, the undesirable behaviors do not serve the client as they did before; and, therefore, (d) the desirable behaviors replace the undesirable behaviors.

Other Indirect Procedures

Two other indirect procedures that may be used include behavioral momentum and the presentation of a sudden, surprising stimulus. These newer techniques can be effective with many children who exhibit undesirable behaviors or who are unlikely to produce the target behaviors with modeling and shaping.

Behavioral momentum is a procedure in which the force of a behavior in progress causes another behavior that may not otherwise be exhibited. In using behavior momentum, you first ask the client to do what he or she is likely to do; as soon as this behavior occurs and it is reinforced, you ask the client to repeatedly and rapidly perform an action that he or she is not likely to perform. The unlikely behavior may be performed because of the force (momentum) of the previous, readily exhibited behavior.

This method has been used to reduce noncompliant behaviors (Mace et al., 1988). For example, assume that a girl does not comply with your request to look at the stimulus picture used in training words. Also assume that she readily will clap her hands when asked to. Then, you could ask her to clap two or three times in succession and immediately ask her to look at the picture. She may then immediately look at the picture. Note that when picture-attending behavior increases, the noncompliance behavior will have decreased. You decreased noncompliance behavior by behavior momentum.

Surprising stimulus presentation also can terminate or prevent an undesirable behavior. A study has shown that sudden loud noise can terminate undesirable behaviors (Charlop, Burgio, Iwata, & Ivancic, 1988). But you may prevent undesirable behaviors by anticipating them and then presenting a sudden and surprising stimulus. For example, a child's imminent crying may be prevented if you suddenly and dramatically pull out a clown or an animated toy just before the crying is about to erupt. You suddenly may turn on the radio, get up from the chair, pull something from a box, or behave in some dramatic fashion. Stimuli that appear so suddenly and dramatically tend to inhibit certain undesirable behaviors.

To prevent undesirable behaviors by sudden stimulus presentation, you must watch the client very closely and observe the early signs of trouble. The stimulus must be presented *before* the response onset; if not, you may reinforce the undesirable response.

Stimuli that *terminate* undesirable behaviors are aversives; but those that *prevent* such behaviors are positive reinforcers. For instance, you say "no" to an undesirable behavior that is promptly terminated. The verbal "no" is an aversive stimulus. To the contrary, when you prevent an imminent crying response by pulling out a clown, you provoke an incompatible response of surprise, curiosity, and so forth. The clown is a positive reinforcer. Be clear about this distinction.

General Guidelines for Reducing Undesirable Behaviors

We have described several procedures of response reduction. Although each of them may reduce responses, you should not think of using an isolated procedure in reducing or increasing behaviors. You must design a comprehensive program of contingency management involving reinforcement for the desirable responses, withdrawal of reinforcers for the undesirable responses, presentation of response reduction consequences for the undesirable behaviors, and others. A combined procedure that simultaneously shapes and reinforces a desirable behavior while withdrawing reinforcers from the undesirable behaviors and presenting them with other response reduction consequences will be the most effective (Hegde, 1998b).

Designing an Effective Response Reduction Strategy

Take the following steps in designing an effective response reduction strategy involving multiple contingencies or procedures:

1. **See if response reduction procedures other than extinction may be omitted altogether.** If the undesirable behavior is not frequent enough to disrupt the treatment process, continue to reinforce the desirable behavior and ignore the undesirable behavior. Use one of the response reduction procedures only when this strategy fails to

bring the undesirable behavior under a manageable level. For example, if reinforcement of correct articulation is doing the job, ignore the incorrect productions. However, if the incorrect productions persist, introduce a more active response reduction procedure (verbal "No," response cost, or time-out).

2. **Use procedures that help prevent undesirable responses.** Model the correct response until the client's productions stabilize. You then would not have to use the response reduction procedures, because the client is successful. Prompt the correct response when the client hesitates; such hesitations may signal an imminent wrong response; you can prevent this by prompting the correct response.

3. **Clearly and narrowly define both the undesirable behavior to be reduced and the desirable behavior to be increased.** For instance, *distorted /s/ productions* is a more clearly and narrowly defined response than *problems of articulation*. Conversely, *production of correct /s/* is a better definition than *improved articulatory skills*. Similarly, *production of part-word repetitions* (and other specific types of dysfluency types) is a more clearly and narrowly defined behavior than *stuttering moment*. Too, *reduced speech rate through syllable prolongation* is a better definition than *controlled rate of speech*. Use response reduction procedures only when you have such clearly defined behaviors on which you can place response contingencies.

4. **Differentially reinforce a desirable behavior that is incompatible with the undesirable behavior (DRI).** For instance, in-seat behavior is incompatible with out-of-seat behavior; any form of cooperative behavior does not coexist with noncooperative behavior; attention replaces inattention; smiling and crying are opposite behaviors. To make the response reduction procedure less aversive, reinforce the incompatible desirable response. When you do this, you will simultaneously increase a desirable behavior and decrease an undesirable behavior. This action will help limit the use of aversive response reduction procedures.

5. **Differentially reinforce a desirable behavior that will secure for the client what the undesirable behavior seems to secure (DRA).** Technically, this means that you teach a desirable behavior that is functionally equivalent to the behavior to be reduced (Carr & Durand, 1985). If it looks like the child is crawling under the table to get your attention, then provide lavish attention to quiet sitting in the chair. Children who are minimally verbal or those who are nonverbal may fuss often because that is the only way they can get their wants satisfied. Teaching mands (requests, demands) may reduce such inappropriate behaviors.

6. **Differentially reinforce the client for reducing the rate of the undesirable behavior (DRL).** If you see systematic reduction in the undesirable behavior, reinforce the child while that behavior is not being exhibited. For example, you might tell a child that he wiggled only once during the last 5 minutes and reinforce when he sits without wiggling.

7. **Differentially reinforce the client for simply omitting the undesirable behavior and for producing any of the many acceptable behaviors (DRO).** For example, in a group, reinforce a disruptive child for not being disruptive; your reinforcers may be made contingent on many and unspecified desirable behaviors.

8. **Use varied consequences to reduce a response** (Charlop et al., 1988). Do not use one type of response consequence constantly. For example, in the same treatment sessions, alternate the use of verbal "no," response cost, time-out, and other consequences that reduce the response rate. Similarly, use varied reinforcers to increase the desirable behavior that will replace the undesirable behavior (Egel, 1981). Verbal praise, tokens backed with many reinforcers, frequent feedback on response accuracy, opportunities for exhibiting high probability behaviors, all may be used in a single session.

9. **See if an interfering response may be used to reinforce correct responses** (Charlop, Kurtz, & Kasey, 1990). For example, a child frequently may leave the seat to go to the chalkboard and scribble on it. Instead of trying to suppress this interfering behavior with a verbal "no" and such other means, you can make short durations of drawing or writing on the chalkboard contingent on sitting for a few minutes and giving correct responses. You will then have turned an annoying, interfering behavior into a reinforcer of desirable target behaviors.

10. **See if behavioral momentum may be effective in decreasing certain undesirable behaviors.** Repeatedly and rapidly evoke a likely behavior, reinforce it, and immediately demand the production of the unlikely target behavior. Reinforce its occurrence as well.

11. **See if the undesirable behavior is a means of escape from therapeutic work you demand of the client.** Some children crawl under a table, leave their seat, or look away from you because they find the treatment aversive. By their undesirable behaviors, children escape from therapy or instruction (Carr & Durand, 1985; Iwata, 1987; Iwata et al., 1990). Treatment may be aversive to clients because of many reasons, but the most frequent reason is that the task is too difficult and the child receives too much punishment and too little reinforcement. Then, simplify the task. Shape the target behavior in small steps so that the child is more successful, and hence, receives reinforcement more often than corrective feedback.

12. **See if a strong, sudden, and surprising stimulus can terminate or prevent an undesirable behavior.** Try to terminate an undesirable behavior by presenting a surprising stimulus. Try to prevent the occurrence of an undesirable response by presenting the surprising stimulus as soon as you anticipate its occurrence.

13. **Use a continuous schedule.** Make sure every instance of an undesirable behavior is followed by the response reduction procedure you have selected. Whether it is response cost, time-out, or verbal stimuli, apply it continuously.

14. **Present or withdraw consequences immediately.** Do not hesitate, wait, or be slow in responding to the undesirable response.

15. **Do not allow escape from the response-reduction procedure.** A crying child being purposely ignored should not get out of the treatment room only to be consoled by the parent waiting outside. This will positively reinforce the crying behavior. Similarly, clients under other response-reduction procedures should not be allowed to leave the treatment scene. If they are, the clients will escape from treatment and get negative reinforcement. (Contrast this with #9; these two are different concepts).

16. **Apply the response-reduction procedure at the earliest sign of the undesirable response.** Do not wait until the undesirable response is completed to apply the procedure. Suppose you wish to reduce a child's behavior of leaving the chair. You should not wait to say "no" until after the child has left the chair and is on the floor. The best time to say "no" (assuming it will be effective) is when you see the slightest movement of the child that suggests an imminent response. In using time-out for stuttering, you should not wait until an instance of stuttering has been completed. Instead, you must watch for the earliest signs of stuttering and apply the procedure.

17. **Dissociate response-reduction procedures from those that reinforce responses.** You should not deliver reinforcers along with or in close proximity with response-reduction procedures. If you do and if it so happens that the reinforcers are stronger than the response reduction procedures, you will have reinforced the undesirable behavior. Some clinicians say "wrong," but immediately smile, touch, or hug the child. These positive responses from the clinician may neutralize the effects of "wrong" or even reinforce the undesirable response.

18. **Minimize the duration of response-reduction procedures.** Time-out should be brief. No response reduction procedure should be applied for too long. If it looks like you have to, you are not using an

effective treatment procedure. Maybe you have a wrong or extremely difficult target for the child; maybe you do not have effective reinforcers to increase the desirable behavior; perhaps you are not administering treatment contingencies properly. Analyze your procedures to make them more effective. If you cannot figure it out, talk to your supervisor, but do not continue with the response reduction procedure.

19. **Remove reinforcers that maintain undesirable behaviors.** If you see the child constantly reaching for your bag on the table, do not continue to reprimand the child; instead, remove the bag and keep it out of the child's reach and sight. See what reinforces the undesirable behavior. If it is something that can be eliminated, do so immediately.

20. **Make sure the client is exposed to more reinforcing consequences than to response-reduction consequences.** Overall, treatment sessions should be much more reinforcing (fun) than aversive to the child. You should be giving more tokens than you withdraw; you should be praising the child more frequently than you reprimand. Of course, to do this, you should be using procedures that help shape the target behaviors.

Aversive Nature of Response-Reduction Procedures

Response-reduction procedures are aversive not only to clients, but also to clinicians. No clinician enjoys applying aversive procedures. Prudent and limited use of response reduction procedures that are only minimally aversive, socially acceptable, and do not involve emotional or physical harm often are necessary in treatment programs. Careless use of aversive procedures can create negative side effects including strong and persistent emotional responses in the clients. See Hegde (1998b) for a more detailed discussion of the negative side effects of response-reduction procedures.

We have argued that in all treatment sessions, the emphasis should be on positive reinforcement procedures. You should design treatment procedures to avoid response-reduction procedures; if this is not possible, the need should be minimal.

Always think of simplifying the desirable target response; find an effective reinforcer for it; target alternative, other, or incompatible responses that will then increase, and will decrease the undesirable behavior. See if extinction will work before you apply more aversive procedures. At the end of the session, count the number of positive reinforcers and response-reducing consequences that you delivered. If you have not applied reinforcing consequences more often than the response-reduction consequences, critically evaluate your treatment procedures. Discuss this with your clinical supervisor. Remember always, that frequent use of response-reduction procedures suggests that something is wrong. Your goal is to avoid response-reduction procedures, if possible; this requires the most effective way of structuring your treatment program and use of the most powerful positive reinforcers.

10

Maintenance of Target Behaviors

You soon will find in your clinical practicum that promoting maintenance of target behaviors in natural settings and over time is a
more challenging job than establishing them in the first place.
Therefore, you must pay at least as much attention to maintenance strategies as you do to response establishment strategies. With persons who
stutter, you may have to work harder on fluency maintenance than on
establishment.

You often will read that generalization is the final goal of treatment.
When a child who learns to produce certain phonemes in the clinic does
not pronounce them at home, you are told that the correct production did
not generalize. Therefore, you are asked to program generalization before
you dismiss a client.

A critical look at generalization shows that it actually, should not be
the final goal of treatment. **Generalization** is a declining rate of response
when untrained stimuli are presented and reinforcers are withheld (Hegde,
1998b). Generalized but unreinforced responses are extinguished. Therefore, if generalization is the final target, we will have to assume that a declining rate of response is the final goal of treatment. No clinician assumes
this. Instead, you are told to have parents and others reinforce generalized
responses produced at home and other nonclinical settings. This action
leads to a contradictory conclusion that generalized responses are reinforced responses. If so, generalization must be redefined as reinforced responses. There is then no difference between treatment and generalization

strategies. Therefore, to avoid all these contradictions, we emphasize that generalization is not the final objective of clinical intervention.

Maintenance of Target Behaviors in Natural Settings

The **final treatment goal is maintenance** of target behaviors. The clinically established communicative behaviors must be produced in conversational speech, in the natural environment, and must be sustained over time. Behaviors that generate favorable consequences are likely to be maintained. If the client reliably produces the behaviors in the clinic but not at home and other settings, then we must have people in those settings do some of the things the clinician did to establish those behaviors. We achieve this by designing a maintenance strategy.

A **maintenance strategy** is an extension of treatment to natural settings (Hegde, 1998b). The main task in implementing a maintenance strategy is to teach people in the life of the client to support and sustain target behaviors. A significant part of the strategy also is to teach the client to manage his or her own behaviors. Therefore, clients, and people who interact with them are the key players in the maintenance strategy.

Maintenance Procedures

To promote maintenance, you must **extend treatment to natural settings**, but there is nothing substantially new in the maintenance techniques, themselves. What is new about the strategy is that the clinician must train others in contingency management at home and at other nonclinical settings.

Treatment strategy changes the client's behavior, but the maintenance strategy changes the behavior of people around the client. If they continue to behave in their usual manner, the client may not maintain the target responses. Therefore, to implement a maintenance strategy, you should learn to work with parents, spouses, siblings, friends, teachers, and colleagues of the client so that they react differently to the client.

Recall that in Chapter 8, treatment in communicative disorders was defined as a rearrangement of a communicative relationship between the client and his or her listeners. You, the clinician, were the initial listener in rearranging that communicative relationship. The final listeners are the people surrounding the client. In both the cases, listeners help change the behavior of the client. Although you know how to change the client's (speaker's) behavior, other listeners do not. To help them learn the techniques of changing the behavior of their particular speaker (your client) is the heart of maintenance strategy.

By training the people in the client's life to manage the reinforcement contingencies, you will be shifting the target behavior control from yourself to others. You also will be shifting the location of response control from the clinic to at least a few natural settings. The basic idea here is that like treatment, response maintenance also is a management procedure.

Besides shifting response control to others, you must take a few other steps as well. Maintenance is a consideration even when you select and teach the target behaviors. As the target behaviors are produced more reliably in the clinical setting, you initiate other, more crucial procedures of response maintenance. Therefore, in a comprehensive maintenance strategy, take the following steps.

Select Useful Behaviors

As pointed out in Chapter 7, behaviors that are **useful to the client** are more likely to be produced and maintained in natural settings. Communicative behaviors that serve the needs of the client are likely to receive reinforcement from others. Therefore, by selecting client-specific, meaningful, and useful behaviors you set the stage for later maintenance strategy.

Reinforce Target Responses in Conversational Speech

Phonemes trained only at the word and phrase levels do not tend to be frequently produced in natural settings where connected speech is expected. Certain other target behaviors, for example, skills of fluency and voice qualities, trained only at the word level, may be ineffective when the client speaks continuously in natural settings. Therefore, the target behaviors must always be monitored in conversational speech in the final stages of treatment.

As early as possible, **move treatment to conversational speech level.** In the treatment of stuttering and voice disorders, move through the simpler levels of words and phrases as rapidly as you can. Spend more clinical time monitoring the target behaviors in conversational speech than in words or phrases. In case of articulation disorders, monitor the correct production of speech sounds in continuous speech. In teaching words to children with disordered language, move to phrases, sentences, and continuous speech as quickly as possible. Do the same in teaching grammatical morphemes, syntactic structures, and pragmatic features.

Shift Reinforcement Schedules

A behavior **reinforced continuously does not resist extinction** as much as the one reinforced intermittently. The longer a behavior resists extinction, the greater the chance that it will come under some reinforcement contingency. This situation then will help maintain the target behavior. Therefore, after having established the target behaviors initially through continuous reinforcement, begin to **reinforce on an intermittent schedule.**

In gradual steps, move from a FR2 to progressively higher ratios. As you decrease the amount of reinforcement, pay close attention to response rates. You may have to lower the ratio, if the response rates decline. In the final stages of treatment when the target responses are monitored in conversational speech, reinforce only sporadically.

Use Social and Conditioned Generalized Reinforcers

Social reinforcers are more prevalent in the natural settings. Therefore, even when you have to use primary reinforcers, **pair them with social reinforcers**, including verbal praise. If the same kinds of reinforcers are encountered in the clinic and natural settings, the responses are more likely to be maintained.

Besides social reinforcers, **use conditioned generalized reinforcers.** A token system with a variety of back-up reinforcers increases the chances of similar reinforcers being encountered in the natural setting. Also, the family members may be able to implement a similar token system at home to sustain the response rates. The job of the client's family members will be easier if they can use an established system of reinforcement.

Spread the Discriminative Stimulus Control

A **discriminative stimulus** is a stimulus in whose presence a response has been reinforced. As a result, the response is likely in the presence of that stimulus. Any stimulus may acquire the power to evoke a response because of its systematic association with reinforcement.

The discriminative stimulus will not continue to evoke the response for very long, if the response is not reinforced. However, an initial response in the presence of a discriminative stimulus gives the opportunity to reinforce that response to sustain it.

The most important discriminative stimuli are persons, physical stimuli, and physical settings. The clinician is the first discriminative stimulus for the target response. By systematically reinforcing the target response, the clinician comes to exert a strong control over it. Soon, the clinical setting also will come to control the target response.

Some dramatic examples illustrate the power of the clinician and the clinical setting in evoking target responses. For instance, parents often are amazed at the amount of fluency their children who stutter exhibit in front of the clinician and in the treatment room. Anywhere else, the children may stutter just as much as they did before treatment. The child who reliably produces words in the treatment room may continue to gesture at home. A woman's hoarseness may all but disappear when she walks into the treatment room. But just as dramatically, her typical untreated voice may disappear as she leaves the clinic. This appearance and disappearance of target behaviors are due to the discriminative stimulus value of the clinician and the treatment room and lack of discriminative stimuli in nonclinical settings.

The task is to spread this discriminative stimulus control exerted almost exclusively by the clinician and the clinical setting to other people in nonclinical settings. When associated with reinforcement, other people and other settings begin to evoke target behaviors. Therefore, to spread the discriminative stimulus value, take the steps:

Ask the client's family members to sit in the treatment room. If they are associated with treatment and reinforcement, the family members may acquire some power to evoke the target responses at home. Whenever possible, the parents and other members of the family should at least observe the treatment sessions. They should do this not from the unseen side of one-way mirrors, but by sitting in the treatment room. This is done to associate their presence with treatment. At this stage, family members do not reinforce or do anything else. In the latter stages of treatment, ask your friends or others who are strangers to the client to observe treatment sessions. Discuss this with parents and clients before you invite other persons to sessions because it raises the issue of confidentiality. You need the permission of adult clients and parents or guardians of minors.

Move treatment to outside the treatment room. The restricted treatment room is useful and often necessary to establish target behaviors, because it provides a controlled environment free of distraction. But the room is so different from a client's everyday environment that the client's learning is restricted to its confines. Therefore, when the client begins to produce the target behaviors in conversational speech, move treatment out of the treatment room. Take a walk with the client outside the clinic. Converse with the client and monitor the production of target behaviors in conversational speech.

If the client's response rate drops dramatically when you move out of the treatment room and you find it hard to control the regression, move back into the treatment room and try again later. If the client sustains responses, then progressively move to different situations. Take the client to shopping centers, restaurants, bookstores, toy stores, and other relevant places and have the client talk to people there. Follow the guidelines in carrying out this procedure:

1. **In the beginning, take the client to less threatening situations.** You may not even ask the client to talk to any strangers the first time you two go outside the clinic. Let the client talk to you in the new environment while you monitor and reinforce the target responses.

2. **Let the client rehearse what he or she will tell a stranger in a new setting.** For example, you might have a client who stutters talk to a bookstore clerk. What the client plans to tell the clerk should be rehearsed with your help so that he or she can speak slowly and fluently.

3. **The first few times, stay close to the client.** If needed, give a subtle signal to trigger the target response. You may touch the client's shoulder as he or she begins to speak to prompt the correct response. In the case of a man who stutters, for example, the touch may mean that he must slow down his rate.

4. **Take note of correct and incorrect productions.** Give subtle and quick reinforcement. This is important, because the strangers the clients talk to will not reinforce. It is your reinforcement in these new situations that will establish the discriminative stimulus value of those situations and listeners.

5. **Gradually increase the distance between you and your client.** As the client begins to talk to strangers, slowly move away from them.

6. **Take the client to progressively more difficult situations.** As the target responses are maintained in each new situation, take the client to a more difficult situation. Reinforce the client in all situations.

Teach Others To Evoke and Consequate Target Behaviors

This technique is the heart of maintenance strategy; it can and must be implemented whether there is initial generalization or not. Treatment will have been extended to the natural environment, if the significant others in the client's life know (a) the exact target behaviors, (b) how to evoke them, and (c) how to enhance them. The target behaviors then have the greatest probability of being maintained.

Take the following steps in teaching others to evoke and administer consequences to target behaviors:

1. **Describe and demonstrate the target behaviors to others.**
   When you invite the family members and others to observe the treatment sessions, describe the target behaviors being taught. Tell them precisely what the client is expected to do. Do not use jargon. Give simple and direct descriptions. For example, while treating a child who stutters, say, "I want Johnny to talk very slowly. Perhaps as slowly as I am talking now. [Model the target rate.] Johnny should stretch his words like this. [Model a few words by prolonging the syllables.] When Johnny stretches his words, he does not stutter that much. When he practices slower speech without stuttering for a while, he can begin to speak a little faster until his speech will sound OK and he will be speaking more fluently."

   While teaching a set of basic words to a child who has a language delay, tell the parents you are teaching a few words, not a "core vocabulary." When you have to use technical terms (e. g., present progressive or prepositions), give examples. Show the parents and other members of the family a list of words, phrases, and sentences you teach the child.

   In treating voice disorders, contrast the desirable and undesirable voice or resonance qualities. In simple terms, describe the relation between vocal abuse and voice problems. With the help of charts and drawings, show them how the vocal mechanism works and how important it is to maintain appropriate vocal behaviors.

2. **Demonstrate how to evoke target behaviors.** Let family members watch you evoke the target behaviors. They should know how to model the target behaviors for the client. Although they are not expected to shape the behavior or model excessively at home, the parents, spouses, and siblings should suggest the target behavior when the client fails to produce it at home. For instance, the family of a person who stutters should model the correct way of slowing the rate of speech. They should do it by stretching the words and not by giving gaps between words. The family members of a child with a language delay or articulation problem should know how to quickly and correctly model words, phrases, and sentences under training.

3. **Teach family members the subtle ways of prompting target behaviors.** When the parents begin their work at home, the need to model extensively will not be crucial. Most likely, the parents will have to prompt the target responses. When prompts do not work, the parents must stop the client, remind the target behavior, and perhaps model as well.

   Parents should give subtle prompts when a failure to produce the target behavior seems imminent. When family members begin to modify the client's behavior in natural settings, loud and obvious signals are not acceptable to clients. Especially when prompts have to be given in the presence of guests and visitors, the prompts must be so subtle that the others present do not notice them. A subtle and brief hand gesture or even a movement of a finger may be all that is needed to slow down the rate of speech, reduce the vocal pitch, increase vocal intensity, and decrease hoarseness of voice. Similar gestures can be devised to remind the client to open his or her mouth to increase oral resonance or to assume a certain articulatory posture. A person sitting next to the client at the dining table may touch the client to prompt the production of a target response. For each specific target response, you must devise such a specific, brief signal.

In training the family members to provide such prompts, you first demonstrate selected unobtrusive signals and teach the client to reliably respond to them in the clinic. Then ask the parents to give those signals frequently at home. Some clients may need a more pronounced stimulus in the beginning. If so, in progressive steps, reduce that obvious stimulus to a brief signal that only the family and the client will know has transpired.

During treatment sessions, give the same signal you ask the family members to use at home. When you take the client out of the treatment room to natural settings, experiment with different types of signals, and find out which one works the best for the client. Ask the parents to use the same signal at home.

4. **Teach family members how to create opportunities for the client to produce the target behaviors.** Often, clients who are communicatively handicapped are reluctant to talk even when their problems have been mostly remediated. Persons who stutter or those with hearing loss may talk less in groups just as they did before treatment, although they are now expected to use their newly acquired skills of fluency or oral language. Treated persons with aphasia also may be reluctant to talk in front of other persons. A child who has just learned to say some words may not speak them. Having gotten used to your client's role as a silent partner, the family and friends may not ask the person with a communicative disability to take part in conversation. Therefore, train family members and other persons to include the client in verbal exchanges. If the family members previously spoke for the client, ask them not to do that. For instance, the child who has learned to make requests should be asked to make relevant requests. The wife of a person who stutters should stop ordering at restaurants for him.

5. **Teach how to reinforce target behaviors.** The client's family, teachers, friends, or colleagues should know how to reinforce the tar-

get behavior productions at home and in other situations. Point out to parents and others the importance of immediate reinforcement and demonstrate how to provide it. Also, tell them it is equally important to stop the client at the earliest sign of a wrong response. Ask them not to wait until a lengthy but wrong response is completed. Show how you do this.

Like prompts that help evoke responses in natural settings, response consequences also should be delivered in a subtle manner. Most clients do not want to be reinforced in front of other persons. A man who stutters does not want his wife to say, "You are very fluent, honey!" in front of formal dinner guests. But reinforcing a stuttering person for speaking fluently in such formal occasions is important. Therefore, a special signal that is not a prompt but a reinforcement may be given discretely. Signals that prompt behaviors are given when the behavior is imminent and signals that suggest approval and praise (reinforcement) are given soon after the target behaviors are produced. If such signals are used often in the company of strangers and acquaintances, and backed up by verbal praise as soon as possible, the signals may act as discriminative stimuli.

Parents and others need not reinforce continuously. By the time maintenance strategies have begun at home, the client will have been reinforced in the clinic on a fairly large intermittent schedule. Therefore, infrequent reinforcement might be effective. Ask family members to increase the frequency of reinforcement only when the correct responses do not seem to be nearly as high as you report for treatment sessions.

6. **Teach how to provide corrective feedback but only minimally.** Generally, parents and others should be trained to reinforce more often than to punish. When wrong responses are produced, it is better to give a swift prompt than to give a punishing signal. For example, it is better to prompt a stuttering person who starts with a fast rate to slow down the rate than to whisper "no!" A hand gesture to slow down is more neutral than such verbal punishers and may be more effective. Therefore, train family members and others to prompt correct responses when incorrect responses seem imminent.

7. **Train family members to stop reinforcing inappropriate behaviors.** Family members may continue to reinforce incorrect or inappropriate behaviors. For example, a previously nonverbal child may continue to get reinforced for gestures at home. When it is clear that the child can use words, parents and others should withhold reinforcers for gestures and other nonverbal behaviors. Reinforcement should be contingent on newly learned desirable behaviors.

8. **Assess whether family members and others are prompting and reinforcing the target behaviors.** Ask them to tape-record a sample conversation or other kinds of exchange and bring it to you. You should ask for such tape-recorded evidence periodically for you to give them feedback on the performance of the family members. If they are making mistakes, you should catch them as soon as possible and give them corrective instructions.

9. **Train family members to conduct home treatment programs.** Although you will most often train parents to promote maintenance of target behaviors you have established in the clinic, you may sometimes ask family to conduct formal treatment sessions at home. For example, while working with small children and infants, you often have to train parents to conduct some portion of treatment at home. Infant language stimulation, early intervention for stuttering and articulation disorders, and intervention for vocal abuse in young children may require a substantial amount of parental work. How to train parents to do this is discussed in a subsequent section on developing home management programs.

   If parents and spouses can be trained to hold brief and parallel training sessions at home, responses may be stabilized at home sooner than otherwise expected. Possibly, parents and spouses who also are therapists even in an informal or limited sense will better promote response maintenance. If parents and spouses cannot do this, at least a few minutes of brief informal sessions at home are highly desirable. When family members agree to do this, they should set aside a time for speech work at home. They should tape-record each session they hold and submit it to you for your feedback.

   Training significant persons in a client's life is perhaps the most challenging and yet the most necessary task in promoting maintenance. You will have to constantly think of new ways of meeting this challenge.

Teach the Client Self-Control

We try to control our behaviors with varying degrees of success. But clients who learn to systematically control their behaviors have constant therapists in themselves. Clients who can monitor their behaviors do not depend much on family and friends to sustain their communicative behaviors. Therefore, **teaching self-control** is an important task in promoting response maintenance.

   From the beginning, ask clients to **judge the accuracy of their behaviors.** Ask the child in articulation treatment to say whether his or her productions were correct or not. In a matter of few training trials, most children can make this judgment. Children who are encouraged to make those judgments frequently begin to monitor their behaviors more closely. They stop as soon as they begin to misarticulate a sound.

Persons getting treatment for stuttering may be asked to judge the occurrence of stutterings, abrupt onset of phonation, a faster than required rate of speech, muscular tension while speaking, and most other target responses. Likewise, they can judge the occurrence of smooth phonation, desired rate, relaxed articulation, and so forth. Speakers who stutter who appreciate the contrast between their stuttered speech and target fluency skills will begin to monitor their speech production. They are likely to stop at the very beginning of a stutter. With further training in self-monitoring, they may stop as soon as they feel tension in their speech musculature and start with greater relaxation. When clients use such tactics, the clinician can reduce the amount of response consequation.

Clients who become proficient in recognizing their own correct and incorrect responses may be **asked to chart their behaviors** along with you. Ask them to make a tally mark on a sheet of paper every time they stutter, articulate a phoneme incorrectly, produce an undesirable vocal characteristic, and so forth. Also, ask them to tally their correct responses. Many children are eager to do it. Other children may be asked to count their correct and incorrect behaviors by placing different colored plastic chips in two cups placed in front of them.

When your clients learn to measure their correct and incorrect behaviors in the clinic, you should ask them to **bring data on their performance** outside the clinic. Measuring their behaviors in outside situations will help them monitor their target responses more closely. Individuals who stutter may be asked to record the frequency of their dysfluencies in situations when tape-recording their speech is not practical. Adult voice clients also may record the frequency of occurrence of hoarseness or hard glottal attacks and so forth. Small, hand-held counters can be used to record the frequency of behaviors.

Another useful strategy of self-control for many clients is to **implant signals that remind them of the target behaviors** in their everyday lives. For instance, clients who stutter or have high-pitched voices may draw arrows pointing downward on small pieces of paper and paste them on telephone receivers, office desks, and other places where they need reminders to reduce the rate of speech or the pitch of their voice.

Clients also may be trained to **select consequences for their own behaviors.** Self-administered consequences can be more immediate than those administered by the clinician. A voice or a fluency client may feel subtle tension in the throat that is a signal for stuttering or hoarseness. The clinician may not be able to respond to this without using a biofeedback unit. But if the client can be trained to pause, relax, and try again, such subtle muscular signals of impending incorrect behaviors will be modified before they occur. This is excellent self-control. Some clients can be trained to self-administer time-out. A man who stutters, for example, may be trained to stop speaking for a few seconds each time he stutters. By doing this, he may be able to reduce his stutterings even when no one is monitoring his fluency and stuttering.

Teach the Client To Prime Others To Administer Consequences

A common problem with contingency management in everyday life is that family members may not notice the production of correct behaviors, or may take them for granted. They may think that their only job is to stop undesirable behaviors. They may not realize that it is more important to encourage the desirable behavior. For instance, parents who are asked to monitor their child's correct and incorrect productions of target phonemes may notice incorrect production more often than correct productions. The child then hears more critical words than encouraging words.

To counter this tendency, you should train the family to prompt and reinforce as often as they can and punish as minimally as they have to. Still, many people in the client's life may be slow to reinforce. Therefore, you should teach clients to prime others to reinforce them. **Priming** is a special way of prompting others to reinforce; it is done by those who wish to receive reinforcement. The clinician asks the parent to reinforce their daughter for her correct production of phonemes. At home, the daughter primes her parents to reinforce her correct productions.

Reinforcement priming is done by drawing other people's attention to one's own behaviors that are expected to be reinforced. Whenever we show off our good behaviors or point out something we did well, we may be priming for reinforcement. We may do it with people who are notorious for ignoring good behaviors in others.

Teach clients to **draw attention to their target behavior productions** and ask the family members to reinforce immediately. Tell the family that you want the client to draw attention. Otherwise, they may think the client is showing off. A girl may let her parents know that she correctly produced a phoneme throughout a segment of conversation. A man who stutters may remind his wife that he has been speaking fluently for several minutes. Or, soon after fluently ordering food in a restaurant, he may draw his wife's attention to his successful but previously troubled performance. A woman with hoarseness may tell her listeners that she has been speaking very softly or very little in an otherwise loud family discussion.

Vocal emphasis on a target language feature may be another way of drawing attention to it. A boy who has learned to produce the regular plural morpheme slightly emphasizes it in his words, phrases, and sentences. This vocal emphasis may draw out the attention of a parent who has ignored the production.

You may train clients to ask their friends and family to remind them with a subtle hint that an undesirable response has been made. A woman with pitch breaks may request her roommate to signal with her finger that pitch breaks occurred. A woman who stutters may ask her husband to stop her whenever she stutters or speaks rapidly.

Give Sufficient Treatment

A simple reason why many clients do not maintain target responses is that they have terminated treatment against your advice or you have prematurely dismissed the client from services. There is not much you can do when clients discontinue therapy for reasons unrelated to your effectiveness. The family may move out of the area or run out of resources to continue treatment. But if the treatment was discontinued because they did not see much progress, you have something to think about. You must change or improve your treatment procedures. This is not an issue of maintenance, because the treatment was not completed. It is a maintenance issue when you prematurely dismiss a client who has been showing good progress.

Clients may be prematurely dismissed because the target responses are produced reliably in the clinical setting. The clinician may not realize that much work still needs to be done. For example, a child who correctly produces phonemes in words may still need help in producing them in conversational speech. A man who has learned to maintain an appropriate vocal pitch in the clinic may still be speaking with his unacceptably high pitch elsewhere. A woman with aphasia may say a few words in the clinic, but may not remember any of them after the treatment sessions. But in all such cases, the clinician may dismiss the client from services, because the target behaviors are produced at some level of response topography in the clinical setting.

When clients are dismissed prematurely, either the target responses have not been trained sufficiently in conversational speech or no maintenance procedures have been implemented. Because maintenance is treatment also, **prematurely dismissed clients will not have received sufficient treatment.** More importantly, treatment may be insufficient regardless of maintenance procedures. In this case, treatment will not have sufficiently strengthened the target behaviors. Also, maintenance procedures may have been started prematurely. Some clients who make rapid progress in treatment may show shaky but quick generalization, creating an illusion that sufficient treatment was given. Therefore, the clinician must **strengthen complex response topographies in the clinic** by intermittent reinforcement. Then the treatment should be gradually extended to natural settings.

Give Booster Treatment

Some clinicians assert that treatment is not successful unless clients are *permanently cured* so that they never need our services for the rest of their lives. Any relapse of stuttering in a treated person often is sharply pointed out by critics who claim there is no successful treatment for stuttering. Voice disorders, too, tend to relapse in some cases and the same argument is made. But a successfully treated disorder may return, and this is not necessarily a negative reflection on the previous success. No successful medical treatment comes with a guarantee that the patient will not catch the same disease again. Similarly, successful treatment of stuttering or any other communicative disorder does not come with a guarantee that clients will be free from the disorder for the rest of their lives.

Communicative disorders that return after successful treatment suggest that the conditions that created the disorder were confronted again by the person who was treated. We may not fully understand these conditions, or if we did, we may have no control over them. This is a matter for further research.

Meanwhile, the clinician can take pride when a disorder is treated successfully, although there is likelihood of relapse. But a careful clinician plans to take care of this eventuality. Therefore, tell your clients, especially the fluency and voice clients, that they may need additional treatment sometime in the future. Assure them that when the problem emerges again, it can be handled successfully. Caution them though, that they should contact you at the earliest sign of relapse. A slight increase in dysfluencies, hoarseness or harshness of voice, undesirable pitch, and so forth must be brought to the clinician's attention. The sooner the process of relapse is caught, the faster the progress in resumed treatment.

Treatment resumed for a client after dismissal is called **booster treatment.** The need for booster treatment shows that we have many problems to solve in the maintenance of treatment gains. But until research solves them, we must have a schedule for booster treatment for every client who needs it.

The need for booster treatment is most acute for persons who stutter. Most children and adults successfully treated for stuttering need booster treatment sometime after they are dismissed from original treatment. Fluency is not maintained in many treated individuals not because the original therapy was useless, but because they did not receive booster treatment. Therefore, plan on giving booster treatment to every person treated for stuttering.

Booster treatment is typically **the same treatment** that was successful initially unless something more powerful has been developed since dismissal. Technical improvements made during the intervening time should be included in booster treatment.

The duration of booster treatment is typically brief. In most cases, a few sessions may be sufficient, especially if the client has returned in the early stage of relapse. If the relapse is substantial, booster treatment may be prolonged.

Some clients need repeated booster treatments spread over a few years. Though discouraging to most clients, if it is explained to them that a few repetitions of treatment is a method of fading out the treatment completely, the clinician is likely to have their cooperation.

Booster treatment is also an opportunity to **strengthen family members' skills** in monitoring the client's target behaviors. It is possible that as the client's target behaviors deteriorated, the family members' monitoring of those behaviors also deteriorated. More important, the target behaviors may have been lost because of the deterioration in the monitoring skills of family members.

Booster treatment is interlinked with follow-up assessments discussed in the final section of this chapter. Extension of treatment to the natural environment, coupled with a schedule of follow-up and booster treatment, are the best the current treatment technology can offer to maintain target behaviors across speaking situations and over time.

Developing Home Treatment Programs

Home treatment programs are different from maintenance programs implemented by families. When families implement a home maintenance program, they deal with behaviors already established by a clinician. In implementing a home treatment program, the **parents may have to establish at least some of the behaviors.** The primary treatment responsibility normally rests with the clinician, but in home treatment programs, that responsibility is assigned to family members.

Home treatment programs are especially recommended for **infants at risk for developing communicative disorders.** Among others, infants who show early signs of mental retardation, potential hearing problems, neurological impairment, language delay, or certain genetic syndromes are candidates for early intervention. Early intervention by professionals may not be practical because of lack of trained personnel, limited clinical facilities, and/or no funds to pay for extended professional help. In such cases, parent training in early intervention may be the only practical course.

Home treatment programs also are needed in cases where **clients receive limited treatment** from a professional with the understanding that the family members will continue some systematic treatment at home. Clients and families who go out of town to consult with a speech-language pathologist who specializes in the treatment of certain disorders are in this category. In such cases, clients of any age may receive home treatment from their family.

Developing home treatment programs requires more information than can be offered here. You must consult other sources for details (McDonald, 1978; McDonald & Gillette, 1986; Odom & Karnes, 1988; Rossetti, 1986; Tjossem, 1976). Only a few basic principles for developing a home training program are summarized in this section.

The clinician should never simply give a written home program and ask the parents to follow it. Therefore, home training programs should be recommended only after the clinician has:

- Thoroughly assessed a client;
- Developed and tried an intervention program that works;
- Trained the parents in a home treatment program, including objective record keeping procedures; and
- Developed plans to make herself or himself available to supervise the family members' work, assess the data supplied by them, modify the treatment program, and retrain the family members when necessary.

A thorough **assessment of the infant or the child** should include an evaluation of communicative behaviors or their potential. In the case of infants, the early signs of speech and language are assessed. Such behaviors as attention, social smile, play, social or emotional responses to other people, interaction with other children, general motor development, physical development, babbling and cooing, early speech sound productions, single-word productions, and use of words in social communication, are among the several aspects of child development that are assessed. Besides, sensory development, intellectual status, and neurological and physical health of the infant also are assessed by psychologists and medical specialists. Unless a team of specialists has made a complete assessment of the child or infant, it may not be appropriate to recommend an extensive home communication treatment program. Most likely, children who need home treatment programs have other disabilities, for which different specialists also will develop home treatment programs. For example, programs for motor, sensory, and physical development may be recommended.

The speech-language pathologist must **develop and experiment with a treatment program** with the infant or the child to make sure it works. Because what works with one infant may not necessarily work with another, the clinician must develop a trial period of treatment to establish effective target behaviors and treatment procedures. The clinician should complete a few days or weeks of systematic work before recommending a program for home use. Continuous data recorded during treatment should be used to assess what an infant has learned in treatment.

The trial treatment is also the opportunity to **train parents in the home treatment program.** Parents should take part in all sessions of trial therapy. They should also take part in the selection of target behaviors and in further refining them as treatment continues. They should know how to move on to more complex targets. By initially watching how the clinician uses the procedures and then implementing those procedures in the presence of the clinician, parents learn to teach communicative behaviors. During the trial treatment, the clinician should teach parents how to record a child's responses and in general record-keeping procedures.

Assessment of treatment data and periodic supervision of parents' work at home is essential to avoid mistakes in implementation. Tape recorded samples of treatment sessions, and preferably, videotaped samples, must be evaluated by the clinician. The clinician should promptly review parents' charts and recording sheets to evaluate changes in an infant's behavior. Frequent telephone contact may be necessary to answer parent questions and to offer suggestions based on submitted data. Periodically, the clinician may visit the home and observe the parents. At this time, the clinician may demonstrate new procedures.

When the data show no significant progress under a home treatment program, **a speech-language pathologist should offer formal treatment.** This may have to be done regardless of home progress, if the communicative disabilities warrant systematic, formal, professional help.

Follow-Up Assessments

Follow up is an assessment of response maintenance over time. It is a **conversational probe** of communicative behaviors. Students in clinical practicum often do not work long enough with the same clients to make follow-up assessments. Each semester of clinical practice, you may be assigned different clients. But follow up is an important part of clinical work. Even if you did not have frequent opportunities to practice follow-up assessments, you must know the procedures. You will be making those assessments when you take a professional position.

An individualized follow-up schedule is prepared before a client is dismissed from treatment. How the client has progressed often dictates how soon and how often follow ups are scheduled. For practical reasons, a client may be dismissed sooner than expected with the understanding that the client will return for an assessment sooner than usual. A strong response rate at a very high level of accuracy maintained in natural settings on repeated measures may suggest that the first follow up need not be too close to dismissal.

Typically, the first follow-up assessment is scheduled **3 months** after a client is dismissed from services. Assuming that the client has maintained the communicative behaviors, the next assessment may be scheduled after 6 months. If the behaviors are maintained, subsequent assessments may be scheduled in yearly intervals. A **3- to 4-year follow up** is needed for speakers who received treatment for their stuttering. A similar schedule may be needed for voice clients. Children who receive treatment for articulation disorders probably do not need such a lengthy follow up. If correct production of articulation is maintained for a year or so, chances of misarticulations returning may not be great. With other clients, such as those with aphasia or progressive neurological and physical diseases, the follow up assessment schedule is based on the client's health and progress in speech or language treatment.

Timely follow-up assessments help determine the **need for booster treatment.** These assessments must be used to prevent significant deterioration in target behaviors by offering booster treatment at the earliest possible time. Therefore, in a typical follow up, **take an extended conversational speech sample.** Make it as naturalistic as possible. If time permits, record the sample in a nonclinical setting as well. Take the client out for a walk and engage in conversation. Use a micro-tape recorder to record the conversation. Give a test only if it samples connected speech and it gives you some unique data. Because such tests are practically nonexistent, an extended conversational speech sample is your best measure.

In sampling language features, you may have to contrive the conversation or direct it in some specific manner to have the client produce those features. Follow the guidelines given in Appendix H on taking conversational speech samples.

Calculate the **percentage correct response rate** for the speech or language sample. Analyze the sample to derive such quantitative data as:

- Percentage dysfluency rate
- Percentage correct production of phonemes
- Percentage correct use of grammatical morphemes and other language features
- Number of words in sentences

- Percentage of speech time a particular voice quality was maintained
- Frequency of pitch breaks per minute of continuous speech
- Percentage of words on which inappropriate nasal resonance was heard
- Percentage of spoken words that were intelligible
- Number of words or syllables spoken per minute.

If the follow-up assessment data suggest that the target behaviors are not maintained or have declined in frequency, **arrange for immediate booster treatment.** Remember, the goal of follow up is to assess response maintenance and to give timely booster treatment to those who need it.

Even with an established follow-up schedule, the client and the family must be told they should contact you for an assessment or consultation as soon as they notice a response deterioration. If they do not understand this, the clients and the family may wait for a scheduled follow up to seek booster treatment. A follow-up schedule is valid only when target behaviors do not deteriorate in the meanwhile.

Much clinical research needs to be done on maintenance of clinically established target behaviors in natural settings. If you approach the problem from the standpoint of extending treatment to nonclinical settings, you may have greater success than if you tried to program generalization. Scheduled follow up and booster treatment and further training of the family members in contingency management during booster sessions are additional features of a sound maintenance strategy.

References

Adler, S. (1993). *Multicultural communication skills in the classroom*. Boston: Allyn & Bacon.

American Speech-Language-Hearing Association. (1983, September). Social dialects. *Asha, 27,* 23–24.

American Speech-Language-Hearing Association. (1985, June). Clinical management of communicatively handicapped minority language populations. *Asha, 27,* 29–32.

American Speech-Language-Hearing Association. (1989, March). Definitions: Bilingual speech-language pathologists and audiologists. *Asha, 31,* 93.

American Speech-Language-Hearing Association. (1993). *1993 omnibus survey results.* Unpublished report.

American Speech-Language-Hearing Association. (1994a, March). Code of ethics. *Asha, 36*(Suppl. 13), 1–2.

American Speech-Language-Hearing Association. (1994b, March). Professional liability and risk management for the audiology and speech-language pathology professions. *Asha, 36*(Suppl. 12), 25–38.

American Speech-Language-Hearing Association. (1996a, Spring). Scope of practice in speech-language pathology. *Asha, 38*(Suppl. 16), 16–20.

American Speech-Language-Hearing Association. (1996b, Spring). Scope of practice in audiology. *Asha, 38*(Suppl. 16), 12–15.

American Speech-Language-Hearing Association. (1997a, Spring). Position statement: Multiskilled personnel. *Asha, 39*(Suppl. 17), 13.

American Speech-Language-Hearing Association. (1997b). *Preferred practice patterns for the profession of speech-language pathology.* Rockville, MD: American Speech-Language-Hearing Association.

Anderson, K. N., & Anderson, L. E. (1994). *Mosby's pocket dictionary of medicine, nursing, and allied health* (2nd ed.). St. Louis: Mosby-Year Book.

ASHA Clinical Certification Board. (1994, March). Standards and implementations for the certificates of clinical competence. *Asha, 36,* 71–78.

ASHA Committee on Quality Assurance. (1990, December). Update. AIDS/HIV: Implications for speech-language pathologists and audiologists. *Asha, 32,* 46–48.

309

ASHA Committee on Service Delivery in the Schools. (1993). Guidelines for caseload size and speech-language service delivery in the schools. *Asha, 35*(Suppl. 10), 33–39.

ASHA Committee on Supervision. (1985, June). Clinical supervision in speech-language pathology. *Asha, 27*, 57–60.

ASHA Governmental Affairs Review. (1990). *Reauthorization of EHA discretionary programs.* Rockville, MD: American Speech-Language-Hearing Association.

ASHA Joint Subcommittee of the Executive Board on English Language Proficiency. (1998). Students and professionals who speak English with accents and nonstandard dialects: Issues and recommendations. Position statement and technical report. *Asha, 40*(Suppl. 18), 28–31.

ASHA Membership and Certification Handbook, Audiology. (1997). Rockville, MD: American Speech-Language-Hearing Association.

ASHA Membership and Certification Handbook, Speech-Language Pathology. (1997). Rockville, MD: American Speech-Language-Hearing Association.

ASHA Professional Services Board. (1984, April). Organization and maintenance of records for clinical service delivery. *Asha, 26*, 39.

ASHA Task Force on Protection of Clients' Rights. (1994, January). The protection of rights of people receiving audiology or speech-language pathology services. *Asha, 36*, 60–63.

Battle, D. E. (1998*). Communication disorders in multicultural populations* (2nd ed.). Stoneham: Andover Medical Publishers.

Benenson, A. S. (1990*). Control of communicable diseases in man* (15th ed.). Washington, DC: American Public Health Association.

Bernthal, J. E., & Bankson, N. W. (1993). *Articulation and phonological disorders,* (3rd ed.). Englewood Cliffs, NJ: Prentice-Hall.

Bloodstein, O. (1987). *A handbook on stuttering.* Chicago: National Easter Seal Society.

Boone, D. R., & McFarlane, S. C. (1998). *The voice and voice therapy.* (5th ed.). Englewood Cliffs, NJ: Prentice-Hall.

Brookshire, R. (1997). *An introduction to neurogenic communication disorders* (5th ed.). St. Louis: Mosby-Year Book.

Burke, F. R. (1990). *Child abuse: Prevention and intervention.* Workshop presented at California State University, Fresno.

California State Department of Education. (1989). *Program guidelines for language, speech, and hearing specialists providing designated instruction and services.* Sacramento, CA: Author.

Campbell, L. (1994). *Clinical practicum and English proficiency.* Paper presented at ASHA Conference on Multicultural Literacy in Communication Disorders. Sea Island, GA.

Carr, E., & Durand, V. M. (1985). Reducing behavioral problems through functional communication training. *Journal of Applied Behavior Analysis, 18*, 111–126.

Case, J. L. (1996). *Clinical management of voice disorders* (3rd ed.). Austin, TX: PRO-ED.

Charlop, M. H., Burgio, L. D., Iwata, B. A., & Ivancic, M. T. (1988). Stimulus variation as a means of enhancing punishment effects. *Journal of Applied Behavior Analysis, 21*, 89–95.

Charlop, M. H., Kurtz, P. F., Casey, F. G., & Greenberg, F. (1990). Using aberrant behaviors as reinforcers for autistic children. *Journal of Applied Behavior Analysis, 23*, 163–181.

Cheng, L. L. (1991). *Assessing Asian language performance* (2nd ed.). Oceanside, CA: Academic Communication Associates.

Cheng, L. L. (1995). *Integrating language and learning for inclusion, an Asian-Pacific focus.* San Diego: Singular Publishing Group.

Chomsky, N., & Halle, M. (1968). *The sound pattern of English.* New York: Harper & Row.

Cole, L. (1992, May). Our multicultural agenda. *Asha, 34,* 38.

Collins, M. J. (1991). *Diagnosis and treatment of global aphasia.* San Diego: Singular Publishing Group.

Davis, G. A. (1993). *A survey of adult aphasia and related language disorders* (2nd ed.). Englewood Cliffs, NJ: Prentice-Hall.

Dublinske, S., & Healey, W. C. (1978, March). P.L. 94-142: Questions and answers for the speech-language pathologist and audiologist, *Asha, 20,* 188–205.

Duffy, J. R. (1995). *Motor speech disorders.* St. Louis, MO: Mosby.

Durand, V. M., & Carr, E. G. (1987). Social influences on "self-stimulatory" behavior: Analysis and treatment application. *Journal of Applied Behavior Analysis, 20,* 119–132.

Egel, A. L. (1981). Reinforcer variation: Implications for motivating developmentally disabled children. *Journal of Applied Behavior Analysis, 14,* 345–350.

Elbert, M., & Gierut, J. (1986). *Handbook of clinical phonology: Approaches to assessment and treatment.* San Diego: College-Hill Press.

Emerick, L. L., & Haynes, W. O. (1986). *Diagnosis and evaluation in speech pathology.* (3rd ed.). Englewood Cliffs, NJ: Prentice-Hall.

Flower, R. (1984). *Delivery of speech-language pathology and audiology services.* Baltimore: Williams & Wilkins.

Goldberg, B. (1994, June-July). Managing diversity: Its common sense. *Asha, 36,* 44–48.

Golper, L. G. (1998). *Sourcebook for medical speech pathology* (2nd ed.). San Diego: Singular Publishing Group.

Hall, P. K., Jordan, L. S., & Robin, D. A. (1993). *Developmental apraxia of speech.* Austin, TX: PRO-ED.

Hamayan, E. V., & Damico, J. S. (Eds.). (1991). *Limiting bias in the assessment of the bilingual child.* Austin, TX: PRO-ED.

Harris, G. A. (1993). American Indian cultures: A lesson in diversity. In D. E. Battle (Ed.), *Communication disorders in multicultural populations* (pp. 78–113). Boston: Andover Medical Publishers.

Hegde, M. N. (1985). Treatment of fluency disorders: State of the art. In J. M. Costello (Ed.), *Speech disorders in adults: Recent advances* (pp. 155–188). Austin, TX: PRO-ED.

Hegde, M. N. (1988). *Principles of management and remediation.* In N. J. Lass, L. V. McReynolds, J. L. Northern, & D. F. Yoder (Eds.), *Handbook of speech-language pathology and audiology* (pp. 377–394). Toronto, Canada: Decker.

Hegde, M. N. (1998a). *A coursebook on scientific and professional writing in speech-language pathology* (2nd ed.). San Diego: Singular Publishing Group.

Hegde, M. N. (1998b). *Treatment procedures in communicative disorders* (3rd ed.). Austin, TX: PRO-ED.

Helm-Estabrooks, N., & Albert, M. L. (1991). *A manual of aphasia therapy.* Austin, TX: PRO-ED.

Hodson, B. W. (1980). *The assessment of phonological processes*. Austin, TX: PRO-ED.

Ingham, R. J. (1984). *Stuttering and behavior therapy: Current status and experimental foundations*. Austin, TX: PRO-ED.

Iwata, B. (1987). Negative reinforcement in applied behavior analysis: An emerging technology. *Journal of Applied Behavior Analysis, 20*, 361–378.

Iwata, B. A., Pace, G. M., Kalsher, M. J., Cowdery, G. E., & Cataldo, M. F. (1990). Experimental analysis and extinction of self-injurious escape behavior. *Journal of Applied Behavior Analysis, 23*, 11–27.

James, S. L. (1990). *Normal language acquisition*. Boston: Little, Brown.

Johns, D. F. (Ed.). (1985). *Clinical management of neurogenic communicative disorders*. Austin, TX: PRO-ED.

Kamhi, A. G., Pollock, K. E., & Harris, J. L. (Eds.). (1996). *Communication development and disorders in African American children: Research, assessment and intervention*. Baltimore, MD: Paul H. Brooks.

Kayser, H. (1995). *Bilingual speech-language pathology: An Hispanic focus*. San Diego: Singular Publishing Group.

Kelly, B. R., Davis, D., & Hegde, M. N. (1994). *Clinical methods and practicum in audiology*. San Diego: Singular Publishing Group.

Kemp, R. J., Roeser, R. J., Pearson, D. W., & Ballachanda, B. B. (1995). *Infection control for the professions of audiology and speech-language pathology*. Chesterfield, MO: Oaktree Products, Inc.

Knepflar, K. J., & May, A. A. (1989). *Report writing in the field of communication disorders: A handbook for students and clinicians* (2nd ed.). Rockville, MD: National Student Speech-Language-Hearing Association.

Langdon, H. W., & Cheng, L. L. (Eds.). (1992). *Hispanic children and adults with communication disorders: Assessment and intervention*. Gaithersburg, MD: Aspen Publishers.

LaPointe, L. L. (Ed.). (1990). *Aphasia and related neurogenic language disorders*. New York: Thieme Medical Publishers.

Lowe, R. J. (1993). *Speech-language pathology and related professions in the schools*. Needham, MA: Allyn & Bacon.

Lubinski, R. (Ed.). (1991). *Dementia and communication*. Philadelphia: Mosby.

Lynch, C., & Welsh, R. (1993, March). Characteristics of state licensure laws. *Asha, 35*, 130–139.

Mace, C. F., Hock, M., Lalli, J. S., West, B. J., Belfiore, P., Pinter, E., & Brown, D. K. (1988). Behavioral momentum in the treatment of noncompliance. *Journal of Applied Behavior Analysis, 21*, 123–141.

Mason, S. A., & Iwata, B. A. (1990). Artifactual effects of sensory-integrative therapy on self-injurious behaviors. *Journal of Applied Behavior Analysis, 23*, 361–370.

Mattes, L., & Omark, D. (1991). *Speech and language assessment for the bilingually handicapped* (2nd ed.). Oceanside, CA: Academic Communication Associates.

McCormick, L., Frome Loeb, D., & Schiefelbusch, R. L., (1997). *Supporting children with communication difficulties in inclusive settings: School-based language intervention*. Boston: Allyn & Bacon.

McCormick, L., & Schiefelbusch, R. L. (1990). *Early language intervention: An introduction* (2nd ed.). Columbus, OH: Merrill.

McDonald, J. (1978). *Environmental language inventory*. Columbus, OH: Merrill.

McDonald, J., & Gillette, Y. (1986). Communicating with persons with severe handicaps: Roles of parents and professionals. *Journal of the Association for the Severely Handicapped, 11,* 225–265.

McMillan, M. O., & Willette, S. J. (1988, November). Aseptic technique: A procedure for preventing disease transmission in the practice environment, *Asha, 30,* 35–37.

Merritt, D. D., & Culatta, B. (1998). *Language intervention in the classroom.* San Diego: Singular Publishing Group.

Meyen, E. L., Vergason, G. A., & Whelan, R. J. (Eds.). (1996). *Strategies for teaching exceptional children in inclusive settings.* Denver, CO: Love Publishing.

Musselwhite, C. R., & St. Louis, K. W. (1988). *Communication programming for persons with severe handicaps.* Austin, TX: PRO-ED.

Nelson, N. W. (1993). *Childhood language disorders in context.* New York: Macmillan.

Odom, S., & Karnes, M. (1988). *Early intervention for infants and children with handicaps.* Baltimore: Paul H. Brookes.

Owens, R. E., Jr. (1991). *Language disorders: A functional approach to assessment and intervention.* New York: Macmillan.

Owens, R. E., Jr. (1992). *Language development: An introduction* (3rd ed.). New York: Times Mirror/Mosby.

Paul-Brown, D. (1994, May). Clinical record keeping in audiology and speech-language pathology. *Asha, 36,* 40–42.

Payan, R. (1984). Language assessment for bilingual exceptional children. In L. M. Baca & H. T. Cervantes (Eds.), *The bilingual special education interface.* St. Louis, MO: Times Mirror/Mosby.

Payne, J. C. (1997). *Adult neurogenic language disorders: Assessment and treatment.* San Diego: Singular Publishing Group.

Payne, K. T., & Anderson, N. (1991). *How to prepare for the N.E.S.P.A.: National examinations in speech pathology and audiology.* San Diego: Singular Publishing Group.

Peterson, H., & Marquardt, T. (1990). *Appraisal and diagnosis of speech and language disorders* (2nd ed.). Englewood Cliffs, NJ: Prentice-Hall.

Reed, V. (1994). *An introduction to children with language disorders* (2nd ed.). New York: Macmillan Publishing Co.

Repp, A. C., Felce, D., & Barton, L. E. (1988). Basing the treatment of stereotypic and self-injurious behaviors on hypotheses of their causes. *Journal of Applied Behavior Analysis, 21,* 281–289.

Roseberry-McKibbin, C. (1995). *Multicultural students with special language needs: Practical strategies for assessment and intervention.* Oceanside, CA: Academic Communication Associates.

Roseberry-McKibbin, C., & Hegde, M. N. (in press). *Comprehensive review of speech-language pathology.* Austin, TX: PRO-ED.

Rosenbek, J. C. (1985). Treating apraxia of speech. In D. F. Johns (Ed.), *Clinical management of communicative disorders* (2nd ed., pp. 276–312). Austin, TX: PRO-ED.

Rosenbek, J. C., LaPointe, L. L., & Wertz, R. (1989). *Aphasia: A clinical approach.* Austin, TX: PRO-ED.

Rossetti, L. (1986). *High-risk infants: Identification, assessment, and intervention.* Austin, TX: PRO-ED.

Schiefelbusch, R. L., & Lloyd, L. L. (Eds.). (1988). *Language perspectives: Acquisition, retardation, and intervention.* Austin, TX: PRO-ED.

Screen, R. M., & Anderson, N. B. (1994). *Multicultural perspectives in communication disorders.* San Diego, CA: Singular Publishing Group.

Seymour, C. M., & Nober, E. H. (1998). *Introduction to communication disorders: A multicultural approach.* Boston: Butterworth-Heinemann.

Silverman, F. (1989). *Speech for the speechless.* Englewood Cliffs, NJ: Prentice-Hall.

Skinner, B. F. (1957). *Verbal behavior.* New York: Appleton-Century-Crofts.

Stoel-Gammon, C., & Dunn, C. (1985). *Normal and disordered phonology in children.* Austin, TX: PRO-ED.

Taylor, O. (Ed.). (1986a). *Nature of communication disorders in culturally and linguistically diverse populations.* San Diego: College-Hill Press.

Taylor, O. (Ed.). (1986b). *Treatment of communication disorders in culturally and linguistically diverse populations.* San Diego: College-Hill Press.

Terrell, S. L., & Terrell, F. (1993). African-American cultures. In D. E. Battle (Ed.), *Communication disorders in multicultural populations* (pp. 3–37). Stoneham, MA: Andover Medical Publishers.

Thompson, C. K. (1988). *Articulation disorders in the child with neurogenic pathology.* In N. J. Lass, L. V. McReynolds, J. L. Northern, & D. F. Yoder (Eds.), *Handbook of speech-language pathology and audiology* (pp. 548–591). Toronto, Canada: Decker

Tjossem, T. D. (Ed.). (1976). *Intervention strategies for high-risk infants and young children.* Baltimore: University Park Press.

Tomblin, J. B., Morris, H. L., & Spriestersbach, D. C. (Eds.). (1994). *Diagnosis in speech-language pathology.* San Diego: Singular Publishing Group.

Trueba, H. T., Cheng, L. L., & Ima, K. (1993). *Myth or reality: Adaptive strategies of Asian Americans in California.* Washington, DC: The Falmer Press.

Trueba, H. T., Jacobs, L., & Kirton, E. (1990). *Cultural conflict and adaptation: The case of Hmong children in American Society.* Washington, DC: The Falmer Press.

Van Keulen, J. E., Weddington, G. T., & DeBose, C. E. (1998). *Speech, language, learning, and the African American child.* Needham Heights, MA: Allyn and Bacon.

Warren, S. F., & Rogers-Warren, A. K. (1985). *Teaching functional language.* Baltimore: University Park Press.

Weeks, M., & Gaylord-Ross, R. (1981). Task difficulty and aberrant behavior in severely handicapped students. *Journal of Applied Behavior Analysis, 14,* 449–463.

Westby, C. E. (1994). *Multicultural issues.* In J. B. Tomblin, H. L. Morris, & D. C. Spriestersbach (Eds.), *Diagnosis in speech-language pathology* (pp. 29–50). San Diego: Singular Publishing Group.

Wilson, D. K. (1987). *Voice problems of children* (3rd ed.). Baltimore: Williams & Wilkins.

Winokur, S. (1976). *A primer of verbal behavior.* Englewood Cliffs, NJ: Prentice-Hall.

Yavas, M. (Ed.). (1994). *First and second language phonology.* San Diego: Singular Publishing Group.

Yorkston, K. M., Beukelman, D. R., & Bell, K. R. (1988). *Clinical management of dysarthric speakers.* Austin, TX: PRO-ED.

A

Glossary of Educational Abbreviations and Acronyms

The following is a list of acronyms, initialisms, and abbreviations commonly used in education. Additional or different acronyms and abbreviations may be used at specific school sites. The names of tests, associations, and universities have not been included in this list.

ADA: average daily attendance
ADD: attention deficit disorder
BICS: basic interpersonal communication skills
CA: chronological age
CALP: cognitive academic language proficiency
CH: communicatively handicapped
DD: developmentally disabled
DIS: designated instructional service
ED: emotionally disturbed—Department of Education
EDGAR: Education Department general administrative regulations
EEEA: Equity and Excellence in Education Act
EHA: Education of the Handicapped Act of 1975 (now known as
            IDEA as amended in 1990)
ESL: English as a second language
FAPE: free appropriate public education
FEP: fluent English proficient
FERPA: Family Education Rights and Privacy Act
FES: fluent English-speaking
HBI: home-based instruction
HI: hearing impaired
IDEA: Individuals with Disabilities Education Act (1990 amend-
            ment of EHA changed name to IDEA)
IEP: Individualized Education Program
IFSP: Individualized Family Service Plan
IMC: instructional materials (media) center
LD: learning disability/learning disabled
LEA: local education agency
LEP: limited English-proficient
LES: limited English-speaking
LH: learning handicapped
LRE: least restrictive environment
LSH: language speech & hearing specialist
MA: mental age
MR: mentally retarded
NES: non-English-speaking
OCR: Office For Civil Rights
OH: orthopedically handicapped
OSEP: Office of Special Education Programs, U.S. Department of
            Education
OSERS: Office of Special Education and Rehabilitative Services
OT: occupational therapy
PDD: pervasive developmental disorder

PL 94–142:   Public Law 94–142, The Education for all Handicapped Children Act of 1975

PL 99–457:   The 1986 amendments to the PL 94–142 which included the Early Intervention Program for Infants and Toddlers (Part H —now Part C)

PLP: present levels of performance

PT: physical therapist

RS: resource specialist

RSP: resource specialist program

SDC: special day class

SEA: state education agency

SED: severely emotionally disturbed

SH: severely handicapped

SST: student study team

B

Glossary of Medical Abbreviations and Symbols

Recording information in a patient's chart is a common form of communication among professionals in the medical setting. It provides a chronological log of patient services. Many abbreviations, acronyms, and symbols are used in recording data. Although there are universal symbols, initialisms, and abbreviations, some may be unique to a specific hospital. To avoid any misunderstanding, if you are unsure of an abbreviation, acronym, initialism, or symbol do not use it; instead, write out the entire word or phrase. Following is a list of some of the commonly used abbreviations, acronyms, and symbols. (Abbreviations for measurements, tests, and professional associations have not been included in this list.)

a.c.:	before meals
ACU:	ambulatory care unit or acute care unit
ACVD:	atherosclerotic cardiovascular disease
Al:	allergy
Amb:	ambulatory
A&O:	alert and oriented
Asp:	aspirate
ATC:	around the clock
b.i.d.:	twice a day
b.i.n.:	twice a night
c̄:	with
Ca:	cancer
CHF:	congestive heart failure
CHI:	closed-head injury
CN:	cranial nerve
CNS:	central nervous system
C/O:	complains of
CPD:	cardio-pulmonary disease
CVA:	cerebrovascular accident
DC (D/C):	discontinue or discharge
DNT:	did not test
DU:	diagnosis unknown
Dx:	diagnosis
FIM:	functional independence measure
Fx:	fracture
h:	hour
h.s.:	hour of sleep or bedtime
HUC	hospital unit clerk
Hx.:	history
IAO:	immediately after onset
ICU:	intensive care unit
Lt. (L):	left
LOS:	length of stay
MS:	mental status
MVT:	motor vehicle accident
NGT:	nasogastric tube
NKA:	no known allergies
n.p.o.:	nothing by mouth
OG:	oralgastric tube
p.c.:	after meals
p.o.:	by mouth
p.r.n.:	as necessary

pt.:	patient
q.:	every
q.d.:	every day
q.i.d.:	four times a day
RO:	renew order
Rt. (R):	right
Rx:	prescription or therapy (treatment)
s̄:	without
SLP:	speech-language pathologist
Stat.:	immediately
TAR:	therapy authorization request
TBI:	traumatic brain injury
t.i.d.:	three times a day
t.i.n.:	three times a night
TPR:	temperature, pulse, respiration
Tx:	therapy (treatment)
WFL:	within functional limits
WNL:	within normal limits
♀	female
♂	male
↑	above or increase
↓	below or decrease
O	absent or no response
∅	no or none
?	doubtful or unknown

C

Sample Clinical Practicum Hour Recording Form

What follows is a general clinical practicum hour recording form. Consult your supervisor for the specific form used in your program.

University Speech and Hearing Center
Clinical Practicum Hours

Student	Supervisor	Semester

Practicum Site	Circle one: Adults	Children

EVALUATION/DIAGNOSTIC HOURS							
Date	Language	Articulation	Voice	Fluency	Other	Staffing	Supervisor Initials
Total							

TREATMENT HOURS							
Date	Language	Articulation	Voice	Fluency	Other	Staffing	Supervisor Initials
Total							

Supervisor's Signature	License #	ASHA CCC Account #

D

Code of Ethics of the American Speech-Language-Hearing-Association (Revised January 1, 1994)

Preamble

The preservation of the highest standards of integrity and ethical principles is vital to the responsible discharge of obligations in the professions of speech-language pathology and audiology. This Code of Ethics sets forth the fundamental principles and rules considered essential to this purpose.

Every individual who is (a) a member of the American Speech-Language-Hearing Association, whether certified or not, (b) a nonmember holding the Certificate of Clinical Competence from the Association, (c) an applicant for membership or certification, or (d) a Clinical Fellow seeking to fulfill standards for certification shall abide by this Code of Ethics.

Any action that violates the spirit and purpose of this Code shall be considered unethical. Failure to specify any particular responsibility or practice in this Code of Ethics shall not be construed as denial of the existence of such responsibilities or practices.

The fundamentals of ethical conduct are described by Principles of Ethics and by Rules of Ethics as they relate to responsibility to persons served, to the public, and to the professions of speech-language pathology and audiology.

Principles of Ethics, aspirational and inspirational in nature, form the underlying moral basis for the Code of Ethics. Individuals shall observe these principles as affirmative obligations under all conditions of professional activity.

Rules of Ethics are specific statements of minimally acceptable professional conduct or of prohibitions and are applicable to all individuals.

Principle of Ethics I

Individuals shall honor their responsibility to hold paramount the welfare of persons they serve professionally.

Rules of Ethics

A. Individuals shall provide all services competently.

B. Individuals shall use every resource, including referral when appropriate, to ensure that high-quality service is provided.

C. Individuals shall not discriminate in the delivery of professional services on the basis of race or ethnicity, gender, age, religion, national origin, sexual orientation, or disability.

---

[1]Reprinted with permission from American Speech-Language-Hearing Association (1994a), Code of Ethics, *Asha, 36*(March, Suppl. 13) pp. 1–2.

D. Individuals shall fully inform the persons they serve of the nature and possible effects of services rendered and products dispensed.

E. Individuals shall evaluate the effectiveness of services rendered and of products dispensed and shall provide services or dispense products only when benefit can reasonably be expected.

F. Individuals shall not guarantee the results of any treatment or procedure, directly or by implication; however, they may make a reasonable statement of prognosis.

G. Individuals shall not evaluate or treat speech, language, or hearing disorders solely by correspondence.

H. Individuals shall maintain adequate records of professional services rendered and products dispensed and shall allow access to these records when appropriately authorized.

I. Individuals shall not reveal, without authorization, any professional or personal information about the person served professionally, unless required by law to do so, or unless doing so is necessary to protect the welfare of the person or of the community.

J. Individuals shall not charge for services not rendered, nor shall they misrepresent,[1] in any fashion, services rendered or products dispensed.

K. Individuals shall use persons in research or as subjects of teaching demonstrations only with their informed consent.

L. Individuals whose professional services are adversely affected by substance abuse or other health-related conditions shall seek professional assistance and, where appropriate, withdraw from the affected areas of practice.

Principle of Ethics II

Individuals shall honor their responsibility to achieve and maintain the highest level of professional competence.

---

[1]For purposes of this Code of Ethics, misrepresentation includes any untrue statements or statements that are likely to mislead. Misrepresentation also includes the failure to state any information that is material and that ought, in fairness, to be considered.

Rules of Ethics

A. Individuals shall engage in the provision of clinical services only when they hold the appropriate Certificate of Clinical Competence or when they are in the certification process and are supervised by an individual who holds the appropriate Certificate of Clinical Competence.

B. Individuals shall engage in only those aspects of the professions that are within the scope of their competence, considering their level of education, training, and experience.

C. Individuals shall continue their professional development throughout their careers.

D. Individuals shall delegate the provision of clinical services only to persons who are certified or to persons in the education or certification process who are appropriately supervised. The provision of support services may be delegated to persons who are neither certified nor in the certification process only when a certificate holder provides appropriate supervision.

E. Individuals shall prohibit any of their professional staff from providing services that exceed the staff member's level of education, training, and experience.

F. Individuals shall ensure that all equipment used in the provision of services is in proper working order and is properly calibrated.

Principle of Ethics III

Individuals shall honor their responsibility to the public by promoting public understanding of the professions, by supporting the development of services designed to furfill the unmet needs of the public, and by providing accurate information in all communications involving any aspect of the professions.

Rules of Ethics

A. Individuals shall not misrepresent their credentials, competence, education, training, or experience.

B. Individuals shall not participate in professional activities that constitute a conflict of interest.

C. Individuals shall not misrepresent diagnostic information, services rendered, or products dispensed or engage in any scheme or artifice to defraud in connection with obtaining payment or reimbursement for such services or products.

D. Individuals' statements to the public shall provide accurate information about the nature and management of communication disorders, about the professions, and about professional services.

E. Individuals' statements to the public—advertising, announcing, and marketing their professional services, reporting research results, and promoting products—shall adhere to prevailing professional standards and shall not contain misrepresentations.

Principle of Ethics IV

Individuals shall honor their responsibility to the professions and their relationships with colleagues, students, and members of allied professions. Individuals shall uphold the dignity and autonomy of the professions, maintain harmonious interprofessional and intraprofessional relationships, and accept the professions' self-imposed standards.

Rules of Ethics

A. Individuals shall prohibit anyone under their supervision from engaging in any practice that violates the Code of Ethics.

B. Individuals shall not engage in dishonesty, fraud, deceit, misrepresentation, or any form of conduct that adversely reflects on the professions or on the individual's fitness to serve persons professionally.

C. Individuals shall assign credit only to those who have contributed to a publication, presentation, or product. Credit shall be assigned in proportion to the contribution and only with the contributor's consent.

D. Individuals' statements to colleagues about professional services, research results, and products shall adhere to prevailing professional standards and shall contain no misrepresentations.

E. Individuals shall not provide professional services without exercising independent professional judgment, regardless of referral source or prescription.

F. Individuals shall not discriminate in their relationships with colleagues, students, and members of allied professions on the basis of race or ethnicity, gender, age, religion, national origin, sexual orientation, or disability.

G. Individuals who have reason to believe that the Code of Ethics has been violated shall inform the Ethical Practice Board.

H. Individuals shall cooperate fully with the Ethical Practice Board in its investigation and adjudication of matters related to this Code of Ethics.

Scope of Practice in Speech-Language Pathology

Ad Hoc Committee on Scope of Practice in Speech-Language Pathology[1]

This scope of practice in speech-language pathology statement is an official policy of the American Speech-Language-Hearing Association (ASHA). It was developed by the Ad Hoc Committee on Scope of Practice in Speech-Language Pathology: Sarah W. Blackstone, chair, Diane Paul-Brown, ex officio; David A. Brandt; Rhonda Friedlander; Luis F. Riquelme; and Mark Ylvisaker. Crystal S. Cooper, vice president for professional practices in speech-language pathology, served as monitoring vice-president. The contributions of the editor, Jude Langsam, and select and widespread peer reviewers are gratefully acknowledged. This statement supersedes the Scope of Practice, Speech-Language Pathology and Audiology statement (LC 6-89), Asha, April l 990, 1-2.

Scope of Practice in Speech-Language Pathology

Preamble

The purpose of this statement is to define the scope of practice of speech-language pathology in order to:

1. delineate areas of services and supports provided by ASHA members and certificate holders in accordance with the ASHA Code of Ethics. Services refer to clinical services for individuals with speech, voice, language, communication, and swallowing disorders, aimed at the amelioration of difficulties stemming from such disorders. Supports refer to environmental modifications, assistive technology, and guidance for communication partners to help persons with these disorders;
2. educate health care, education, and other professionals, consumers, payers, regulators, and members of the general public about treatment and other services and supports offered by speech-language pathologists as qualified providers;
3. assist members and certificate holders in their efforts to provide appropriate and high quality speech-language pathology services and supports to persons across the life span with speech, voice, language, communication, and swallowing disabilities;

---

[1]American Speech-Language-Hearing Association (1999). Scope of practice in speech-language pathology [On-line]. Available: www.asha.org. Reprinted with permission.

4. establish a reference for curriculum review of education programs in speech-language pathology.

The scope of practice defined here and the areas specifically set forth are part of an effort to describe the broad range of services and supports offered within the profession. It is recognized, however, that levels of experience, skill, and proficiency with respect to the activities identified within this scope of practice vary among the individual providers. It may not be possible for speech-language pathologists to practice in all areas of the field. As the ASHA Code of Ethics specifies, individuals may only practice in areas where they are competent based on their education, training, and experience (American Speech-Language-Hearing Association, 1994). However, nothing limits speech-language pathologists from expanding their current level of expertise. Certain clients or practice settings may necessitate that speech-language pathologists pursue additional education or training to expand their personal scope of practice.

This scope of practice statement does not supersede existing state licensure laws or affect the interpretation or implementation of such laws. It may serve, however, as a model for the development or modification of licensure laws.

The schema in Figure 1 depicts the relationship of the scope of practice to ASHA's policy documents of the Association that address current and emerging speech-language pathology practice areas; that is, preferred practice patterns, guidelines, and position statements.

Finally, it is recognized that speech-language pathology is a dynamic and continuously developing practice area. Listing specific areas within this scope of practice does not necessarily exclude other, new, or emerging areas. Indeed, changes in service delivery systems, the increasing numbers of persons who need communication services, and technological and scientific advances have mandated that a scope of practice for the profession of speech-language pathology be a dynamic statement. For these reasons this document will undergo periodic review and possible revision.

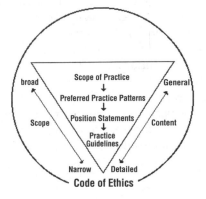

Figure 1. Conceptual Framework of ASHA Policy Statements

The documents depicted in this diagram together serve as a guide to professional practice in speech language pathology.

Statement

The goal of the profession of speech-language pathology and its members is provision of the highest quality treatment and other services consistent with the fundamental right of those served to participate in decisions that affect their lives.

Speech-language pathologists hold the master's or doctoral degree, the Certificate of Clinical Competence of the American Speech-Language-Hearing Association, and state licensure where applicable.

These professionals serve individuals, families, groups, and the general public through their involvement in a broad range of professional activities. They work to prevent speech, voice, language, communication, swallowing, and related disabilities. They screen, identify, assess, diagnose, refer, and provide treatment and intervention, including consultation and follow-up services, to persons of all ages with, or at risk for, speech, voice, language, communication, swallowing, and related disabilities. They counsel individuals with these disorders, as well as their families, caregivers, and other service providers, related to the disorders and their management.

Speech-language pathologists select, prescribe, dispense, and provide services supporting the effective use of augmentative and alternative communication devices and other communication prostheses and assistive devices.

Speech-language pathologists also teach, supervise, and manage clinical and educational programs, and engage in program development, program oversight, and research activities related to communication sciences and disorders, swallowing, and related areas.

They measure treatment outcomes, evaluate the effectiveness of their practices, modify services in relation to their evaluations, and disseminate these findings. They also serve as case managers and expert witnesses. As an integral part of their practice, speech-language pathologists work to increase public awareness and advocate for the people they serve.

Speech-language pathologists provide services in settings that are deemed appropriate, including but not limited to health care, educational, community, vocational, and home settings. Speech-language pathologists serve diverse populations. The client population includes persons of different race, age, gender, religion, national origin, and sexual orientation. Speech-language pathologists' caseloads include persons from diverse ethnic, cultural, or linguistic backgrounds, and persons with disabilities. Although speech-language pathologists are prohibited from discriminating in the provision of professional services based on these factors, in some cases such factors may be relevant to the development of an appropriate treatment plan. These factors may be considered in treatment plans only when firmly grounded in scientific and professional knowledge.

As primary care providers of communication treatment and other services, speech-language pathologists are autonomous professionals; that is, their services need not be prescribed by another. However, in most cases individuals are best served when speech-language pathologists work collaboratively with other professionals, individuals with disabilities, and their family members. Similarly, it is recognized that related fields and professions may have some knowledge, skills, and experience that could be applied to some areas within this scope of practice. Defining the scope of practice of speech-language pathologists is not meant to exclude members of other professions or related fields from rendering services in common practice areas.

The practice of speech-language pathology includes:

1. Providing screening, identification, assessment, diagnosis, treatment, intervention (i.e., prevention, restoration, amelioration, compensation) and follow-up services for disorders of:

   - speech: articulation, fluency, voice (including respiration, phonation, and resonance)
   - language (involving the parameters of phonology, morphology, syntax, semantics, and pragmatics; and including disorders of receptive and expressive communication in oral, written, graphic, and manual modalities)
   - oral, pharyngeal, cervical esophageal, and related functions (e.g., dysphagia, including disorders of swallowing and oral function for feeding; orofacial myofunctional disorders)
   - cognitive aspects of communication (including communication disability and other functional disabilities associated with cognitive impairment)
   - social aspects of communication (including challenging behavior, ineffective social skills, lack of communication opportunities);

2. Providing consultation and counseling, and making referrals when appropriate;
3. Training and supporting family members and other communication partners of individuals with speech, voice, language, communication, and swallowing disabilities;
4. Developing and establishing effective augmentative and alternative communication techniques and strategies, including selecting, prescribing, and dispensing of aids and devices and training individuals, their families, and other communication partners in their use;

5. Selecting, fitting, and establishing effective use of appropriate prosthetic/adaptive devices for speaking and swallowing (e.g., tracheoesophageal valves, electrolarynges, speaking valves);
6. Using instrumental technology to diagnose and treat disorders of communication and swallowing (e.g., videofluoroscopy, nasendoscopy, ultrasonography, stroboscopy);
7. Providing aural rehabilitation and related counseling services to individuals with hearing loss and to their families;
8. Collaborating in the assessment of central auditory processing disorders in cases in which there is evidence of speech, language, and/or other cognitive-communication disorders; providing intervention for individuals with central auditory processing disorders.
9. Conducting pure-tone air conduction hearing screening and screening tympanometry for the purpose of the initial identification and/or referral of individuals with other communication disorders or possible middle ear pathology.
10. Enhancing speech and language proficiency and communication effectiveness, including but not limited to accent reduction, collaboration with teachers of English as a second language, and improvement of voice, performance, and singing;
11. Training and supervising support personnel;
12. Developing and managing academic and clinical programs in communication sciences and disorders;
13. Conducting, disseminating, and applying research in communication sciences and disorders;
14. Measuring outcomes of treatment and conducting continuous evaluation of the effectiveness of practices and programs to improve and maintain quality of services.

Refer to the Reference List for the most recent ASHA documents on these topics.

Reference List

General

American Speech-Language-Hearing Association. (1993). Definition of communication disorders and variations. *Asha, 35*(Suppl. 10), 40–41.
American Speech-Language-Hearing Association. (1993). Preferred practice patterns for the professions of speech-language pathology and audiology. *Asha, 35*(Suppl. 11), 1–100.
American Speech-Language-Hearing Association. (1994). Code of Ethics. *Asha, 36* (Suppl. 13), 1–2.

Speech: Articulation, Fluency, Voice

American Speech-Language-Hearing Association. (1992). Position statement and guidelines for evaluation and treatment for tracheoesophageal fistulization/puncture. *Asha, 34*(Suppl. 7), 17–21.

American Speech-Language-Hearing Association. (1992). Position statement and guidelines for vocal tract visualization and imaging. *Asha, 34*(Suppl. 7), 31–40.

American Speech-Language-Hearing Association. (1993). Position statement and guidelines for oral and oropharyngeal prostheses. *Asha, 35*(Suppl. 10), 14–16.

American Speech-Language-Hearing Association. (1993). Position statement and guidelines on the use of voice prostheses in tracheotomized persons with or without ventilatory dependence. *Asha, 35*(Suppl. 10), 17–20.

American Speech-Language-Hearing Association. (1995, March). Guidelines for practice in stuttering treatment. *Asha, 35*(Suppl. 14), 26–35.

Language

American Speech-Language-Hearing Association. (1975). Meeting the needs of children and adults with disorders of language: the role of the speech-language pathologist and audiologist. *Asha, 17*(4), 273–277.

American Speech-Language-Hearing Association. (1982). Definition of language. *Asha, 24*(6), 44.

American Speech-Language-Hearing Association. (1982). Position statement on language learning disorders. *Asha, 24*(11), 937–944.

American Speech-Language-Hearing Association. (1989). Issues in determining eligibility for language intervention. *Asha, 31*(3), 113–118.

American Speech-Language-Hearing Association. (1991). Guidelines for speech-language pathologists serving persons with language, socio-communicative and/or cognitive-communicative impairments. *Asha 33*(Suppl. 5), 21–28.

American Speech-Language-Hearing Association Task Force on Central Auditory Processing Consensus Development. (1995). *Central auditory processing: Current status of research and implications for clinical practice.* Rockville, MD: ASHA.

Oral, Pharyngeal, Cervical Esophageal, and Related Functions

American Speech-Language-Hearing Association. (1987). Ad hoc committee on dysphagia report. *Asha, 29*(4), 57–58.

American Speech-Language-Hearing Association. (1989). Report: Ad hoc committee on labial-lingual posturing function. *Asha, 31*(11), 92–94.

American Speech-Language-Hearing Association. (1990). Knowledge and skills needed by speech- language pathologists providing services to dysphagic patients/clients. *Asha, 32*(Suppl. 2), 7–12.

American Speech-Language-Hearing Association. (1991). The role of the speech-language pathologist in assessment and management of oral myofunctional disorders. *Asha, 33*(Suppl. 5), 7.

American Speech-Language-Hearing Association. (1992). Position statement and guidelines for instrumental diagnostic procedures for swallowing, *Asha*, *34*(Suppl. 7), 25–33.
American Speech-Language-Hearing Association. (1993). Orofacial myofunctional disorders: knowledge and skills. *Asha*, *35*(Suppl. 10), 21–23.

Cognitive Aspects of Communication

American Speech-Language-Hearing Association. (1982). Serving the communicatively handicapped mentally retarded individual. *Asha*, *24*(8), 547–553.
American Speech-Language-Hearing Association. (1987). The role of speech-language pathologists in the habilitation and rehabilitation of cognitively impaired individuals. *Asha*, *29*(6), 53–55.
American Speech-Language-Hearing Association. (1988). The role of speech-language pathologists in the identification, diagnosis, and treatment of individuals with cognitive-communicative impairments. *Asha*, *30*(3), 79.
American Speech-Language-Hearing Association. (1989). Report: Interdisciplinary approaches to brain damage. *Asha*, *31*(10), 238–239.
American Speech-Language-Hearing Association. (1990). Interdisciplinary approaches to brain damage. *Asha*, *32*(Suppl. 2), 3.
American Speech-Language-Hearing Association. (1991). Guidelines for speech-language pathologists serving persons with language, socio-communicative and/or cognitive-communicative impairments. *Asha*, *33*(Suppl. 5), 21–28.
American Speech-Language-Hearing Association. (1995). Guidelines for the structure and function of an interdisciplinary team for persons with brain injury. *Asha*, *37*(Suppl. 14), 23.

Social Aspects of Communication

American Speech-Language-Hearing Association. (1990). Interdisciplinary approaches to brain damage. *Asha*, *32*(Suppl. 2), 3.
American Speech-Language-Hearing Association. (1991). Guidelines for speech-language pathologists serving persons with language, socio-communicative and/or cognitive-communicative impairments. *Asha*, *33*(Suppl. 5), 21–28.

Augmentative and Alternative Communication

American Speech-Language-Hearing Association. (1989). Competencies for speech-language pathologists providing services in augmentative communication. *Asha*, *31*(3), 107–110.
American Speech-Language-Hearing Association. (1991). Augmentative and alternative communication. *Asha*, *33*(Suppl. 5), 8.
American Speech-Language-Hearing Association. (1991). Report: Augmentative and alternative communication. *Asha*,. *33*(Suppl. 5), 9–12.

(See also prosthetic/adaptive devices)

Prosthetic/Adaptive Devices

American Speech-Language-Hearing Association. (1992). Position statement and guidelines for evaluation and treatment for tracheoesophageal fistulization/ puncture. *Asha, 34*(Suppl. 7), 17– 21.

American Speech-Language-Hearing Association. (1992). Position statement and guidelines for vocal tract visualization and imaging. *Asha, 34*(Suppl. 7), 31–40.

American Speech-Language-Hearing Association. (1993). Position statement and guidelines for oral and oropharyngeal prostheses. *Asha, 35*(Suppl. 10), 14–16.

American Speech-Language-Hearing Association. (1993). Position statement and guidelines on the use of voice prostheses in tracheotomized persons with or without ventilatory dependence. *Asha, 35*(Suppl. 10), 17–20.

(See also augmentative and alternative communication)

Instrumental Technology

American Speech-Language-Hearing Association. (1992). Position statement and guidelines for instrumental diagnostic procedures for swallowing. *Asha, 34*(Suppl. 7), 25–30.

American Speech-Language-Hearing Association. (1992). Position statement and guidelines for vocal tract visualization and imaging. *Asha, 34*(Suppl. 7), 31–40.

Aural Rehabilitation

American Speech-Language-Hearing Association. (1984). Competencies for aural rehabilitation. *Asha, 26*(5), 37–41.

American Speech-Language-Hearing Association. (1990). Aural rehabilitation: An annotated bibliography. *Asha, 32*(Suppl.1), 1–12.

Hearing Screening

American National Standards Institute. (1989). *Specifications for audiometers* (ANSI S3.6.-1989). New York: Acoustical Society of America.

American National Standards Institute. (1991). *Maximum permissible ambient noise levels for audiometric test rooms* (ANSI S3.1-1991). New York: Acoustical Society of America.

American Speech-Language-Hearing Association. (1990). *Guidelines for screening for hearing impairments and middle-ear disorders.* Asha, 32(Suppl. 2), 17–24.

American Speech-Language-Hearing Association. (1991). Issues in ethics: Clinical-practice by certificate holders in the profession in which they are not certified. *Asha, 33*(12), 51.

Communication Instruction

American Speech-Language-Hearing Association. (1979). Standards for effective oral communication programs. *Asha, 21*(12), 1002.

American Speech-Language-Hearing Association. (1983). Social dialects (and implications). *Asha, 25*(9), 23–27.

American Speech-Language-Hearing Association. (1993). The role of the speech-language pathologist and teacher of voice in the remediation of singers with voice disorders. *Asha, 35*(1), 63.

Supervision

American Speech-Language-Hearing Association. (1985). Clinical supervision in speech-language pathology and audiology. *Asha, 28*(6), 57–60.

American Speech-Language-Hearing Association. (1989). Preparation models for the supervisory process in speech-language pathology and audiology. *Asha, 32*(3), 97–106.

American Speech-Language-Hearing Association. (1992). Supervision of student clinicians. *Asha, 34*(Suppl. 9), 8.

American Speech-Language-Hearing Association. (1992). Clinical fellowship supervisor's responsibilities. *Asha, 34*(Suppl. 9), 16–17.

Research

American Speech-Language-Hearing Association. (1992). Ethics in research and professional practice. *Asha, 34*(Suppl. 9), 11–12.

Sample Clinical Interview

Interviewing the Parents of a Child Who Stutters

The following is a sample interview with parents of a 5-year-old child who stutters. Note the kinds of questions asked and the types of information sought by the clinician. Also, note how the clinician answered many questions the parents had about stuttering, its causes, and treatment.

Clinician: When did you first think that there may be something wrong with Brian's speech?

Mrs. Thomas: About a month ago, on a Sunday morning, I noticed that Brian was repeating a lot. I remember asking him what he wanted to eat for lunch that day. Brian started to say something like "I want a hot dog for lunch," but he had a lot of trouble saying it.

Clinician: What exactly did he do?

Mrs. Thomas: Well, he started like "I-I-I-I-I wa-wa-wa-want a hot d-d-d-d-dog, Mom." He was trying too hard to say it. I could see a lot of struggle to get it out.

Clinician: You had not heard that kind of problem in Brian's speech before?

Mr. Thomas: My wife has not heard it, but I have. About two months ago, when I was reading a story to him, he wanted to interrupt me to ask a question about the story. I don't remember what exactly he said at that time, but I remember him repeating a lot. Periodically I have heard him repeat a bit too much, but I thought it may be a passing thing. I remember him asking me once "What t-t-t-time is it Dad?"

Clinician: Have you seen an increase in repetitions?

Mr. Thomas: I think so. During the last month or so, his speech problems have increased. He is repeating more and getting stuck more often. Now it takes him longer to get out of a block. And that too, only after some struggle.

Clinician: What do you mean by a block?

Mrs. Thomas: His mouth and face look like he is trying hard to say something, but nothing comes out. His lips are quivering, mouth is sometimes open, at other times tightly shut. You can see the struggle to say something but he is not saying anything. This is what scares me the most.

Clinician: Did anything unusual happen around the time you first noticed his repetitions or more recently when you noticed an increase in them?

Mr. Thomas: No, not really. Things have been pretty routine at home.

Clinician: Has he been sick lately?

Mrs. Thomas: No, Brian has always been a healthy boy.

Clinician: What about your health when you were carrying Brian?

Mrs. Thomas: I was fine during pregnancy and the delivery was normal. The baby was healthy. We did not notice any problem until this stuttering came about.

Clinician: What about his speech and language development? Was there any reason to be concerned?

Mrs. Thomas: No. In fact, Brian began to speak earlier than my other son Chad, who is 4 years older than him. We thought he was quite advanced in his speech. He usually talked a lot and learned new words fast.

Clinician: So everything has been normal until you began to notice his stuttering.

Mr. Thomas: We may have missed something, but that is our impression.

Clinician: I want to go back to Brian's stuttering. You said that he repeats a lot. Does he prolong a sound? Have you heard him say something like "I want sssssome sssssoup, please?" I prolonged the *es* sound in both the words. Does he prolong sounds like that?

Mrs. Thomas: Oh, yes. He does it all the time. This morning, while eating a new kind of cereal, he said "It is rad, Mom," but he prolonged the *a* sound. It was more like "raaaad."

Clinician: Does Brian repeat words and phrases? Does he say "I-I-I want it or let-let-let me do it or he-was he-was he-was coming" and things like that?

Mr. Thomas: Yes, we have heard him do that. Sometimes he repeats a word or a bunch of words many times before he moves on to the next word. Yesterday I heard him say to his brother "Why are you - why are you - why are you - why are you do- do - doing it?."

Clinician: Does he use what we call interjections like *uh* or *um* or *er*? As you know, most speakers have them, but I wonder how much Brian interjects.

Mrs. Thomas: I think he interjects a lot. In fact, Brian drives me up the wall with his *uhs* and *ums*. He starts a lot of sentences with ums. This morning he said "Um - um - um what am I - I - I g-g-g-going to have um - um - um - um for breakfast, Mom." Sometimes he keeps going with ums.

Clinician: What about interjected words like *well*, *OK*, and phrases like *you know*, *I mean*, and *you see*?

Mrs. Thomas: He uses them some of the time. We hear more *ums* and *uhs* than what you just described.

Clinician: Does Brian show any facial grimaces when he stutters? Some people who stutter blink their eyes, wrinkle their noses and foreheads, purse their lips, wring their hands, swing their arms, and move their legs. Does Brian do any of these?

Mrs. Thomas: Yes, he does a few of those. I have seen him blink his eyes and wrinkle his nose and forehead. His hands and feet also move when he stutters. His mouth is distorted when he has a bad block. He also looks away from you when he stutters.

Clinician: Does Brian stutter all the time or only some of the time?

Mr. Thomas: His stuttering varies. One day we may hear just a few problems and the next day he may stutter on most of the words he speaks. He may be quite fluent in the morning but struggling to say his name in the afternoon. I find this puzzling. Is this true of other children who stutter, too?

Clinician: Yes, it is. A basic characteristic of stuttering is that it varies across time and speaking situations. Stuttering may be more when speaking on complex or unfamiliar topics. Dialogues in which one must take quick turns to talk and be silent also are difficult for stutterers.

People who stutter are more fluent while talking aloud to themselves or when they are speaking in monologue. Stuttering also varies depending on the kinds of persons those who stutter face. Persons who stutter may be very fluent talking to pets and babies. Many adult stutterers talk to their subordinates with increased fluency but when they confront their bosses, fluency may break down abruptly. Does Brian stutter more with some people and less with others?

Mr. Thomas: He is more fluent with his younger sister Michelle, who is 3 years old. He has the most trouble with me, somewhat less with his mother. I would say his stuttering is about average when he talks to his older brother.

Mrs. Thomas: But his worst stuttering comes out when he talks to a stranger or in a new place. I took him to Chad's school the other day. One of the teachers there talked to Brian, who blocked on every word he tried to say. The poor kid couldn't say his name. It was a heartbreaking scene for me. Also, his stuttering is worst when he talks to some of the kids in the neighborhood.

Clinician: Many folks who stutter avoid certain words. Older children and adults use substitutes for difficult words. Do you know of any words that Brian avoids saying?

Mrs. Thomas: I think I do. The other day Brian wouldn't say *John*, who is a friend of Chad. Brian kept saying "Your friend called" but wouldn't say who it was. When Chad asked about four times "Who was it?," Brian finally said "J-J-J-John" and stuttered very badly on it. Of late, I have not heard him say "Hi" to people because he can't get it out. Another puzzling thing about his problem is that he can sing songs and not have a trace of trouble. Is this also typical?

Clinician: Yes, it is! Most persons who stutter have no trouble singing.

Mr. Thomas: It's amazing! Though Brian has certain words on which he stutters frequently, he can say those very same words fluently. I suppose this is also characteristic of stuttering.

Clinician: That is also true. Stuttering on words is a matter of probability. Stuttering is more probable on some words than on other words. But even the words on which the stuttering probability is the highest may be, on occasion, spoken fluently. Therefore, it is not a question of not being able to say the words. As you know very well, Brian can say every word that he stutters on. He knows exactly what to say, he just cannot say it smoothly and easily.

Mrs. Thomas: That makes sense.

Clinician: I want to talk a little bit about the family history. Is there a history of speech disorders in the family? Are you aware of a speech problem on either side of the family?

Mr. Thomas: When I was a kid, I used to stutter. I do not believe that my father ever stuttered, but an uncle of mine did.

Clinician: Do you know when you began to stutter and how severe was it?

Mr. Thomas: I am not sure, but I think I began to stutter when I was about 4. I think it was pretty bad, because I still remember having a lot of trouble in grade school. I remember the painful teasing and the frustration of getting blocked in front of the class and things like that.

Clinician: Did you receive treatment? Do you remember what it was?

Mr. Thomas: I did go to a speech therapist, but not very regularly. I can't remember much about what she did with me.

Clinician: When did your stuttering disappear, if it has. So far, you have not stuttered here.

Mr. Thomas: I do not stutter any more. I think my stuttering was at its peak during my years in intermediate school. High school was different. I began to be more fluent, although I was not taking speech therapy at that time. The problem became less noticeable when I started college, and stuttering disappeared in subsequent years. Is this common?

Clinician: To some degree. Persons who stutter may recover from it at any age, although recovery is more common in preschool children. Also, children who begin to stutter after age 7 also have a better chance of recovery. Children whose stuttering persists through the ages of 5 and 6 are likely to be chronic stutterers. During the early childhood years, girls who begin to stutter recover more often than boys of the same age. Roughly, some 30 percent of stutterers recover from it without much professional help. We call this spontaneous recovery. Mrs. Thomas, how about on your side of the family?

Mrs. Thomas: I do not believe there was any stuttering in my side of the family. I can't be sure, though. I did read in a newspaper article that stuttering runs in the family. Is this true?

Clinician: To a certain extent, stuttering tends to run in the family. The blood relatives of a person who stutters have a greater chance of stuttering, compared to the blood relatives of persons who do not stutter. We call this the familial incidence of stuttering. But the higher familial incidence also is related to the sex ratio. You know that there are more male stutterers than female stutterers.

Mrs. Thomas: Yes, I have wondered about that. I have seen only one woman who stuttered in my life, but many male stutterers. But how does it relate to the familial incidence?

Clinician: The familial incidence is related to the sex of one or more persons labeled as stuttering found in the family. If a male stutterer is found in a family, the familial incidence for that family may be higher, compared to the incidence in the general population. However, if a female stutterer is found in a family, the familial incidence may be the highest. This means that although females are less likely to stutter, a female who stutters poses the maximum risk to the members of her family. In fact, the brothers and sons of a female who stutters run a very high risk of developing stuttering. Sisters and daughters of a male *or* female who stutters do not run that much of a risk. Of all the people, the sons of stuttering mothers run the greatest risk of developing stuttering.

Mr. Thomas: Does it mean that stuttering is hereditary?

Clinician: Some experts believe that stuttering is genetically transmitted, although the exact mechanism of transmission is not known. However, we must remember that all stutterers do not have relatives who stutter. Therefore, we cannot conclude that stuttering is inherited in all cases. Most experts believe that both heredity and environment play a role in the development of stuttering.

Mrs. Thomas: If it is inherited, is it more difficult to treat?

Clinician: No, there are no data that suggest that. Research has shown that almost all individuals who stutter improve with treatment and many improve to a significant extent. Early treatment of stuttering is especially effective and I am glad that you brought Brian in this early.

Mr. Thomas: Well, that is good news for Brian and for us!

Examples of Dysfluency Types and Calculation of Dysfluency Rates

There is some variability in scoring different forms of dysfluency types. Some clinicians measure only *stutterings,* and not specific types of dysfluencies. What follows is a general list of dysfluencies and their examples. Consult your clinical supervisor about the measurement of dysfluencies or stuttering.

Dysfluency types	Examples
REPETITIONS:	
Part-word repetitions	"What *t-t-t* time is it?"
Whole-word repetitions	"*What-what-what* are you doing?"
Phrase repetitions	"*I want to-I want to-I want* to do it."
PROLONGATIONS:	
Sound/syllable prolongations	"*Lllllllet* me do it."
Silent prolongations	A struggling attempt to say a word when there is no sound.
INTERJECTIONS:	
Sound/syllable interjections	"*Um...um* I had a problem this morning."
Whole-word interjections	"I had a *well* problem this morning."
Phrase interjections	"I had a *you know* problem this morning."
SILENT PAUSES:	
A silent duration within speech considered abnormal	"I was going to the [*pause*] store."
BROKEN WORDS:	
A silent pause within words	"It was won[*pause*]derful."
INCOMPLETE PHRASES:	
Grammatically incomplete utterances	"*I don't know how to* . . . Let us go, guys."
REVISIONS:	
Changed words, ideas	"I thought I will write a letter, card."

HOW TO CALCULATE PERCENT DYSFLUENCY RATES

Measure the frequency of all types of dysfluencies exhibited in a sample. Count the number of words spoken in the sample. Calculate the percent dysfluency rate as shown:

$$\frac{\text{Number of words spoken}}{\text{Number of dysfluencies}} \times 100$$

Types of Dysfluency	Frequency
Part-word repetitions	19
Whole-word repetitions	12
Phrase repetitions	22
Silent prolongations	34
Sound prolongations	26
Sound/syllable interjections	21
Word interjections	13
Phrase interjections	16
Broken words	10
Silent pauses	17
Incomplete phrases	9
Revisions	2
Total of all types	**201**
Number of words spoken	978
Percentage dysfluency rate	**20.5**

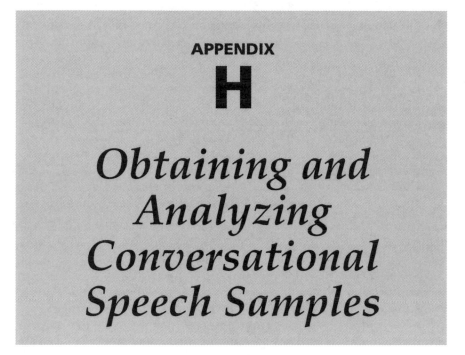

Obtaining and Analyzing Conversational Speech Samples

The conversational speech sample provides data essential to the evaluation of your clients articulation, fluency, voice, and language. The information offered suggests guidelines for obtaining and analyzing conversational speech samples of children and adults.

Obtaining Speech Samples

1. **Obtain a representative sample of your client's speech.**
Obtain a minimum of 100 utterances. An extended sample of 300 to
500 utterances is preferred. It is necessary to sample conversation in
a variety of environments with different individuals. Ask clients to
submit a taped sample of their speech at home, work, or school. Tell
them that while taping, they should be doing most of the talking.
With very young children or children with severely limited speech
and language, you may need to sample speech over several sessions.
If you are unable to adequately sample a child's speech, ask the parent to maintain a record of the child's speech for one week. If the
child is reluctant to talk with you, obtain a sample of the child's
speech while he or she talks with the parent. Schedule another session in which you may evoke speech from the child. Explain to the
parent that you want them to talk with the child as they normally
would while you are out of the room. Record the conversation.

2. **Video tape-record the sample, if possible.** With video, you
will be able to review nonverbal behaviors, later. In addition to
speech, you will be able to note eye contact, gestures, attention to
tasks, and so on. You also may observe if your change in posture or
position affects the client's communicative behaviors.

3. **Audio tape-record the sample.** Do this even if you are video
recording. Attach a small clip-on microphone to your client's collar if
he or she will be sitting in the same place throughout the sample. (This
usually results in better quality recording of the client's voice.) Have a
paper and pen available to note any relevant nonverbal behaviors.

4. **Check your recording equipment.** Before beginning your session, make sure your equipment is operating correctly. Check batteries, electrical plugs and outlets, and tapes. Turn equipment on
before beginning your sample.

5. **Have a variety of materials available.** Different children, adolescents, and adults have different interests. Have various types and
sizes of toys available to children (e.g., large and small blocks,
trucks, and dolls). Have different types of pictures available (e.g.,
pictures of sports activities, children playing, and people crying,
laughing, and yelling).

6. **Have materials that are culturally and linguistically
appropriate for the child.** Know the cultural background of the
child before you select the stimulus materials. Follow the guidelines
specified in Chapter 6.

7. Engage adults and adolescents in conversation. You usually do not need to use stimulus materials for such clients. Often the interview will allow you to obtain one conversational sample. Later you can ask the client to speak on the phone, talk with the secretary, or speak with another clinician. You occasionally may need to use such stimulus materials as pictures with adolescents.

8. Try to engage children in conversation before introducing books and toys. Many children will talk to the clinician if they are given the chance. Do not bring out toys and books until after you first have tried to engage the child in a conversation. Talk with a child about least and favorite school activities, cartoons, movies, vacations, friends, pets, teachers, birthdays and other special occasions, and so forth. Discuss likes and dislikes about siblings and events that make them very happy, mad, or sad. (If a child's speech is unintelligible, you may have to use props to try and understand his or her speech.)

9. Avoid using books. Unless you plan to have a client retell a story, do not use books. Children want to look at the pictures or read the books, rather than describe what is happening in the pictures.

10. Keep questions to a minimum. Use such open-ended statements as *"Tell me about your classes,"* and *"What shows do you watch on Saturday morning?"* Avoid asking such closed-end questions as *"Are you taking a math class?"* or *"Is your birthday coming soon?"*

11. Tell something about yourself. For example, if you know a child has a sister, talk about your sister first: *"My sister really made me upset yesterday. She wouldn't let me watch the TV show that I wanted to watch."* Talk about a recent movie you know the child has seen. Talk about an interesting scene in the movie to stimulate talking on the child's part.

12. Allow children to direct the conversation. You may present a subject or activity and the child may have a completely different idea of what he or she wants to discuss. Follow the child's lead in beginning communications. You can always direct the conversation later to sample additional language structures.

13. Give opportunities for the client to exhibit different language structures. Direct the conversation to allow the client to talk about past, present, and future occurrences. Sample the use of pronouns, declaratives, negation, interrogatives, and so on.

14. Allow pauses in the conversation. Do not worry if there are periods of silence in your client interaction. Allow your clients plenty of time to respond to questions. Give them time to continue the conversation.

15. **Relax and have fun with children.** Children like such absurdities as boxes that "talk," balls that bounce to the moon, and puppets that have squeaky voices.

Analyzing Speech Samples

1. **Transcribe the conversational speech sample as soon as possible.** Allow sufficient time to record all necessary information.

2. **Transcribe the sample using standard English orthography.** It is unnecessary to transcribe an entire sample phonetically. Transcribe unintelligible utterances and misarticulated words phonetically.

3. **Note the context in which speech is produced.** Include in your transcription events preceding each of the client's utterances. For example, if you showed a picture, asked a question, discussed an event, or performed an action, include this as part of your transcription: Clinician: bounced the ball. Client: "Pretty ball."

4. **Include in your analysis mean length of utterance and syntactic, morphologic, semantic, and pragmatic use.** As much as possible, give percentage of occurrences. Describe how many production opportunities (obligatory contexts) were present for a particular feature and in how many of those opportunities the feature was used correctly. For instance, a child may have had 20 opportunities to produce the regular plural morpheme but may have produced it correctly in only 10 of them. This means the child's correct production of the regular plural morpheme is 50%. Try to give such quantitative data for language structures of interest.

5. **Analyze voice characteristics** including pitch, rate, and intensity. These may be statements of clinical judgments unless a disorder is noted.

6. **Analyze fluency.** Describe all dysfluency forms and calculate total percentage of dysfluencies.

7. **Compute speech intelligibility.** Overall speech intelligibility may be computed using the total conversational speech sample, rather than sample for language analysis. Some language analysis programs exclude unintelligible utterances from the analysis. Note if any articulation errors produced at the conversation level are different from or in addition to those noted in single word productions.

8. **Save the conversational speech analysis** to compare with later samples.

APPENDIX

I

Sample Probe Recording Sheet

This shows a probe recording sheet. The example demonstrates the probe procedure in which the trained (T) and untrained (U) responses (preposition *on* in phrases) are alternated to find out the percent correct probe response rate. For additional information on probes see Hegde (1998b).

Client: Les Likely   Clinician: Mimi Doit
Age: 8   Date: [specify]
Disorder: Language   Session No. 7
Target Behavior: Preposition   Reinforcement: Verbal; for
    on in phrases   the trained responses only

Target Behaviors	Scoring
1. Juice on table (T)	+
2. Pillow on sofa (U)	+
3. Dog on floor (T)	+
4. Man on horse (U)	−
5. Woman on bike (T)	+
6. Boy on skateboard (U)	+
7. Girl on roof (T)	−
8. Cookie on counter (U)	+
9. Pot on stove (T)	+
10. Pen on desk (U)	−
11. Clock on wall (T)	+
12. Ball on chair (U)	+
13. Teddy on bed (T)	+
14. Book on shelf (U)	+
15. Hat on head (T)	+
16. Baby on shoulders (U)	+
17. Spot on shirt (T)	+
18. Wrinkle on face (U)	−
19. Cat on tree (T)	+
20. Bird on tree (U)	+

Note: (+) = Correct   (−) = Incorrect
Percentage Correct Probe Response Rate: 70

In this example, 10 trained exemplars were intermixed with 10 untrained exemplars. Responses given to trained exemplars were reinforced and those given to untrained exemplars were not. In calculating the percentage correct probe response rate, responses given to only the untrained exemplars are considered. The client's responses to 7 of the 10 untrained exemplars were correct, yielding a 70% correct probe response rate for the production of preposition *on* in phrases.

Sample Treatment Plan

Treatment plans provide a comprehensive program of treatment, from the beginning of treatment to dismissal. Treatment plans are developed before beginning treatment and can be modified, if necessary, as treatment progresses. Following is a sample of a treatment plan. For additional discussion and examples of treatment plans, see Hegde (1998a, 1998b).

University Speech and Hearing Clinic
Treatment Plan

Name: Sal Uda

Address: 312 N. South #111

City: Martinsville, 64812

Telephone: XXX-XXXX

School: Preschool

Date of Birth:[specify]

File no.: 900111-3

Diagnosis: Articulation

Semesters in Therapy: 1

Date of Report: [specify]

Background Information

Sal Uda, a 4-year-old-male, began his first semester of speech treatment at the University Speech and Hearing Clinic on [date]. Sal's speech and language were evaluated on [date]. The evaluation revealed an articulation disorder characterized by substitutions, omissions, and reduced intelligibility. See his folder for a diagnostic report. Treatment was recommended to train correct production of misarticulated phonemes to increase speech intelligibility.

Based on inconsistent production during assessment, the production of the following phonemes was selected for the initial treatment: /p/, /m/, /s/, /k/, and /g/. Production of each phoneme was baserated with 20 stimulus words administered on modeled and evoked discrete trials. Sal's correct production of the target phonemes on modeled and evoked baserate trials were as follows:

/p/ : 15%

/m/ : 10%

/s/ : 22%

/k/ : 18%

/g/ : 14%

Treatment was begun after obtaining the baserates. The following general treatment procedures will be used during the semester. The procedures will be modified as suggested by Sal's performance data. These changes will be described in the final summary report.

Treatment Procedure

Training for each target phoneme will begin at the word level. When Sal's probe response rate at the word level meets a 90% correct criterion, training will be initiated on two-word phrases. A similar probe criterion will be used to shift training to sentences and then to conversational speech.

Intermixed probes on which trained and untrained words, phrases, or sentences are alternated will be administered every time Sal meets a tentative training criterion of 90% correct response rate on a block of 20 evoked training trials. Sal will be trained to meet this criterion at each level of response topography (words, phrases, sentences).

Initially, the clinician will provide stimulus pictures, but Sal will be required to find at least five pictures in magazines or draw two pictures representing the target sound and bring them to the clinic sessions. After he correctly produces the target sound on five consecutive trials, he will paste the pictures in a book to be used for both clinic and home practice.

Training will begin at each level with discrete trials and modeling. The clinician will show Sal a picture, ask a question ("What is this?") and model the response (word or phrase). Sal will then be required to imitate the clinician's production. When Sal correctly imitates the target sound on five consecutive trials, modeling will be discontinued. The clinician will show Sal a picture and ask "What is this?" to evoke a response.

At the modeled and evoked word levels, verbal reinforcement will be administered on an FR1 schedule for correct productions. At the phrase and sentence levels, a FR4 will be used. At the conversational level verbal reinforcement will be delivered on an approximate VR5 schedule. All incorrect productions at each level will immediately be interrupted by saying "stop."

Modeling will be reintroduced if Sal gives two to four incorrect responses on the evoked trials. Shaping with manual guidance will be used as necessary.

All productions will be charted by the clinician. Sal also will chart productions with an X under the "happy face" or X under the "sad face." At the end of each session, Sal will assist the clinician in recording his progress on a graph.

It is expected that different target sounds will reach the training criterion at different times. Therefore, the clinician expects to train several sounds at different response topographies in each session. Some sounds may be trained at the word level, while others may be trained at the phrase or even sentence level. When the initially selected target sounds meet the criterion of 90% correct probe rate in conversational speech in the clinic, new target sounds will be baserated and trained.

Maintenance Program

After Sal produces the target sound with 90% accuracy at the evoked word level, his mother will be asked to participate in treatment. Initially, she will observe the treatment procedure, and then she will present stimulus items and chart correct and incorrect productions. She will be trained to immediately reinforce the correct productions, stopping Sal at the earliest sign of an inaccurate production.

After Sal's mother identifies correct and incorrect responses with at least 90% accuracy in the clinic session, she will be trained to work with him at home. The mother will begin with such structured activities as reciting from a list or "reading" from the book he is developing in treatment. Assignments will progress to monitoring and recording speech during dinner and phone conversations with Sal's grandmother. She will be trained to prompt and then praise the correct productions in conversational speech. Sal, the clinician, and Sal's mother will review tape-recorded home assignments. The mother will be given feedback on the procedures implemented at home.

When Sal produces the target sound with 90% accuracy in conversation in the sessions, he will be taken out of the clinic to practice correct productions in nonclinic situations. The clinician will take Sal for a walk on campus and talk with him. Subsequently, he may be taken to the campus bookstore, library, cafeteria, and other places. Eventually, his speech may be monitored informally in shopping centers and restaurants.

When Sal's speech is 98% intelligible and he produces most of his speech sounds at least 90% correct, he may be dismissed from treatment. A follow-up visit will be scheduled for 6 months after dismissal. Based on the initial follow-up results, booster treatment, treatment for persistent errors, or additional follow ups will be planned.

Marla Model, Student Clinician

Barbara Sierra, M.S., CCC/SLP
Clinical Supervisor

K

Sample Lesson Plan

Lesson plans describe what the clinician intends to do in a treatment session. Lesson plans may be brief or detailed depending on the site and your supervisor. In all cases, lesson plans should give enough information so your supervisor can understand and evaluate them. For various kinds of treatment and lesson plans, see Hegde (1998a).

UNIVERSITY SPEECH AND HEARING CLINIC
LESSON PLAN

Client: Erik Sounds   Date of birth: [specify]
Clinician: Julie Matters   Supervisor: Wendy Marks
Date: [specify]

Objective: Production of initial /l/ with 90% accuracy at word level in nonimitated training trials.

Procedures: I will present pictures of words representing /l/ in the initial position. In the beginning, I will model the correct productions. When Erik imitates at 90% accuracy in at least 10 trials, I will skip modeling and ask him to name the pictures. I will reinforce each correct production with verbal praise. I will stop Erik every time he begins to produce an incorrect response by saying "no" or "stop." Toward the end of the session, Erik will begin to plot his progress on chart.

Results:

Objective: Correct production of /f/ in conversational speech with 95% accuracy in all word positions.

Procedures: I will ask Erik to talk about the baseball game he is going to next week. If he has difficulty thinking of things to say, I will prompt him with pictures of baseball games. I will reinforce his correct production on a FR5 schedule. I will react to his incorrect production as described before. I will ask him to self-correct all incorrect /f/ productions in conversational speech.

Results:

APPENDIX
L

Sample Diagnostic Report

The formats and contents of diagnostic reports vary depending on the professional setting and disorders. For a variety of examples of diagnostic reports, see Hegde (1998a).

UNIVERSITY SPEECH AND HEARING CLINIC
DIAGNOSTIC REPORT

NAME: Susan Murmer
BIRTHDATE: [specify]
AGE: 21
ADDRESS: 44 W. Wilson
CITY: Lothar
TELEPHONE: 000-0000
REFERRED BY: Dr. Marie Meyr

DATE OF EVALUATION: [specify]
DIAGNOSIS: Voice Disorder
EXAMINER: Dawn Goode
SUPERVISOR: Faye Kremtolf
INFORMANT: Self
OCCUPATION: Student
FILE NO: 98032-51

STATEMENT OF PROBLEM

Susan Murmer, a 21-year-old female, was seen for a speech and language evaluation at the University Speech and Hearing Clinic on [date]. Susan was referred to the university clinic by Dr. Marie Meyr, an otolaryngologist. Susan reported difficulty speaking for long periods of time. Susan said that Dr. Meyr had diagnosed vocal nodules.

BACKGROUND INFORMATION

Susan's medical history was unremarkable, with the exception of the recent diagnosis of vocal nodules. In a report dated [*specify*], Dr. Meyr stated the presence of "bilateral vocal nodules in the classic position." Dr. Meyr recommended surgical intervention for removal of the nodules; however, Susan chose not to follow the recommendations. Subsequently, Dr. Meyr recommended voice evaluation and treatment at the University Speech and Hearing Clinic.

Susan reported that she majored in economics and was active on a livestock judging team. She stated that judging took place from October to April, during which time she practiced 3 to 4 hours daily. On judging days, Susan was required to use her voice almost continually for 7 hours. She reported that she must use a louder than normal intensity level during judging. According to Susan, her voice did not interfere with her ability to communicate with others; however, she was concerned about the sound of her voice and how quickly her voice fatigued. She reported that in [*date*], while yelling, she experienced a sharp pain in the laryngeal area. This experience had frightened her and she sought medical help.

Susan further reported that her voice sounds much better in the mornings and on days when she does not speak much. But often, by evening her voice is hoarse and tired.

OBSERVATIONS AND ASSESSMENT RESULTS

Oral Peripheral Examination: An oral peripheral examination revealed relatively symmetrical facial features and adequate labial and lingual movement. Palatal structures were within normal limits. Adequate velopharyngeal functions were noted. The soft palate elevated symmetrically on phonation of /a/. Velopharyngeal closure was acoustically judged to be within normal limits. Normal muscular function was demonstrated during rapid articulatory movement.

Hearing: A pure tone audiometric screening was performed at 15 dB HTL for the frequencies 500, 1000, 2000, and 4000 Hz. Bilateral responses were obtained for all frequencies.

Articulation: Articulation was evaluated during Susan's spontaneous speech and reading of the "Rainbow Passage." Speech was 100% intelligible. No articulation errors were noted.

Language: An analysis of a 100-utterance language sample did not reveal any deviations. The mean length of utterance was 7.5 words and 8.0 morphemes. All language structures were correctly used.

Fluency: The conversational speech sample was used to assess fluency and dysfluencies. Susan's dysfluency rate was 3% and consisted mainly of syllable and word interjections. Her rate and types of dysfluencies were not of clinical significance.

Voice: A conversational speech sample of 250 words was obtained to evaluate overall vocal quality. Vocal quality was characterized by inappropriately loud intensity, hoarseness, low pitch, and pitch breaks. Frequent hard glottal attacks and throat clearing were observed throughout the assessment session.

Susan spoke in a loud voice during the evaluation. Sound level meter measurements revealed speech consistently exceeding 60 dB. When asked to lower her intensity, Susan did so for four or five words, then gradually increased her intensity. Susan said that she used a loud voice in other environments. She stated that her roommate had told her not to bother to use the telephone because her voice was so loud she didn't need one.

Chest and clavicular breathing were observed throughout the assessment. Maximum duration of phonation and breath support were measured by having Susan prolong the phoneme /a/. Susan exhibited the ability to sustain /a/ for 5, 7, and 6 seconds over three separate trials, well below the optimal level of 16 seconds. Three separate trials were used to measure Susan's ability to sustain the cognates /s/ and /z/. The average ratio for these trials was 0.70, which was below the expected level of 1.0 for normal speakers. A reading sample also revealed inefficient breath support. In reading, 80% of Susan's phrases deteriorated into glottal fry or hoarseness by the second word of the phrase.

Habitual pitch was measured using the Visi-Pitch™. Habitual pitch during conversational speech was 196 Hz, with a pitch range of 57.8 Hz to 988 Hz. The higher frequencies were noted during pitch breaks. Variable pitch and frequent pitch breaks were noted frequently during spontaneous speech. Optimal pitch was determined to be 262 Hz. Susan could increase her pitch using feedback from the Visi-Pitch. When pitch was raised, hoarseness was eliminated until pitch again decreased.

Rate, resonance, and inflection were evaluated during conversation. These vocal parameters were considered normal.

SUMMARY OF FINDINGS

Susan Murmer's otolaryngologist has diagnosed bilateral vocal nodules. The current voice assessment suggests a history of vocal abuse, and that her voice is inappropriately loud and characterized by hoarseness, low pitch, and frequent pitch breaks. Susan exhibited inefficient breath support during phonation and employed several vocally abusive speech behaviors.

RECOMMENDATIONS

It is recommended that Susan Murmer receive speech-language pathology services for treatment of her voice disorder, a minimum of two sessions per week. Treatment should focus on eliminating vocally abusive behaviors, increasing breath support, and increasing pitch. It is also recommended that Susan return to her otolaryngologist for a follow-up visit after 3 months of voice treatment at this clinic.

_____

Dawn Goode, Student Clinician

_____

Faye Kremtolf, M.A., CCC/SLP
Clinical Supervisor

M

Discrete Trial Treatment Procedure and Recording Form

Discrete trials are often needed in the initial stages of treatment. They are most useful in teaching articulation and language targets.

DISCRETE TRIAL TREATMENT PROCEDURE

In the discrete trial treatment procedure, you may use two to six training stimuli at any one time. The following example shows how to train the present progressive *ing* using modeling and six exemplars (training stimuli). Skip modeling according to the criteria described in the text. See Hegde (1998b) for details.

1. Place the stimulus picture in front of the client. For example, place the picture of a *boy running* in front of the client.

2. Ask a question designed to evoke the correct response. Ask "What is the boy doing?"

3. Immediately model the correct response. "Say, *the boy is running.*"

4. Wait a few seconds for the client to respond.

5. If the response is correct, immediately reinforce the client. If the response is incorrect (the present progressive omitted), say "No" and use other response reduction procedures (response cost, time-out).

6. Record the response on your recording sheet.

7. Pull the stimulus picture away from the client to mark the end of the trial.

8. Start the next trial by again placing the picture in front of the client.

DISCRETE TRIAL TREATMENT RECORDING SHEET

In the following example, the clinician trained a person with aphasia in naming five photographs or pictures and recorded the responses on the recording sheet. On discrete trials, modeling was introduced and withdrawn as shown.

Client: Wendy Nullnem   Clinician: Arnold Chatters
Age: 65   Date:
Disorder: Aphasia   Session No. 5
Target Behavior: Naming   Reinforcement:
Continuous/Verbal

Target Responses											% Correct
	1	**2**	**3**	**4**	**5**	**6**	**7**	**8**	**9**	**10**	
1. "Tom"	m+	–	+	–	–	+	–	+	+	+	—
(Husband)	+	+	e–	–	m+	+	e+	+	+	+	m 71% / e 83%
2. "Jenny"	m+	+	–	+	–	+	+	+	+	+	—
(Daughter)	e–	–	m+	+	e+	+	+	–	+	+	m 83% / e 62%
3. "Cup"	m–	+	–	+	–	+	+	+	–	+	
	+	+	+	+	e+	–	+	+	–	+	m 71% / e 66%
4. "Water"	m+	+	–	+	+	–	+	+	+	+	—
	+	e–	–	m+	+	+	+	e+	+	+	m 86% / e 60%
5. "Phone"	m–	+	+	+	+	+	e–	–	m+	+	—
	e–	+	–	+	+	–	+	+	+	+	m 85% / e 58%

Note: (+) = Correct response   (–) = Incorrect or no response
       m = Modeled trial   e = Evoked trial, no modeling
       Total Number of trials: _____
       Total % Correct Responses: _____

APPENDIX
N

Daily Progress Notes

Progress notes are recorded after each treatment session to document client progress. Following is a sample of progress notes using "SOAP notes" (subjective, objective, assessment, plan).

CITY HOSPITAL SPEECH-LANGUAGE PATHOLOGY AND AUDIOLOGY DEPARTMENT

Name of patient:
Date of birth:
Clinician(s)

Date	Progress Notes	Initials

9/23/91 John appeared alert today. He greeted the
clinician with a smile. The client responded to
20 yes/no questions with 70% accuracy. He
produced simple CV words @ the imitation
level with 80% accuracy. John demonstrated
progress in both treatment tasks today.
Response to yes/no questions ↑ 60% to 70%
(in 20 trials). Imitative productions ↑ from
75% to 80% for CV words. Continue current
activities.

LPG SPIIIII

Date	Progress Notes	Initials

9/24/91 John greeted the clinician $\bar{c}$ a smile, but appeared tired—his eyes closed occasionally during the 30 minute session. Client responded to yes/no questions $\bar{c}$ 70%. Imitative tasks for CV words was 60%. John demonstrated ↓ in both tasks today. As noted, he seemed tired. Thsi was discussed $\bar{c}$ nurse who repeated that John had not slept well. Rec. continue current activities, but re-ceval if John's behavior/health changes.

LPG SPIIIII

Sample Progress Report

Progress reports summarize services offered to a client. They usually contain information on the client's background, treatment objectives and procedures, results or the outcome to date, and recommendations. The formats of progress reports vary depending on professional settings, disorders, and the professional or the agency that receives them. For a variety of progress reports, see Hegde (1998a).

SIERA SPEECH AND HEARING CENTER

Speech-Language Progress Report

[Date]

Richard Smith, M.D.
3030 E. Fairview Ave., #24
Oceanview, CA 93711

PATIENT: John North
DOB:
PERIOD COVERED: From: To:
NUMBER OF SESSIONS ATTENDED:
LENGTH OF SESSIONS:

Dear Dr. Smith:

John North, a 3-year, 3-month-old boy was seen for a speech and language evaluation on (*date*). The evaluation revealed significantly delayed speech and language with verbal apraxia. At that time, John was basically nonverbal with the exception of a few single syllable word approximations. He had less than 15 functional words. As a result of the evaluation, John was enrolled in speech-language treatment. He received treatment approximately twice a week from (*dates*).

SUMMARY OF TREATMENT

Goal 1: Production of the following sounds with at least 90% accuracy in conversational speech in the clinic and home setting: /p, b, m, n, t, d, k, g/, and /s/.

Treatment: Treatment began at the phoneme level for each sound and progressed to the word, phrase, and conversation level after a criteria of 95% accuracy was met at each level. Tactile, auditory, and visual stimulation initially were used to train sound production. Verbal praise and token gain and loss were used during treatment.

Progress: This goal has been met.

Goal 2: Production of the following language features in continuous speech during structured treatment activities with 90% accuracy: present progressive, regular plural morphemes, possessives, regular past tense inflections, and prepositions.

Treatment: John was presented with stimulus pictures representing each word in the phrase. The clinician modeled each phrase and John was required to touch each card as he imitated the clinician (e.g., *boy is jumping*). John was praised for his correct productions. Incorrect productions were interrupted and the clinician modeled the correct production.

Progress: John met the goal for the following structures: present progressive, plurals, possessives, and the prepositions "in," "on," and "under." John continues to work on the regular past tense.

IMPRESSIONS AND RECOMMENDATIONS

John has made excellent progress in his speech and language treatment sessions. His willingness to try to interact with others and the reinforcement of successful communication have had a positive effect on his behavior and social development. Excellent parental support and participation from his mother has encouraged carryover into other environments. John is now able to communicate using a larger vocabulary of single words and simple sentences of two to three words. It is recommended that John continue to receive speech-language services two times per week. Treatment will emphasize:

1. Continued training on the regular past tense.

2. Production of the following sounds: /f, w, ng, y, sh/, and /l/.

3. Increased mean length of utterance.

4. Parent training to work with John at home.

I hope this information is helpful. Please contact me if you have questions.

Yours sincerely.

Susan Frances, M.A., CCC-SLP
Speech-Language Pathologist

Sample Final Summary

The final summary is written at the end of a treatment period (such as at the end of a semester). It provides information on the client's treatment, progress, and recommendations for continuing treatment. The format and contents of final summaries vary depending on the professional setting, the disorder, and the professional or the agency that receives them. For a variety of final summaries, see Hegde (1998a).

UNIVERSITY SPEECH AND HEARING CLINIC
Final Summary

Client: John J. John

Address: 444 E. Southdrive

City: Grayson

Telephone: 000-0000

Occupation: Student

Period Covered:

From: To:

Clinic Schedule

Sessions per week: 2

Number of clinic visits: 22

Birthdate: [specify]

Clinic File No.: 910077

Diagnosis: Stuttering

Semester in Clinic: 1

Date of Report: [specify]

Length of sessions: 1 hour

Total clinic hours: 22 hours

STATUS AT THE BEGINNING OF TREATMENT

John J. John, a 25-year-old male, began his first semester of treatment at the University Speech and Hearing Clinic. John reported that he stuttered. He said it interfered with his part-time job as a store clerk and that people occasionally made fun of his speech. He reported that he had received speech therapy when he was 9 and 10 years old, but that he always continued to stutter.

Two conversational speech samples were analyzed before beginning treatment. Language, voice, and articulation were subjectively evaluated and judged to be normal. The first sample, obtained in the clinic, contained 1,400 words with a dysfluency rate of 18%. The second sample was recorded by John when he talked with his wife at home. This sample revealed a dysfluency rate of 16%. Both samples contained part-word repetitions, whole word repetitions, interjections of words and phrases, pauses, and prolongations. A complete diagnostic report dated [specify] is placed in the folder.

SUMMARY OF TREATMENT

Treatment involved training fluent speech through the use of a management of airflow, easy vocal onset, and reduced rate of speech through vowel prolongation. A detailed treatment program written for John may be found in the folder.

Initially, each of the fluency skills were trained separately. John was asked to inhale a larger than the usual amount of air, immediately exhale a small amount of air through his mouth, and begin saying the word in a soft and easy manner. He was asked to prolong the vowels and speak at a reduced rate. This process usually resulted in stutter-free speech.

Stutter-free speech was trained starting with words and phrases. In gradual steps, treatment progressed to controlled sentences and conversational speech. In all treatment sessions, the criterion of fluency required of John was 98% or better. Both dysfluencies and errors in fluency skills (e.g., failure to inhale or exhale, abrupt phonatory onset, rapid rate) were measured in all sessions. When John maintained at least 98% fluent speech at any level of training for either a block of 50 utterances (phrases, sentences) or for a duration of 10 minutes or more, the training was moved to the next level of response topography. If John's dysfluency rate increased when moved to a higher level of training, he was returned to the lower level.

At the earliest sign of an incorrect response or a dysfluency, John was asked to "Stop." In the initial stages, he was told what went wrong. For example, the clinician said: "You forgot to breathe in"; "You did not breathe out"; "You were about to stutter," and so forth. Later on, he was asked simply to "Stop." Correct productions of target behaviors resulting in stutter-free speech were verbally reinforced at the end of the response chain. Initially, a continuous schedule was used; gradually, the amount of reinforcement was reduced to an approximate VR5 schedule at the conversational level.

John was trained to chart the correct use of target behaviors and all dysfluencies. After John demonstrated accurate monitoring of responses and 98% fluency at each level, home assignments were given for that level. John's wife observed four sessions in which she was trained to monitor his fluent speech by stopping and reinforcing him as the clinician did. John and his wife were recommended to practice the skills of fluency for at least 20 minutes each day. John's wife was asked also to monitor his speech in most speaking situations.

To promote maintenance, the clinician accompanied John to the campus book store and cafeteria where he talked to other persons. The clinician monitored John's speech by giving subtle hints to prompt the target responses and provided verbal reinforcement whenever practical. Various probes were taken to document changes in his dysfluency rate.

RESULTS

By the end of the semester, John's dysfluency rate in conversational speech with the clinician at the clinic was 98%. However, a 10-minute conversational speech sample recorded at his home with his wife showed a fluency rate of 94%. A probe of his speech with his boss at work showed a fluency rate of 92%.

RECOMMENDATIONS

It is recommended that John continue treatment for his stuttering. The treatment next semester should emphasize maintenance of fluency at home, office, and other settings.

_____

Dana Monroe, Student Clinician

_____

Greg Hallstoni, M.S., CCC/SLP
Clinical Supervisor

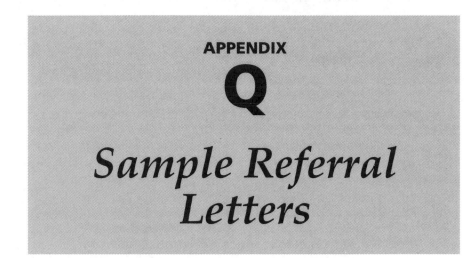

APPENDIX

Q

Sample Referral Letters

Speech-language pathologists write many kinds of referral letters to other professionals. Three common kinds are illustrated on the following pages. See Hegde (1998a) for additional examples.

SAMPLE REFERRAL LETTER 1

The following sample illustrates the kind of letter a speech-language pathologist might write to another professional to acknowledge the referral of a client for speech-language services.

[*date*]

John Jones, M.D.
228 N. Way, Suite 101
Bloomington, CO 78123

Dear Dr. Jones:

Thank you for referring Sal Uda to our Clinic. He was seen for a speech and language evaluation on [*date*]. Sal was accompanied to the evaluation by his mother who expressed concern over her son's lack of speech intelligibility.

Results of the assessment revealed a severe articulation disorder, with multiple sound substitutions and omissions. Receptive language was age appropriate; however, expressive language was delayed. Sal was cooperative during the evaluation and easily stimulable for the sounds he misarticulated and omitted.

I recommended that Sal begin treatment for his speech and language disorder. He will be seen two times per week for one hour each visit.

Enclosed is a copy of Sal's speech and language evaluation report. If you have any questions, please contact me at 555-5555.

Sincerely,

Dorothy Ozzz, M.A., CCC/SLP
Speech-Language Pathologist

SAMPLE REFERRAL LETTER 2

The following sample illustrates the kind of letter one speech-language pathologist might write to another to make a referral.

[*date*]

Donna Jones, M.S.
Speech-Language Pathologist
Melvin Communication Clinic
Melvin, Alaska

Dear Ms. Jones:

Robert Fine, a 67-year-old man, who suffered a stroke nearly four months ago was diagnosed with apraxia and aphasia, characterized by moderate auditory comprehension and severe verbal expression deficits. At the time of assessment, his conversational speech consisted primarily of several automatic phrases.

  Robert has received treatment at our clinic for the past three months. He has demonstrated significant progress. He is able to express himself in 6- to 7-word utterances. He accurately uses many language structures including nouns, various verb tenses, modifiers, plurals, possessives, and some prepositional phrases.

  Although Robert has made good progress, he needs continued treatment to stabilize his conversational speech skills in extraclinical situations. Because he is moving to your town, I am referring him to your clinic. Robert is highly motivated to continue treatment. He would be an excellent candidate for your treatment program. I hope you will consider accepting Robert as a client. If you have questions, please contact me at 888-8888.

Sincerely,

Georgia Shurr, M.S., CCC/SLP

SAMPLE REFERRAL LETTER 3

The following sample illustrates the kind of letter a speech-language pathologist might write to a physician (or another professional) to refer a client.

[*date*]

Jean Jayne, M.D.
333 W. Hills, Suite 101
Beverly, NM 20111

Dear Dr. Jayne:

I saw Jerry Blank in my office for a voice evaluation on [date]. He requested an evaluation because he felt that his voice was "too deep." During the evaluation he reported chronic hoarseness and occasional pain in the laryngeal area.

During the voice evaluation, Jerry exhibited a harsh, breathy voice with frequent pitch breaks. He had difficulty sustaining phonation. His intensity sometimes became inaudible towards the end of phrases.

I recommended that Jerry have a laryngeal evaluation. He reported that you were his otolaryngologist and would be making an appointment with you. According to Jerry's request, I have enclosed a copy of his voice evaluation.

If you have questions, please contact me.

Sincerely,

Micron MacGregor, M.S., CCC/SLP
Speech-Language Pathologist

Discrete Trial Baseline Procedure and Recording Sheet

The trial baserating procedure is illustrated on the following page. The example shows how to baserate the correct production of speech sounds at the word level. You can adapt it to baserate other target behaviors including language structures.

DISCRETE TRIAL BASELINE PROCEDURE AND RECORDING SHEET

Client: Thomas Tucks   Clinician: Belinda Speaks
Age: 10   Date:
Disorder: Articulation   Session No. 1
Target sound: Initial /s/ in words   Reinforcement: Noncontingent

	Trials	
Target Behaviors	Evoked	Modeled
1. Sun	−	−
2. Soup	−	−
3. Seed	−	−
4. Soap	−	+
5. Sink	−	−
6. Sock	−	+
7. Suit	−	−
8. Cent	−	−
9. Salt	−	−
10. Sign	−	−
11. Salad	−	−
12. Sofa	−	−
13. Soda	−	−
14. Swing	−	−
15. Syrup	−	−
16. Sunrise	−	−
17. Sweater	−	−
18. Circle	−	−
19. Sand	−	−
20. Sandwich	−	−

Note: (−) = Incorrect; (+) = Correct.
Incorrect production of word-initial /s/ on evoked trials: 0%.
Incorrect production on modeled trials: 90%.
(The target phoneme was correctly produced in 2 out of 20 modeled trials).

Index